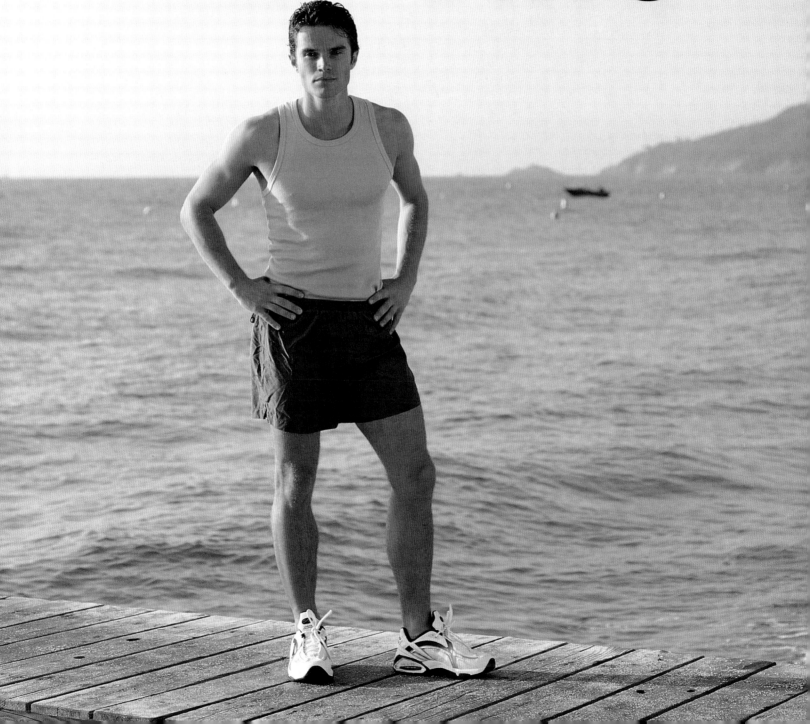

Matt Robe...

fitness for life

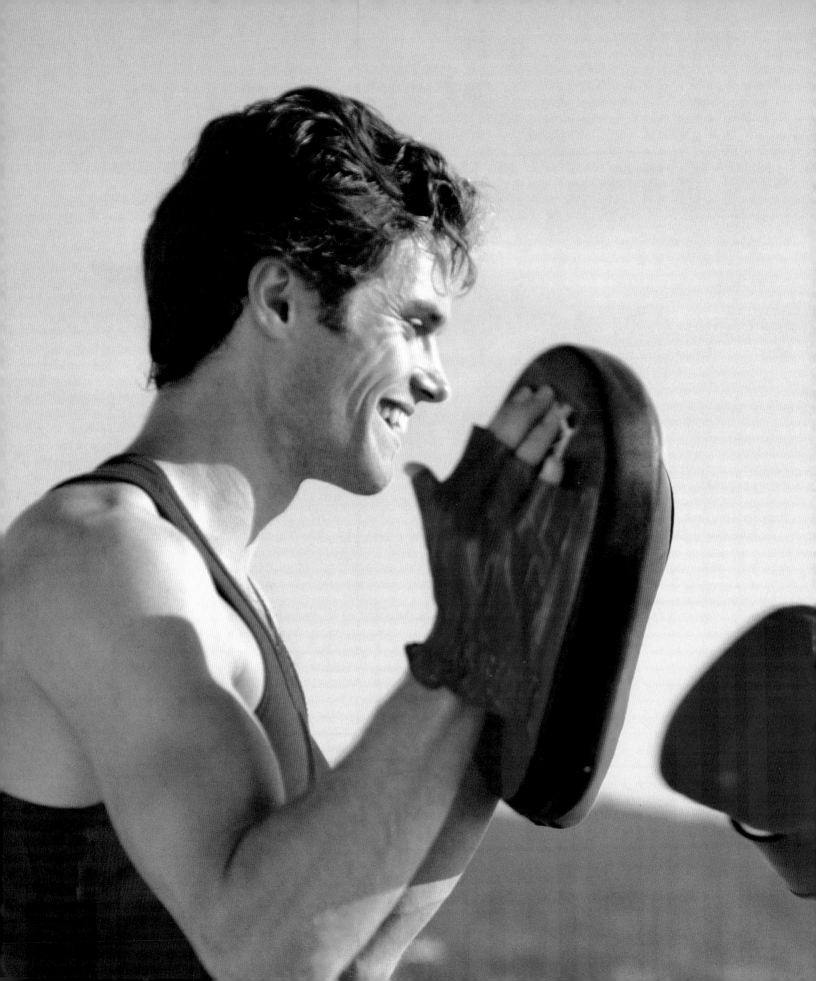

Matt Roberts
fitness for life

**Photography by
John Davis**

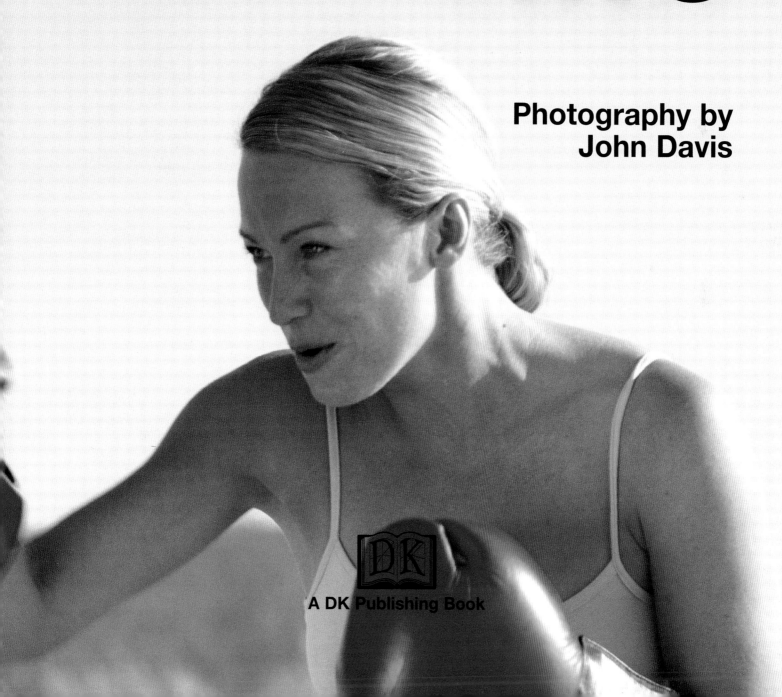

A DK Publishing Book

DK

LONDON, NEW YORK, MUNICH, MELBOURNE, DELHI

To Mike
Thinking of you and wishing you well

project editor Nasim Mawji
project art editors Paul Reid and Darren Bland at cobaltid
managing editor Gillian Roberts
senior art editor Karen Sawyer
US editor Gary Werner
category publisher Mary-Clare Jerram
art director Tracy Killick
dtp designer Louise Waller
production manager Sarah Coltman

First American Edition, 2002
This paperback edition, 2004
04 05 10 9 8 7 6 5 4 3 2
Dorling Kindersley is represented in Canada by
Tourmaline Editions Inc., 662 King Street West, Suite 304
Toronto, Ontario M5V 1M7
Copyright © 2002 Dorling Kindersley Limited, London

Text written by Jon and Matt Roberts
Text copyright © 2002 Matt Roberts Personal Training

Always consult your doctor before starting a fitness and nutrition program if you have any health concerns.

A CIP catalogue record for this book is available from the National Library of Canada

ISBN 1-55363-036-X

Color reproduced by Colourscan, Singapore
Printed and bound by Mondadori Printing S.p-.A, Verona-Italy

Discover more at
www.dk.com

contents

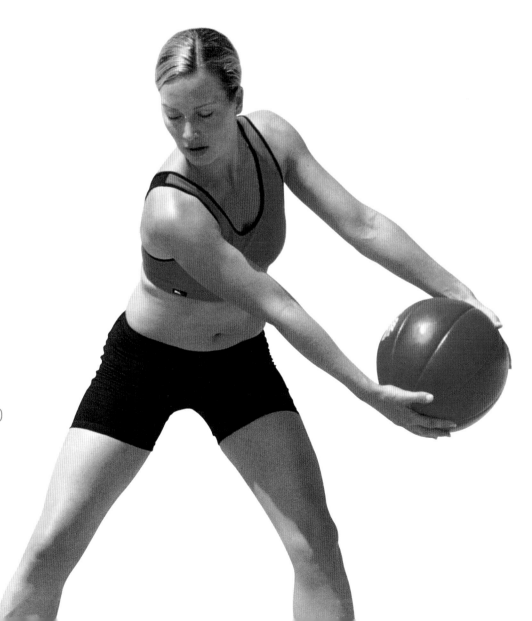

introduction

The aim of this, my second book, is to provide answers to questions and solutions to problems. It will serve as a reference book when you want to know which exercises work which muscles or understand how different training techniques affect the body in different ways. As a personal trainer, I believe it's important to understand how your body responds to exercise – that way you can set yourself realistic goals and actually work with your body to achieve them.

Our fitness goals change, and they are different for everyone. With this in mind, I have designed 20 specially tailored programs. They can help you to do anything from lose weight or build muscle, to tone your butt, get back into shape after pregnancy, or even run a marathon. And because you complete a fitness test before you embark on a program, you will always be working at the right pace for your fitness level.

No fitness program would be complete without sound nutritional guidelines and advice. The chapter on healthy eating therefore outlines the importance of a balanced diet that keeps energy levels up and fits in with your life rather than dominating it. Where relevant, individual programs advise on other adjustments to your diet that will help you to achieve your goal.

▶ **set health and fitness goals**
As I always say, "If you don't know where you are going, how will you know when you have arrived?"

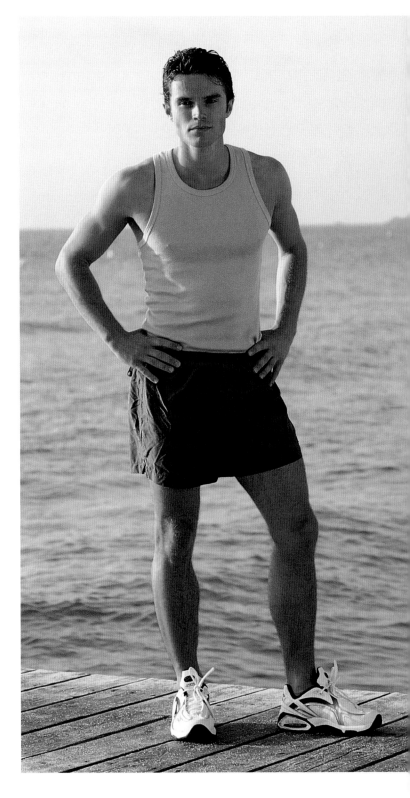

So often fitness books don't relate to real people. This is the exception that does. One of the most exciting experiences of creating the book was working with our case studies. I put five people, men and women, through different programs and charted the progress of each individual with photographs and training journals along the way. Their fantastic achievements are proof that the programs really work.

The health and fitness industry is continuously growing. There are more exercise classes on offer, more fitness instructors, more personal trainers, a wider range of equipment available and more gyms than ever before. With all this choice, there is bound to be confusion. Exercise classes can be an enjoyable way to get and stay in shape, so in the exercise class directory I have assessed the more popular ones on offer today. Here, I tell you what to expect from a class and what results you can hope to achieve if you attend regularly.

Making the Right Choices guides you through the maze of buying exercise equipment for the home, and choosing a gym and personal trainer. A lot of people call themselves personal trainers but actually know very little about the important principles of nutrition and exercise. There are good trainers out there, but it's essential to find one who is well qualified and who can help you to set and achieve realistic personal fitness goals.

Your health and fitness routine should be an integral part of your life – and you should enjoy it. It shouldn't dominate your life but definitely enhance it. This book can do just what the title suggests and help you to achieve fitness for life.

I hope this book will serve as a useful and long-standing reference to the world of health and fitness, and that it will enable you to aspire to new and unexpected fitness goals.

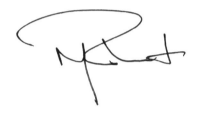

▶ **running in the surf**
One of the high points of putting this book together was the outdoor photography. Exercise doesn't have to confine you to the gym.

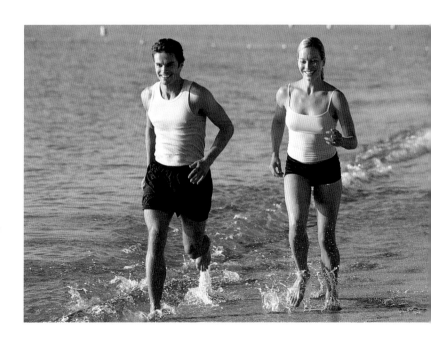

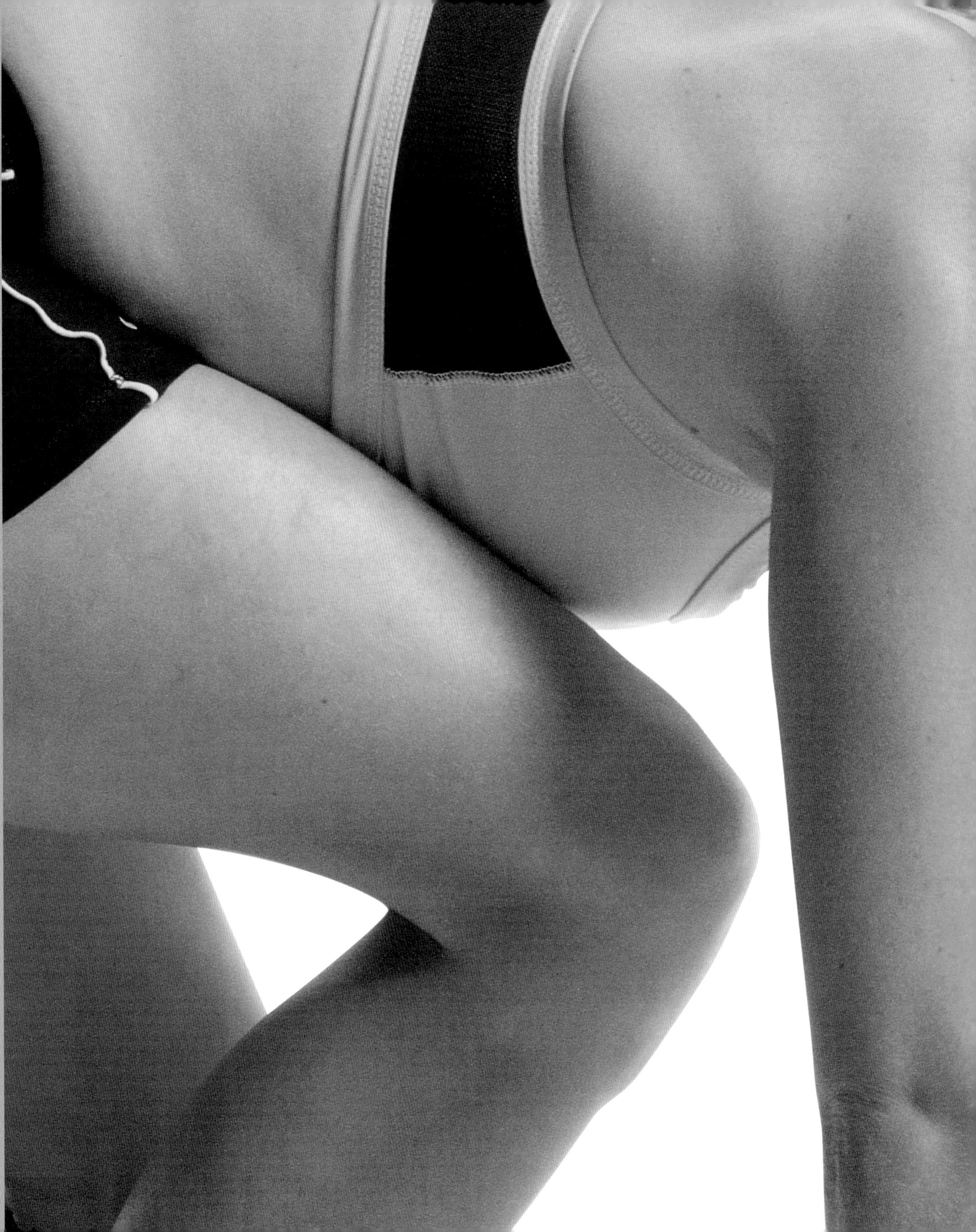

getting started

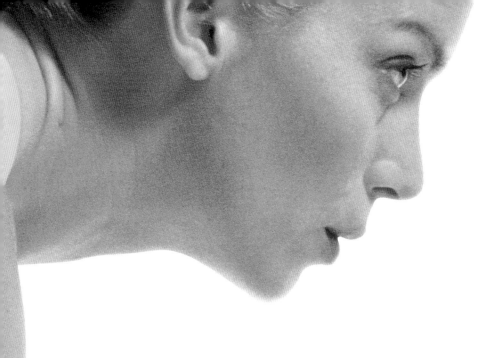

getting started

It's important to understand how the body works before embarking on an exercise program or making lifestyle changes. This chapter explains how different body systems work together in harmony to keep you alive and healthy. It also explains how you can maintain and strengthen them by getting regular exercise and eating a healthy, balanced diet. Once you understand how your body responds to exercise and diet, you can set yourself realistic and achievable health and fitness goals. First, complete the nutrition and physical questionnaires on pages 20–23 to establish your starting point and current level of fitness.

the human body

The human body is an amazing organism. It is made up of many different body systems, each with its own specific function. All of these body systems support each other and work together to keep us alive and healthy. The better we take care of our bodies, the better they will serve us and the more resilient they will be.

the musculoskeletal system

The body's muscular and skeletal systems are apparently far from perfect in design. Human beings started off on all fours, evolved into cave dwellers hunched over fires, and today we walk around upright on two legs. As our bodies have evolved, a structure that was once admirable for its purpose seems to have become less suitable. If you asked a structural engineer to design the human body, taking into consideration the everyday tasks it needs to be able to perform, the mobility of the joints and the weight the structure has to bear, he almost certainly would not design the human skeleton as we know it.

And yet with all these imperfections, people function remarkably well. The skeleton provides the framework for the muscles, and one of the functions of the muscles is to protect it. The muscles work with the skeleton and enable every movement, from the smallest twitch of a little finger to hitting a ball with a tennis racket, which requires coordination and power. The skeletal muscles also support the body and are responsible for maintaining posture; without them you wouldn't be able to stand upright or hold your head straight.

bones

The human skeleton consists of many bones, each one made up of living tissue that constantly grows and renews itself. Bone marrow in the center of each bone produces most of the body's red blood cells.

Your bones can reveal details about your sex, weight, height, and even your diet. Taking care of your bones when you are younger – by eating a balanced diet that is rich in calcium and by getting regular exercise – reduces your risk of developing bone diseases such as osteoporosis and osteoarthritis later in life.

joints

Where two bones meet, a joint is formed. Joints are covered with lubricated cartilage, which enables smooth movement. Some joints have a greater range of movement than others. Where joints are less mobile, bones are attached by strong ligaments, and they generally provide more stability, which is the case in the feet, spine, and wrists, for example. The most complex joint is the shoulder. It is a ball and socket joint, and has the greatest range of motion because it can move in any direction as well as rotate. The knee is the largest joint. It is a hinge joint – as is the elbow – and this means that it can bend upward and downward along a single plane, in the same way a hinged door moves. Hinge joints can rotate slightly.

muscles

Muscle makes up about half of the weight of the body. All of the voluntary movements you make depend on your relaxing and contracting your skeletal muscles (*see right*). Muscles can't push, they can only pull, so often they are arranged on each side of a joint to produce opposing movements. In the arm, for example, the bicep contracts to pull the lower arm up, while the tricep is relaxed. The tricep contracts to bring the lower arm down, and the bicep is relaxed.

Muscles are attached to bones by tendons: I liken the structure to the cables on a suspension bridge. The muscles on each side of the body should be equally strong to keep the structure in good balance. If the cables on one side of the suspension bridge were stronger than on the other side, the bridge would bend and weaknesses would appear. The same happens in the human body. If a group of muscles on one side of the body is tighter than those on the other side, weaknesses develop. Muscle imbalances can develop if, for example, you always carry a heavy bag on the same shoulder, or sit every day in an awkward position at your desk.

One of the most common places to feel the effects of such an imbalance is in the lower back. If the hamstrings are tight and the quadriceps weak, tension accumulates in the lower back and you experience pain there. The most common cause of this is spending long periods seated and also being inactive. Getting regular exercise and constantly stretching the muscles to ensure they are flexible will help to prevent muscle imbalances.

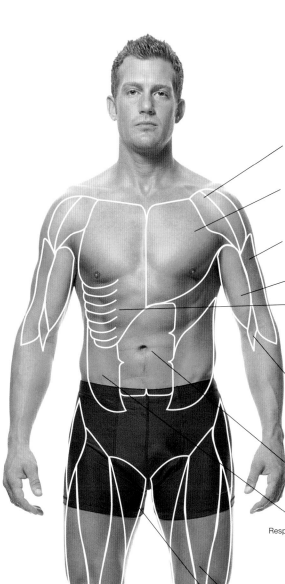

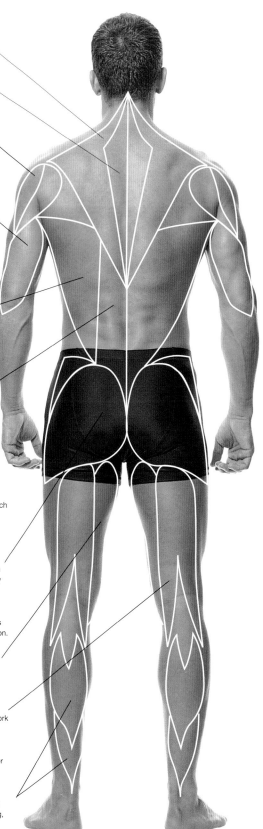

Trapezius
Used in the shrugging action when you pull your shoulders up toward your ears.

Rhomboid
Enables rowing movements and protects the spine.

Deltiods
Used in any large arm movements and in the lifting action.

Pectorals
Used to move the arms across the body and in the pushing action.

Tricep
Allow you to straighten your arms against pressure and to push.

Bicep
Responsible for bending the arms and moving the hand toward the face.

Intercostal muscles
Assist in breathing.

Latissimus dorsi
Responsible for lowering the arms toward the body against a pressure.

Brachialas
Assists the biceps in bending the arm and helps grip strength.

Erector spinae
Enables backward movement of the spine and protects the lower spine.

Rectus abdominus
Enables forward movements of the spine and maintains posture.

Oblique abdominal
Responsible for any diagonal torso movements such as bending to the side.

Gluteus maximus
Used to pull the leg back, as when running, or in any action that pushes the body upward or away from resistance.

Quadriceps
Used to straighten the leg and in actions such as walking, getting up out of a chair, jumping and so on.

Adductor
Used to pull the leg inward toward the body.

Hamstrings
A group of muscles at the back of the thigh that work to bring the heel toward the butt.

Anterior tibialis
Pulls the foot upward when walking or running, for example.

Gastrocnemius and soleus
The calf muscles; used in pushing the foot down and for stabilizing the foot when standing, walking, or running.

getting started

how different body systems work

One of the most important factors in achieving a fit and healthy body is ensuring that each of the body's complex systems is strong and able to function as efficiently as possible. The digestive, cardiovascular, and nervous systems all perform unique roles in the body, but their interrelationship means that they work in harmony to keep you healthy. If one system functions poorly, your whole body suffers as a result.

the digestive system

The function of the digestive system is to break down food by complex physical and chemical processes so it can be absorbed into the bloodstream as nutrients and used to fuel the body. The digestive system is made up of the mouth with its salivary glands, esophagus, stomach, liver, gall bladder, pancreas, and small and large intestines including the colon. Waste products are excreted at the anus. Thirty feet (9m) of muscular tubing extend between the mouth and the anus.

The digestive process is easily affected by your emotional state, in particular stress, but also by the speed with which you eat, your diet, the quality of the food that you take in, and the chemical environment of your digestive system.

Digestive stress is a term that is increasingly used and is, unsurprisingly, often stress-induced. The higher your stress levels, the more acidic your digestive system, and the less efficiently your body can break down food and absorb its nutrients. People often eat poorer quality food – convenience and processed foods – when they are stressed and busy, and eat quickly and on the run. As a result, the quantity of good, high value nutrients that pass into the bloodstream to fuel the cells is reduced. This adds to the stress in the body; with less available energy, it can't function as efficiently.

in the mouth

The mouth is where the first stage of digestion takes place. Food is moistened and broken down into smaller particles by saliva, which is produced in the salivary glands under the tongue and in the cheek, and by chewing. Often people simply don't chew their food thoroughly enough, which puts

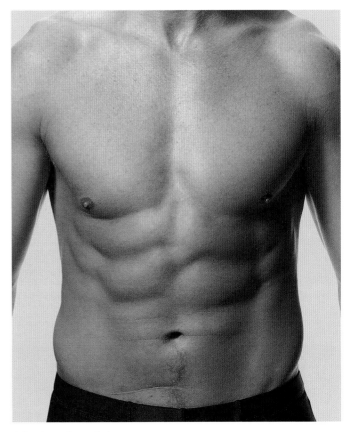

▲ **body systems in harmony**
It is good to have an understanding of how the different body systems work together to keep you alive and healthy. Take care of your body so that it can serve you well. You'll feel and look better, too.

additional stress on the digestive system. When food is not broken down properly in the mouth, the body has to work harder to extract nutrients from it.

My team and I did a study with a group of professional people who all had symptoms of digestive disorder ranging from lethargy to poor concentration. With analysis we found that their digestive systems were stressed and acidic, and did not break down their food efficiently. We made no changes to their diets, simply asking them to drink 2 quarts (2 liters) of water a day and make a conscious effort to chew their food thoroughly until it was of a pulpy consistency.

After six weeks we reevaluated the group. With just these two changes, every single person had dramatically improved digestive efficiency and increased energy levels.

the stomach

Once food has been chewed into a mass in the mouth, it is swallowed and takes seconds to travel down the esophagus into the stomach. Once there, food is broken down further by contractions and gastric juices, which are designed to be very acidic; the digestive process has begun. This stage is especially important for the digestion of proteins because many of the enzymes that break down proteins are in the stomach.

Food stays in the stomach for up to four hours until the resulting mixture, called chyme, is released into the small intestine. The rate at which this happens depends on the type of food eaten. For example, low-alkaline foods pass through very quickly; but red meat, which is more acidic, takes much longer and also produces high levels of acid in the process. Wholesome, unprocessed, low-alkaline foods tend to put very little stress on the digestive system, and high levels of acid do not need to be produced in the stomach to digest them. The stomach also responds to emotions. If you are stressed, more acid will be produced and your digestion will be affected.

the small intestine

This is the most important section of the process of digestion and absorption. In the first section of the small intestine, the duodenum, the semi-digested food comes into contact with

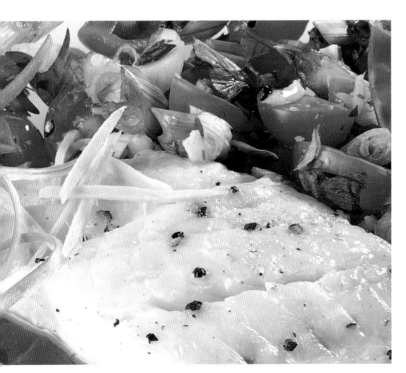

three different digestive substances that break it down further.

• Bile. This comes from the liver and is stored in the gall bladder. It breaks down fats so that they can be digested and absorbed into the bloodstream.

• Pancreatic juices. These are produced in the pancreas and are alkaline-based. Their purpose is to neutralize the acidity of the chyme, which comes from the stomach. Foods that are highly processed or difficult to digest, for example red meat, put extra strain on this part of the digestive process. The small intestine has to work harder to break them down and extract nutrients. Pancreatic juices also contain enzymes that break down fats, proteins, and carbohydrates into their component parts so that they can then be absorbed into the bloodstream.

• Intestinal juices. These are produced in the small and large intestines and contain more digestive enzymes. A diet that is high in processed foods can affect the level of these juices as processed foods have a flushing, leaching effect on the system and can affect the body's ability to extract nutrients from food as efficiently as it should.

the large intestine

Undigested food passes into the large intestine. This is essentially the waste product gathering ground. As a result of poor digestion or in times of stress, undigested food and waste can accumulate in the large intestine. This can lead to a buildup of gases that can cause bloating, flatulence, and stomach pains. Feces are stored here before they pass through to the colon and are eventually expelled from the body.

the digestive system in balance

When the whole of the digestive system is in balance, food is broken down quickly and easily, and the body is able to extract the nutrients it needs to fuel itself and function efficiently. An unbalanced diet, stress, processed foods, inactivity, and poor general health – either singly or in combination – can affect the body's ability to digest food efficiently. This can burden the body with unnecessary stress, causing poor concentration, lethargy, and skin problems . It may also put you at higher risk of developing more serious illnesses.

◀ **enjoy your food**
Wholesome, unprocessed foods put less strain on the digestive system. You owe it to your body to eat a healthy, balanced diet, but this doesn't mean that food has to be tasteless or boring. Experiment with new ingredients and different cuisines to keep your diet lively.

getting started

the cardiovascular system

This consists of the heart, blood, blood vessels, and lymphatic system. Your heart is the most important and amazing muscle in your body. Medical advances have drastically reduced the incidence of heart conditions such as valve disease (once the biggest cause of heart failure), yet in industrialized countries, coronary artery disease is still the biggest cause of death in the over 35s. The main reason for this increase in heart disease is our own self-abuse. Smoking, eating high cholesterol foods, excessive alcohol intake, and being overweight; diabetes, high blood pressure, unresolved stress, and low levels of physical activity all weaken the cardiovascular system.

Your heart is simply a pump. In a resting state it pumps approximately six to seven quarts (6–7 liters) of blood around the body every minute. As blood passes through the lungs it picks up oxygen that is transferred through the alvioli (small air sacs) into the blood vessels for distribution around the body. Blood also rids itself of waste carbon dioxide in the lungs, and this is expelled when you exhale. As your activity level increases, your body needs more oxygen, and the volume of blood flow per minute increases. As you breathe more rapidly, you bring more oxygen into your lungs. Once the oxygen is being carried by the blood cells it can be conveyed to your active muscles and internal organs – including your brain which needs the most oxygen – and to the heart itself.

You need to understand what can go wrong with your heart in order to protect it, and this will help to ensure that you enjoy a long, active, and healthy life. A significant factor that contributes to heart disease is atherosclerosis. This occurs when there is excess fat and cholesterol in the blood, and fatty deposits build up in the artery walls as a result. This causes the interior of the arteries to become narrowed, which increases pressure in them, reduces blood flow, and can ultimately block them entirely. This can lead to chest pains known as angina and then heart attack. Ultimately the heart will stop working altogether – cardiac arrest – which normally means death.

Research has shown that, because of its beneficial effects on the circulation, regular exercise can also reduce your risk of deep vein thrombosis. People have become more familiar with this term since a link was established between the condition

▶ **find different ways to exercise**
Regular exercise that involves coordination and uses large dynamic moves not only improves your aerobic capacity, it helps to stimulate other vital body systems, too.

and long-haul flying. Deep vein thrombosis occurs when a blood clot forms and obstructs the flow of blood in a blood vessel; this can eventually block the blood vessel completely. In some cases, particles from the clot may break away and become lodged elsewhere in the body. If a clot reaches the lungs, it can be fatal.

The ultimate aim in preventing heart disease is to combine a healthy cardiovascular system with a healthy blood profile. This means that the blood that is pumped around the body is rich in nutrients that fuel the body and help it to function at optimum efficiency. A strong cardiovascular system on its own cannot prevent cardiovascular disease if your body is suffering

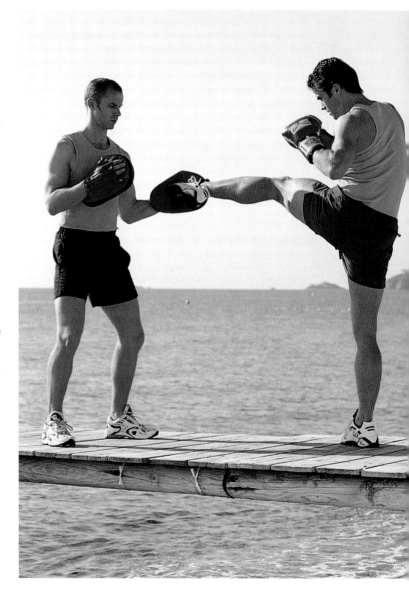

the effects of a poor diet. If the arteries are "furred up" from a high-fat, high-sugar diet, even the strongest heart would have problems pumping blood around the body.

blood pressure

This is the pressure of the blood on the walls of the arteries. The two figures in a blood pressure reading give the systolic and the diastolic pressures. Systolic pressure measures the pressure when the heart is contracting, and diastolic pressure when it is relaxed. Hypertension, a consistently elevated blood pressure, is affecting more and more people these days. It is generally caused by the buildup of fats on the inside of the artery walls which thickens and narrows them, impeding the flow of blood through them. This causes pressure to build up in the arteries and puts the heart under more strain because it has to work harder to pump blood around the body. A strong link has been established between hypertension and stress, and although you might not experience any symptoms, your risk of heart attack and stroke is greatly increased. Good nutrition, in particular a low-fat, low-sodium diet, and regular exercise combined with good rest and sleep patterns can help to reduce hypertension considerably.

Although the main health concerns arise from high blood pressure, low blood pressure (although rare) can also be a problem. This is when the blood flows through the arteries with less force than it should. The condition is less dangerous than having high blood pressure, but still means that the body can't function at optimum efficiency. It needs a healthy blood pressure to ensure that it can deliver blood, and the nutrients in it, to the whole body. Low blood pressure can result in poor circulation. Symptoms are feeling light-headed, or having cold or numb fingers and toes. Low blood pressure associated with iron deficiency anemia can be improved by making sure than you include plenty of iron-rich foods (*see page 31*) in your diet.

the nervous system

This is undoubtedly the most complex of the body's systems: it controls every voluntary and involuntary action. The brain receives nerve impulses in response to external and internal stimulation and sends messages in the form of chemical and electrical signals to the different parts of the body.

This network of nerve pathways is highly advanced and can adapt to new situations, but it is also incredibly delicate; it's important to take care of it, because damaged nerve tracts

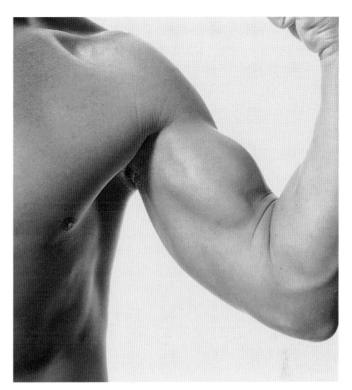

▲ muscle power
Work your muscles. Exercise can strengthen the muscles, but it can also help to improve reaction times – quick reaction times improve performance in most sports.

can't recover completely. However, nerves have a remarkable ability to grow, develop, and adapt as they are tested, which is why, over time, training methods become progressively easier and faster to perform. Muscle strength is not dictated solely by muscle growth. When you use your muscles to exercise or just to become more active, there is increased nerve stimulation and, as a result, increased electrical activity within the nerves. The effect is to utilize more muscle fibers. It is this stimulation that can increase muscle strength without increasing muscle size. Exercise trains the body to respond quickly in different situations, which improves the message signaling between the brain and other parts of the nervous system.

Disease, viruses, blood circulation problems, alcohol, and recreational drugs all affect your nerves and interfere with the chemical messages sent from the brain. This is why reactions may be impaired after drinking alcohol or taking drugs.

Research has shown that a combination of regular exercise and a healthy diet can reduce the likelihood of stroke. Aerobic exercise is particularly important as it improves circulation and encourages increased blood flow to the brain.

getting started

the importance of setting goals

Most people "hit the wall" or fail at exercise regimes or programs, not for lack of focus or motivation, but more because they have no firm direction. It is not enough vaguely to want to exercise to get in a little better shape, or to diet to lose some weight. Although these approaches may be effective in the short term and will have positive health benefits, they simply aren't focused enough. Before you embark on any health routine or fitness program, it is imperative that you set yourself clear – and realistic – goals.

how to set goals

Be tough on yourself. It all comes down to your health in the end, and only you can make the decision to improve, neglect, or disregard it totally. It might help to think back to any previous exercise regimes or diet programs that were unsuccessful and consider why they failed. Perhaps they were impractical, and couldn't fit into your life. What was the stumbling block?

Examine your performance when considering how well you've managed to stick with fitness programs in the past. I use the word "performance" because the aim is to evaluate your previous attempts in just the same way that you might evaluate a work project. Why should your own health plan be any different in terms of importance, effort, and commitment from something related to work? You might manage to get out of bed to go to work every day without any major problems, yet fitting in a workout or resisting a chocolate croissant is a huge effort that seems impossible to make. Is your work really more important than your health? Sometimes it can be hard to see how you can incorporate fitness into your life, but it's important to strive toward a balance, because being fit and healthy has benefits for every aspect of your life. Treat your commitment to your own health and fitness like an important work project, and devote to them the time they deserve.

▶ **work toward an achievable goal**
Focus on your short-term goals to help you achieve your long-term goal. No program can deliver instant results; it's the short-term goals that will keep you motivated along the way.

My clients vary enormously, and their goals are equally varied, but what they do have in common is a specific goal plan, or training journal, that helps them to achieve their ultimate aims. Whether the goal is to be fit for a grueling concert tour, a physically demanding movie role, a marathon, or an Olympic final, each person has sat down with me and planned a goal-driven route toward their chosen aim.

My favorite cliché stands true: "if you don't know where you are going, how will you know when you have arrived?". It couldn't be more appropriate now. Today is the time to start planning for your future health and fitness.

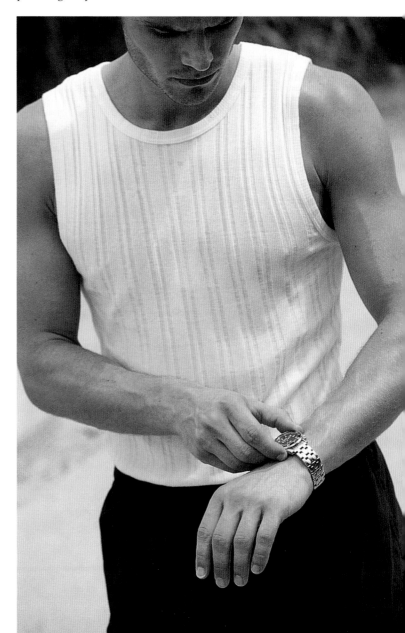

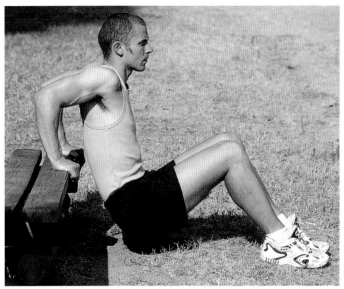 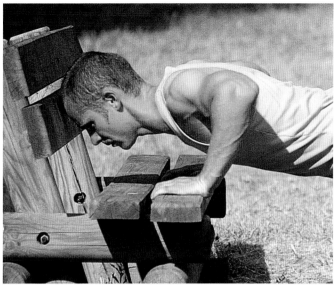

▲ **be more active**
Leave your car at home and walk, get off the bus a stop early, or take your workout outdoors, as in the park program (*see pages 188–89*).

▲ **find time to exercise**
Your health and fitness regime is important – make it a positive and enjoyable part of your life.

setting long-term goals

Your first step in planning is to buy a new journal and write down your goal for the future. Your long-term goal should be no further away than a year at most. Ideally, try to choose a goal that is achievable within three to six months because that is a more manageable timescale. Longer than that, and I often find that people get distracted or lose interest.

Begin by writing in your journal the specific goal you are aiming to achieve, the date it will be assessed, and the parameters for success and failure. Setting goals is also about understanding the realms of possibility. A common goal for many people is losing weight, but it would be pointless setting yourself a goal to, for example, lose 55lb (25kg) in 10 weeks when losing 5lb (2.5kg) a week is clearly neither healthy nor sensible. Be realistic about what is possible; poor goal setting leads to disappointment and failure.

The programs in this book will guide you and help you to set yourself achievable goals; the structured workout plans will help you to push your body, but not to overdo it; and the nutrition and diet advice will give your body the nutrients it needs to perform at its best. Your long-term goal should be a clear and specific target for you to aim toward. Be precise. Exactly how much weight will you lose? How fast will you run your race? What will your exact waist size be? It is essential to commit yourself to this goal and treat it as if it were the most

important personal project that you have ever set yourself. If you don't take it seriously, you will start to make excuses for why you won't succeed. Remember that you are setting this goal for yourself and nobody else.

setting short-term goals

In your journal, work from day one to the final day of your long-term goal, and set yourself short-term goals. Write out weekly or daily targets that can be checked off as you meet them and progress through your program. Your short-term targets should set goals for your workouts, rest times, and diet, and should be as precise and clear as possible. So, for example, you might set targets to work with progressively heavier weights, to do more repetitions, to increase your running distances or to drink more water or less coffee or tea. The programs will set your short-term exercise goals for you, and some set specific diet goals, too. Writing them down in your journal will help you to stick with your program and achieve your ultimate goal. Each time a goal starts to slip, add it back into your list of short-term goals alongside any new ones. You should probably have three or four short-term objectives to fulfill each week, besides your exercise plan, which gives you daily goals. It's worth taking the time to set out your short-term goals. Treat them like a business plan or a route map to your destination. They help to ensure your success.

getting started

keeping focused

Even with the strongest resolve, we all succumb to moments of weakness, and we all find the same excuses when we fail:"I will make up for it tomorrow," "I didn't have time,""I had to have a drink because everyone else was having one,""I'll pick it up again next week."They are common excuses that we all use to justify not doing the things that seem to involve simply too much effort. But, if you make enough of these excuses in the short term, they will prevent you from achieving your ultimate goal in the long term. With a written goal-driven plan for your program, you are far more likely to succeed.

motivating yourself

You may give in to the occasional bout of laziness. It's not that you don't want to achieve the targets that you've set yourself, but sometimes you can lose sight of your long-term goal. You can't be perfect all the time (life would be just too boring), but most of what you do has a positive or negative consequence for you, and to some degree a healthy lifestyle is about balancing the two to achieve equilibrium.

Having said that, there are times when it may not be possible to stick with a training program that demands a good deal of commitment. A trauma such as a bereavement or other personal tragedy might mean that you have to set your program aside temporarily. It's important to keep things in perspective – it's all part of maintaining a balanced approach to your fitness program. Sometimes simply growing tired of the goal you are striving toward can be enough to weaken resolve. Or perhaps you miss the life you lead before you embarked on your program. Maybe your children take up a lot of your time and you just want to rest when they go to bed. Maybe you don't really believe that you can ever have the body that you want and all of the effort is for nothing.

▶ **take stock**
Be firm but kind with yourself. Take your goals seriously, but keep things in perspective. A slip-up is a minor setback that can always be overcome; it shouldn't be an excuse for giving up.

Self-doubt can be terribly undermining. If you don't really believe you can achieve your goal, you are doomed to failure before you've even begun. You'll never know what you can achieve unless you try, and you don't give yourself a real chance at success unless you have set yourself clear and realistic goals. If you feel that you don't have time for a fitness program because of work, the children, or family obligations, for example, start putting your own needs first. In fact, you'll find that regular exercise will probably help you to perform better at work, give you more energy so you can enjoy your children, and make the time you spend with your family richer and more satisfying.

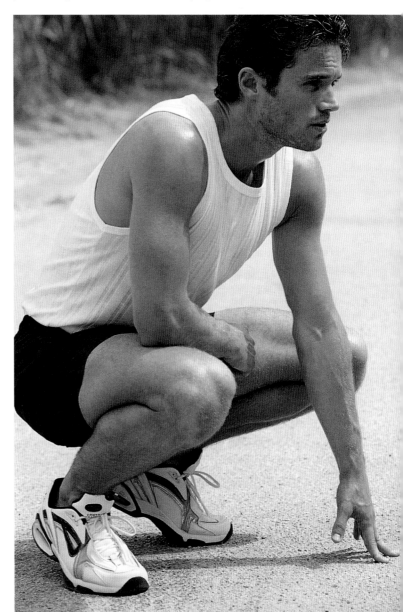

reassessing your goals

Of course, there will be times when you won't be able to work out – and it would be unrealistic to expect you to be able to stick to a program one hundred percent of the time. When you do miss a short-term goal, you can still make up for it. Assess what you've missed and add extra work to your schedule when necessary. So, for instance, if you miss a session where you might have concentrated on aerobic training, compensate by doing more aerobic work next time you train. If you miss one day of training over a month, don't worry. If you miss one or two sessions a week, you may need to reassess your long-term goal. If you eat breakfast five days out of seven you are doing quite well and need not be concerned; if you are eating breakfast two days a week and it is only an apple, you have a slight problem that must addressed.

You can always reassess your goals – whether long-or short-term – if you find that despite, your most valiant efforts, you still can't meet them. In this case, your short-term goals must now become your long-term goals and you must focus on achieving them in the foreseeable future. Otherwise, you will lose sight of your long-term goal, and it will become more and more difficult to attain. This doesn't undermine the importance of setting long-term goals. It merely emphasizes how valuable it is to set realistic and achievable ones, and to understand your own limits and motivation levels.

building resolve

The first steps on the path to a healthier life are the most difficult. Subsequent steps become easier and easier. If you feel yourself starting to falter, think back to other challenges you have met in your life, and remember how even the most difficult things often seem less daunting in retrospect.

It's easier to stay motivated if you have the support of the people around you: your friends, family, and work colleagues. There will always be someone who can't wait to tell you a story of past failure, or to suggest a better exercise routine or a more effective diet. The trick is to stay focused on your own program, and keep your personal goal in sight.

You give yourself a greater chance of success if you can enlist the support of at least one person who understands what you are doing. Spend some time with the person you think will be the most supportive, and talk through your program with them. Try to highlight the areas that you feel will need the most work and where you anticipate needing

Goal: to lose 15 lbs in 2 months			
Date:	11/12	11/14	11/17
Chest press	(35kg/16reps/2 sets)	(40kg/14reps/2 sets)	(40kg/15reps/2 sets)
Lat pull-down	(40kg/16reps/2 sets)	(40kg/16reps/2 sets)	(45kg/14reps/2 sets)
Leg curl	(25kg/16reps/2 sets)	(30kg/14reps/2 sets)	(30kg/16reps/2 sets)
Ball squats	(x25)	(x30)	(x30)
Lat raise	(10kg/12reps/1 set)	(10kg/12reps/2 sets)	(10kg/14reps/2 sets)
Notes:	Felt tired, good workout	Cardio 85%MHR ran 20 mins good workout	Had body fat measured and had lost 2%

▲ make a plan
Set yourself clear, realistic goals, and monitor your progress as you work toward them. Keep a training journal (see pages 218–19) and make a note of how you feel at the end of each workout.

the most encouragement. It's often surprising how much of a positive influence a friend can be, and how much they will be prepared to do to ensure that you keep on course. It may be your partner, a friend, a member of your family, or even a someone you work with – anyone who you feel cares enough to see you achieve your goal. Make this person your ally so that they have a personal stake in your achievement. You never know: you may be doing the same for them one day.

Once your support network is in place and you've chosen your program, you are ready to take the first steps toward changing your health and fitness level for the rest of your life. But always remind yourself of your personal goals and how much it means to you to achieve them. Remember who the program is for … you!

getting started

nutrition questionnaire

This questionnaire is designed to make you think about your diet and how well your body responds to it. It also assesses hydration levels and your body's acid/alkaline balance, which can affect your energy levels and general health. For the results, see page 215.

1 How much water do you drink each day?

a Less than 1 pint (½ liter)
b 1 pint–1 quart (½–1 liter)
c More than 1 quart (1 liter)

2 How many cups of coffee or tea do you drink each day?

a More than 4
b 2–4
c 1 or fewer

3 How many sugary or carbonated drinks do you normally have each day?

a More than 4
b 2–4
c 1 or fewer

4 How many pieces of fruit do you eat each day?

a 0–1
b 1–3
c More than 3

5 How many portions of fresh vegetables do you eat each week?

a 2–4
b 4–7
c more than 7

6 Do you eat a nutritious, healthy breakfast every day?

a Never
b Sometimes
c Always

7 How often do you eat after 8 o'clock in the evening?

a Regularly
b Occasionally
c Never

8 How many of your daily meals contain red meat?

a 2 meals
b 1 meal
c 0 meals

9 How many of your daily meals contain wheat in any form? (eg, bread, pasta)

a 3 meals
b 2 meals
c 1 meal

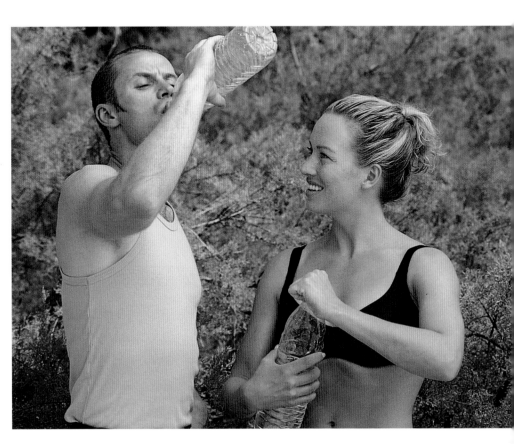

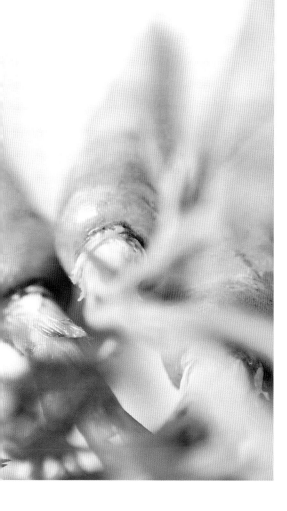

13 How many units of alcohol do you drink each week? (a unit is a glass of wine, a single measure of spirits, or half a pint of beer)

a Male: 21 units or more
Female: 16 units or more

b Male: 14–20 units
Female: 8–15 units

c Male: less than 13 units
Female: less than 7 units

14 Do you suffer from bloating after eating?

a Often
b Sometimes
c Never

15 Do you chew your food thoroughly?

a No
b Yes

16 Do you suffer from constipation or diarrhea?

a Often
b Sometimes
c Never

17 Do you suffer from heartburn or acid reflux?

a Often
b Sometimes
c Never

18 Do you suffer from ulcers or gastritis?

a Often
b Sometimes
c Never

10 Do you suffer from stomach pains when you are emotionally upset or stressed?

a Often
b Sometimes
c Never

11 Do you suffer from stomach or abdominal pains either before or after eating meals or snacks?

a Often
b Sometimes
c Never

12 Do you suffer from indigestion or regularly take antacids?

a Often
b Sometimes
c Never

19 Do you suffer a loss of energy in the middle of the afternoon?

a Often
b Sometimes
c Never

20 Do you crave sweet foods such as chocolate?

a Often
b Sometimes
c Never

21 Are you a fast eater? Do you gobble your food?

a Yes
b No

22 Do you go longer than four hours without eating?

a Often
b Sometimes
c Never

23 How many of your daily meals or snacks consist of bread, potatoes, white pasta, or white rice?

a 3 or more
b 1–2
c 0

getting started

physical questionnaire

The tests below assess your aerobic fitness, strength, flexibility, and body proportions. They will help you to evaluate your current level of physical fitness. You should complete this questionnaire before embarking on any of the programs. For the results, see page 215.

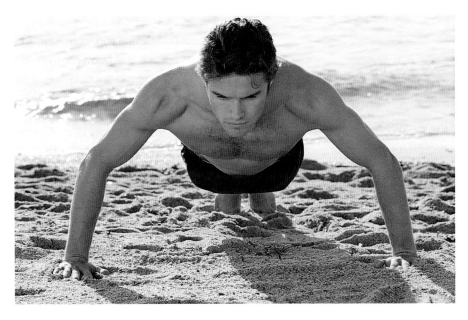

3 One-minute push-up test This tests your upper body strength. Do as many full push-ups or easier half push-ups (*see page 85*) as you can in one minute. Whichever you choose, always use the same push-up to test in the future. If you cannot do a full minute of push-ups, count the number you complete before your technique suffers.

Full push-ups

a Male: 9 or less
Female: 4 or less
b Male: 10–30
Female: 5–15
c Male: 31 or more
Female: 16 or more

Half push-ups

a Male: 29 or less
Female: 24 or less
b Male: 30–50
Female: 25–40
c Male: 51 or more
Female: 41 or more

1 Body Mass Index (BMI) evaluation This assesses your weight in relation to your height and gives an indication of how healthy your current body shape is. Divide your weight in kilograms by your height in meters squared (1lb = 0.45kg 1ft = 30.48cm).

So, if you weigh 52kg and are 1.72m tall, first calculate your height squared (1.72 x 1.72 = 2.96), then divide 52 by 2.96 to give you a BMI of 18.

a Male: 26.1 or more
Female: 26.1 or more
b Male: 21–26
Female: 21–26
c Male: up to 20.9
Female: up to 20.9

2 Three-minute step test This tests your cardiovascular fitness. Use a step or bench that is 16 inches (40 cm) high and step up and down at a rate of 30 steps per minute. Do step-ups (*see page 109*) for 3 minutes, breathing normally throughout. Stop and take your pulse for 15 seconds (*see page 55*), then multiply the figure by 4 to give your number of heartbeats per minute.

a Male: 157 or more
Female: 167 or more
b Male: 131–156
Female: 141–166
c Male: 120–130
Female: 128–140

getting started

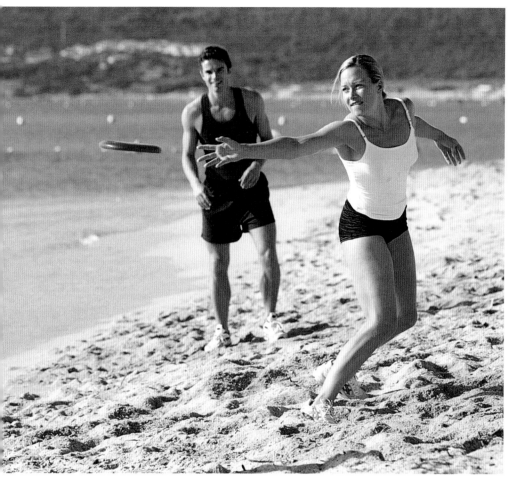

6 **Hip-to-waist ratio** This test assesses your body shape and fat distribution. Measure the hips (just below the top of the pelvis), then measure your waist (over your belly button). Divide your waist measurement by your hip measurement (you can use either metric or imperial measurements).

a Male: above 0.95
  Female: above 0.86
b Male: 0.81–0.94
  Female: 0.71–0.85
c Male: below 0.8
  Female: below 0.7

4 **One-minute crunch test** This tests the strength of your abdominals, or stomach muscles. Do as many basic crunches (see page 102) as you can in one minute. Stop and start if you need to, but keep your technique correct.

a Male: 24 or less
  Female: 24 or less
b Male: 25–45
  Female: 25–45
c Male: 46 or more
  Female: 46 or more

5 **Sit and reach test** This assesses your spine and leg area flexibility. Sit with your back against a wall and your legs together, extended in front of you. Reach forward and measure how far down your legs your fingertips can touch.

a Thighs
b Bottom of knee cap
c Shin and beyond

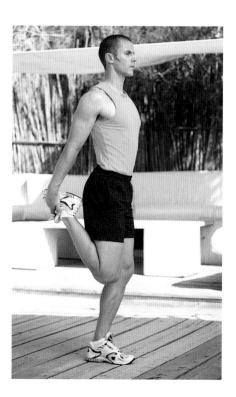

getting started

23

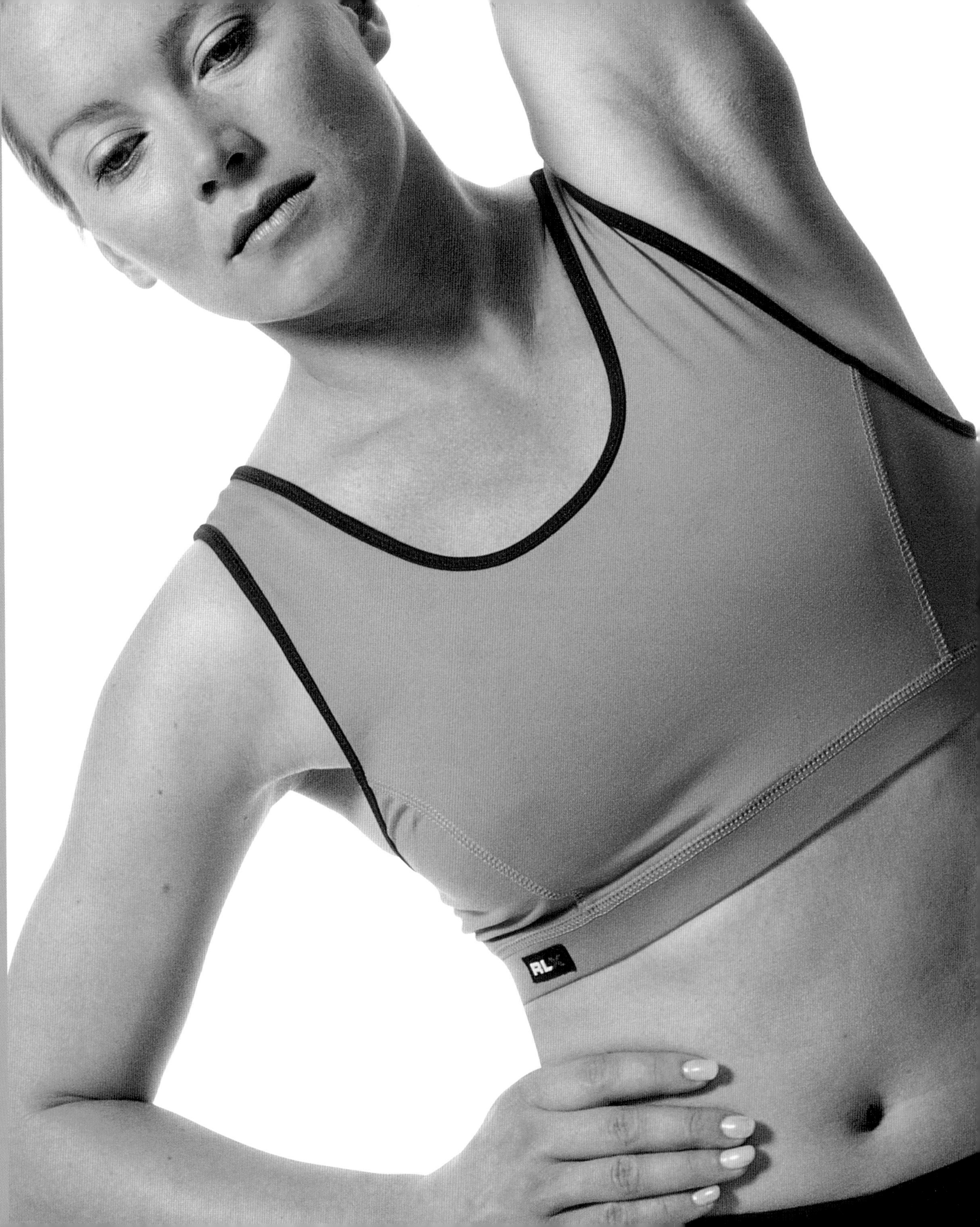

healthy
eating

Any health and fitness program needs to be supported by sound advice on diet and nutrition. Even if you work out regularly, you will never achieve a good level of health and fitness unless you nourish your body with the wholesome foods it needs to look after itself and maintain energy levels. Applying the ins and outs of good nutrition shouldn't dominate your life. It should enable you to take pleasure in what you eat.

what is a healthy diet?

As soon as the word diet is mentioned, most people think of weight loss. Really, your diet is simply the food you choose to eat. Having said that, we do need to consider weight loss when we talk about diets. For a big part of the Western world, the modern diets we eat, together with inactive lifestyles, are combining to produce people who are fatter than at any other time. How can this be the case when there are so many low-fat products available and we are more aware of fat than we have ever been? The answer does not lie in fat alone. Everyone needs a diet that provides the body with enough energy and nutrients in the form of healthy food to fuel itself and optimise its strength.

popular diets

A healthy diet is also for life. It is of little use if you can make healthy changes for only a short period of time, and then get bored with them. In the search for the perfect diet many different ways of eating have been analyzed and promoted as the answer to modern dietary problems. Of all the diets on offer today, my team and I would not advocate following a single one – in particular those that recommend excluding specific food types. However, I never simply dismiss a diet. My dietitian, physiologist, and I analyze each one. Here are our findings on some of today's more popular diets.

the high-protein diet

This diet advocates a high intake of protein from meat, poultry, fish, eggs, and cheese and a low intake of carbohydrate. The theory behind it is that high carbohydrate diets raise the insulin level in the blood and insulin promotes fat storage, so this leads to obesity and ill health. Protein is an essential nutrient in the body and is used for growth, repair, and regulatory processes. Any excess protein can be used as an energy supply for the body. But protein is not the body's preferred source of fuel.

▶ **eat well, live well**
It is simply common sense to eat plenty of fresh fruit and vegetables and lots of nutritious foods that satisfy all of the body's requirements.

The body uses carbohydrates (sugars and starches) to maintain blood glucose levels. Glucose is used by the cells, and the brain, for fuel. If our carbohydrate intake is low, the body has to get the fuel from somewhere else, so it uses protein to make glucose. It also breaks down fat differently to produce an alternative fuel source known as "ketone bodies." If carbohydrate intake is too low, the body becomes so desperate for carboyhydrate that it actually goes into starvation mode. It produces excessive amounts of ketone bodies, which can upset the body's acid base balance and force minerals like potassium, as well as fluid, out in the urine. This excess fluid loss explains the initial rapid weight loss. Other side effects of this diet include feeling light-headed, fatigue, dizziness, nausea, and a stale, unpleasant taste in the mouth.

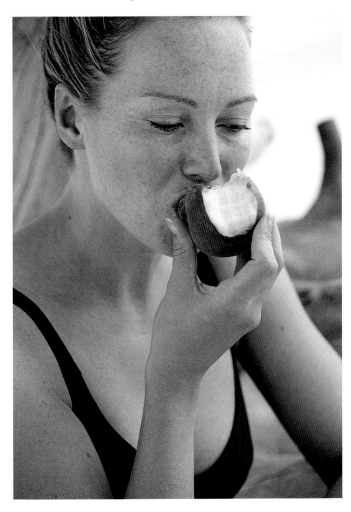

time to digest, because (the theory goes) the body cannot cope with different digestion requirements at the same time.

Unfortunately, my team and I have not been able to verify the theory. The only reason we can suggest that this diet helps people to lose weight is the restriction it imposes on the way you eat and the fact that it restricts fatty and sugary foods and encourages you to eat more fruit and vegetables. Staying faithful to the diet while also living a normal life is so difficult that you end up eating far less and far smaller portions. As a result you manage to lose weight.

the mediterranean diet

This is often cited as being the healthiest diet. Certainly when you look at the rate of heart disease in the Mediterranean countries it is far lower than that in the UK, US, and other parts of Europe, which suggests that the diet does have some positive health benefits.

But the traditional Mediterranean diet has a high fat content. It uses a lot of olive oil and, as a result, the percentage of fat in the diet is much higher than is recommended in the Western diet; yet generally, people who follow it enjoy better health. This is perhaps because the fats in the diet are what I term good fats, namely monosaturated fats. By contrast, the typical Western diet includes high levels of what I call bad fats, namely saturated fats. The Mediterraneans also eat high levels of fresh fruit and vegetables. Traditionally, people shop daily and prepare food from raw ingredients, so it is always fresh. The general trend in the rest of the West is to eat more processed foods. Culturally, the Mediterraneans eat their food at a leisurely pace and often enjoy it with a glass of wine. This means that food is broken down properly in the mouth before being swallowed and also allows adequate time for digestion. By contrast, elsewhere many peoples' lives tend to be faster, more stressful, and provide less time for meals. This diet is also one that has few of the foods that are high in refined sugar.

On the negative side, the Mediterranean diet is big on starchy carbohydrates, such as pasta and bread, and high in calories. Although the high fat content in the diet is good fat, an inactive lifestyle will mean the calories are stored as fat, leading to a fatter body even if there is less risk of heart disease compared to the traditional Western diet. Avoid this diet if you want to lose weight; but if you are active with no weight problem, it will do you no harm. However, my diet (*see page 33*) utilizes its strengths while eliminating its problems.

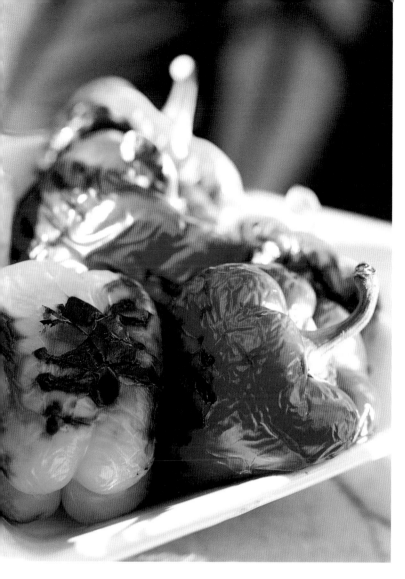

▲ **the mediterranean diet holds some answers**
The Mediterranean diet includes plenty of fresh fruit and vegetables, but it is also high in fat and starchy carbohydrates. This means that, combined with an inactive lifestyle, it may promote weight gain.

food combining

The basis of food combining is that you should never eat certain foods together because this has an adverse effect on your body's ability to digest them properly. On a food combining diet the principle is to never eat carbohydrate and protein in the same meal – they must be eaten at separate meals. This way of eating automatically makes what we consider a normal meal very difficult. For example, spaghetti bolognese becomes a meal you are not allowed; the same goes for potatoes with fish or meat, a baked potato filled with cheese, and quiche Lorraine.

The theory behind this diet is that different foods need different amounts of time to digest. You should eat only those meals that are made up of foods that take the same amount of

healthy eating

components of a healthy diet

To function optimally, the body requires a large range of different nutrients. The aim of a good, healthy diet is to provide the body with these nutrients and fuel it so that vital functions and systems such as energy production and the immune system can perform their roles under any circumstances. Each different nutrient that exists in your diet has a unique role to play in the body yet interacts with all the other nutrients. If any particular nutrient is lacking in the diet, it means that an essential function in the body will underperform. Without the essential nutrients – carbohydrates, fats, protein, fiber, vitamins, and minerals – and water as well, the body quickly slows down, and this is where many of the fashionable diets that advocate omitting certain food groups from the diet fall down. With the demands of modern life, eating a healthy, balanced diet couldn't be more important.

carbohydrates

The main function of carbohydrates is to provide the body with a source of energy or fuel. The body breaks them down into glucose, which it uses as an energy supply. Carbohydrates are particularly important as an energy source for the brain. They are divided into simple carbohydrates and complex carbohydrates, which are made up of starches and dietary fiber.

simple carbohydrates

These are made up of units, or molecules, of sugar and in most cases are sweet in taste. These sugars come from fruit, some vegetables, milk, and sucrose, or table sugar (from sugar cane and sugar beet). Sucrose is added to foods such as ice cream, cookies, chocolate, and cakes, and also to most carbonated soft drinks. Simple carbohydrates provide you with quick-release energy, which means that your body can break them down quickly. This is why you experience a quick energy burst after eating foods with a high simple carbohydrate, or sugar, content. These foods are also classified as high glycemic.

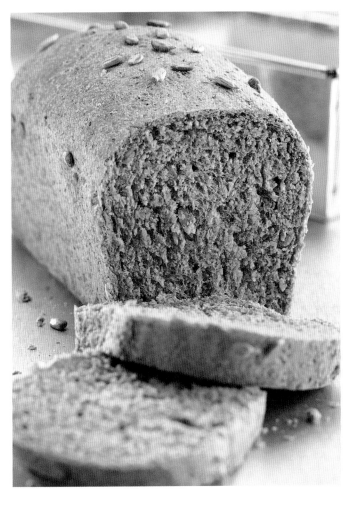

▲ **wholemeal bread**
Try making the switch from white bread, which is made from processed white flour, to wholemeal bread. It is made from flour that includes the whole grain, has more nutrients, and provides slow-release energy.

complex carbohydrates

These consist of starches and dietary fiber. They have a more complicated structure than simple carbohydrates and, as a result, the body takes longer to break them down. That is why you won't experience a sudden burst of energy after eating them. Instead, the energy release is slower and longer lasting. Sources of complex carbohydrates include grains and grain products such as bread and pasta; fruit, vegetables, beans, and dairy products. Within starches, I make a distinction between "heavy" carbohydrates such as white bread, white rice, white pasta, and potatoes, and "light" carbohydrates such as wholemeal bread, brown or wild rice, vegetables, pulses, and grains. Heavy carbohydrates either have a high glycemic value and so cause the body to produce high levels of insulin, or they are more difficult for the body to digest and slow the digestive process.

Dietary fiber is also classified as a carbohydrate. It comes from the structural part of plants, and the body can't digest it. Dietary fiber enables the passage of digestible foods through the small and large intestines and so helps to avoid problems such as constipation. Good sources of dietary fiber include vegetables, fruit, pulses, and wholegrains.

carbohydrates and insulin response

Fifty years ago the typical diet was higher in starch and dietary fiber and lower in added sugars than it is today. There is some evidence that quickly digested carbohydrate-rich foods, such as most sugary, refined carboydrates and heavy carbohydrates like white rice and potatoes, cause blood glucose levels to rise quickly and provoke a rapid insulin response. On the other hand, carbohydrate-rich foods that are digested slowly – light carbohydrates such as wholemeal bread, brown rice, pulses, and vegetables – do not raise blood glucose levels in this way and stimulate a more gradual insulin response. If you eat more light carbohydrates, your body produces less insulin over the day and you may find that your appetite is better regulated as a result. High levels of insulin in the body also prevent the body from utilizing fat as an energy source, therefore making it more difficult to lose body fat.

fats

In many ways people in the West have become obsessed by fat. Very often when you want to lose weight or eat more healthily, you attempt to eliminate all fat from your diet. In fact, if you consider some of the healthiest diets in the world, the Mediterranean diet, for example, they are actually quite high in fat. This is because fats can be conveniently divided into good fats and bad fats. Good fats are essential to the body because they assist in both energy production and immune function; they also improve skin and hair condition. Bad fats are of no benefit to the body.

good fats

The good fats are the unsaturated fats: polyunsaturated oils and fats and the monounsaturated oils and fats. Generally, these fats are liquid at room temperature, and if not stored correctly, can spoil quickly due to their relative chemical sensitivity. The body needs these fats as a source of energy and also to help it extract energy from other food sources. These fats are found in olive oil, nuts, eggs, linseed oil, and sunflower seeds, and oily fish such as mackerel, fresh tuna, salmon, and sardines.

Good fats help energy production and speed up the metabolism. They strengthen the immune system, assist in the transportation of vitamins, help purify the blood and help fight against heart disease, cancer, arthritis, and other joint problems.

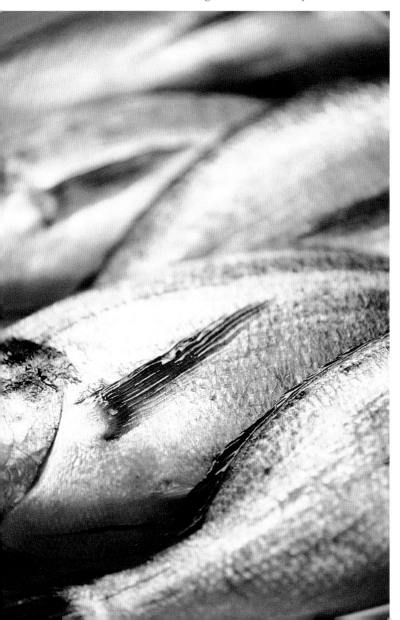

◄ oily fish
Try to make oily fish a big part of your weekly diet. They provide a rich array of nutrients and essential fats, which have countless health benefits for the whole body.

bad fats

The bad fats are saturated fats. Generally, these are hard or solid at room temperature. They are often used in processed foods. These fats offer no real benefit to the body at all and help increase the level of LDL's (low density lipoproteins) in the body. Bad fats can cause clogging of the arteries (just like hard water deposits in pipes) and thicken the blood, which contributes to high blood pressure and increases the risk of heart attack. These fats come from fatty meat, butter, hard margarine, cheese, and pastries.

Bad fats slow down the metabolism, encourage the buildup of cholesterol in the body, thicken the density of the blood, and are linked with high blood pressure and heart disease.

visible and invisible fats

Fats come in two other forms: visible fats and invisible. Visible fats are the ones that you can see, such as butter, margarine, oils, and the fat on meat. Invisible fats are the fats that slip into the diet without your knowing, such as fats in cookies, cakes, processed snack foods, nuts, cheese, and other dairy or animal products. All of these fats can be broken down into good and bad fats; it's just knowing which foods contain which type.

hydrogenated fats

Many of the margarines available contain oils that have been hydrogenated – treated to turn a liquid fat into a hard fat. This hydrogenation process changes the chemical structure of good fats so that they have more of the characteristics of bad fats. For this reason, no matter what the base oil, we would classify it as a bad fat. These fats are fine in small amounts, but use moderation because so many of them are hidden in processed foods. When making your choice of margarines and spreads, look for those labeled "no hydrogenated fats."

protein

Protein is the building block of the body. The continuous rebuilding, growth, and repair that goes on in the body is all down to protein and the amino acids that make it up. Without protein in the diet, the body cannot look after itself and vital body maintenance slows down. Excess protein in the diet can also be used as energy, but should never be used as the main energy source, as in high-protein diets (*see page 26*).

Meat is a good source of protein, but it is also possible to get protein from nonmeat sources. These also tend to be low in saturated fat (cheese is the exception) and include nuts, seeds, eggs (preferably free range), soya, tofu, beans, pulses, and cheese. If you do not eat meat, it is important to have as wide a variety of proteins as possible because there are not many nonmeat sources that contain all the essential amino acids. Therefore, eat as many different sources as you can so that your body receives what it needs to function optimally.

minerals

The minerals your body requires for good health can be readily obtained from a balanced diet. Minerals are important for the maintenance and growth of healthy bones and teeth; the transport of nutrients to and within cells; and controlling the composition of body fluids. They also work as catalysts for enzymes in the production of energy within the body and maintain a healthy blood profile and quality.

▼ **packed with vitamins and minerals**
Green vegetables are generally rich in vitamins A and C. Eat them in their raw state, or cook them very lightly so they retain more nutrients.

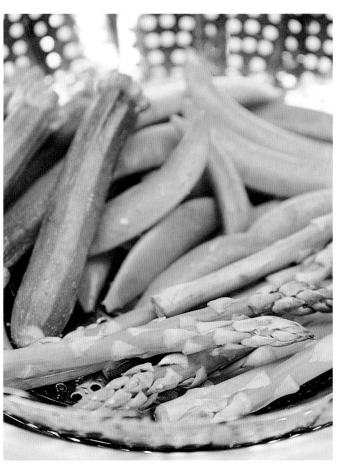

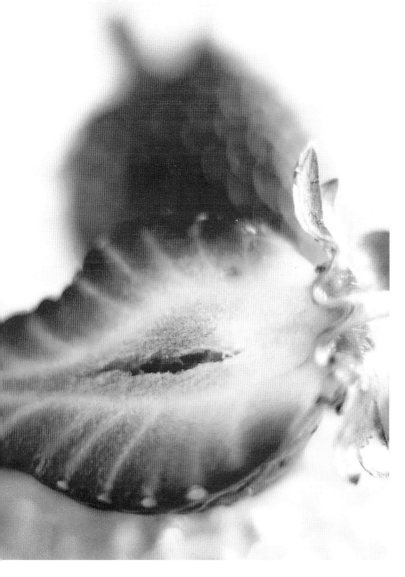

◀ **strawberries**
Try adding a few strawberries to your fruit salad in the morning, or include them in a smoothie with other fresh fruit. They provide an excellent source of vitamin C and are low in calories.

phosphorous: forms teeth and bones, maintains pH balance of blood; good sources: fish, poultry, cheese, eggs, yogurt

potassium: regulates blood pressure, nerve and muscle function; good sources: juices, fruit, nuts, pulses, vegetables, red wine

selenium: important for antioxidant enzymes made in body; good sources: nuts, seaweed, fish, wholegrains, meat

sodium: regulates body water balance, nerve function; good sources: common salt, wholemeal bread

zinc: promotes healthy nerves, brain tissue, immune system; good sources: meat, liver, eggs, beans, miso, pumpkin seeds

vitamins

Your body needs vitamins to regulate bodily functions, maintain bones, skin, blood, and nerves and keep it strong. Try to include as many as possible of the following vitamins by including the foods in your diet. The chart below tells you the function in the body and good sources for each vitamin.

vitamin A: essential for good eyesight, healthy skin, and body tissue; good sources: gleafy dark green vegetables, milk, cheese, fish, liver

vitamin B: essential for energy production, detoxifying alcohol, the metabolism of amino acids, healthy red blood cells and nerve function; good sources: meat, wheatgerm, eggs, peanuts

vitamin C: necessary for the maintenance of healthy connective tissue, assists immune function, effective anti-oxidant, aids body repair; good sources: citrus fruit, tomatoes, green peppers, leafy dark green vegetables, strawberries

vitamin D: helps maintain bones, assists calcium supply in the blood; good sources: dairy products, cod liver oil, oily fish, eggs

vitamin E: strong antioxidant in the body, maintains health of skin, may help to slow the aging process; good sources: leafy dark green vegetables, seeds, nuts, avocados (smaller amounts in cereals, fruit, meat)

vitamin K: essential blood clotting function; good sources: gleafy dark green vegetables, cereals, meat, yogurt, eggs

The following are considered to be essential minerals that are important for good health. Try to eat the mineral-rich foods listed here ias a regular part of your diet:

calcium: forms teeth and bones, helps blood clotting; good sources: milk, cheese, dark green vegetables, pulses

chloride: transports nutrients; good sources: most vegetables

copper: helps the production of hemoglobin, improves blood quality and condition of skin and hair; good sources: liver, fish, nuts, mushrooms, prunes

chromium: regulates insulin production and metabolism; good sources: pulses, wholegrains, meats, brewer's yeast

iron: forms red blood cells and healthy blood; good sources: wholegrains, pulses, leafy dark green vegetables, dried fruit, oily fish, red meat

magnesium: forms body tissues and bone; good sources: pulses, leafy dark green vegetables, fish, seeds, nuts, cocoa

supplements

There debate over the need for supplements in the diet continues. Dietitians say that most people can get all of the nutrients they need from a healthy, balanced diet – and this should certainly be your intention. Taking supplements should never be an excuse for a poor diet. There are just so many nutrients and beneficial phytochemicals (substances found in plants) and antioxidants that can't be packaged in a pill.

However, life today is faster and more stressful than ever before, and this can take its toll on the body. It can also make it harder to control food intake and eating choices, and the quality of our diet tends to worsen as a result.

People also eat more mass-produced food than ever, which is grown on depleted ground that, because of demand, has no time to replenish its nutrients. Some argue that, as a result, this food is less nutritious.

So, sometimes the body does need extra help to ensure that it functions as close to optimally as possible. I do not condone the use of high levels of single nutrients, but what my team and I find is that many people do require more help from certain minerals such as magnesium, potassium, and zinc and very often require extra levels of antioxidants.

variety in your diet

There was a time when the food that people ate was dictated by the seasons. Such variety was good for the body because it was ensured a range of nutrients from different foods in prime condition. These days we can buy most fruit and vegetables all year round so we don't have to change our diet in that way. Yet, even with increased choice, many people put the same foods in their shopping carts from one week to the next. A recent study showed that most weekly grocery purchases vary by less than 10 percent throughout the year.

There is no need – and it would be difficult – to go back to seasonal shopping, although many people argue that it is a healthier and more natural way to eat. But you should try to introduce as much variety into your diet as possible to ensure that you eat a more balanced diet and provide your body with a broader spectrum of nutrients.

seasonal diets

When it is cold, the body responds to an instinctive desire to gain body fat to keep warm. This is why you may find yourself craving starchy carbohydrates – for example, bread, pasta, and

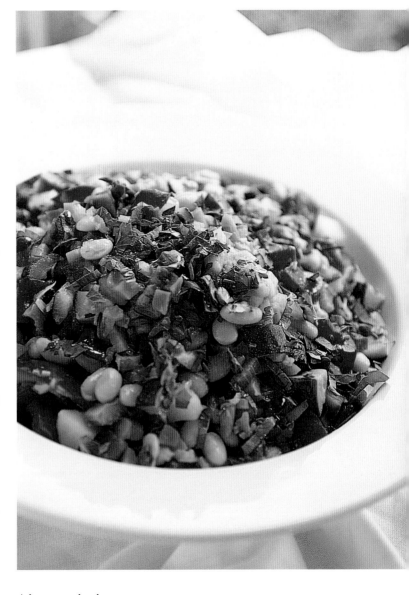

▲ **beans and pulses**
A rich source of nutrients, beans and pulses are low in fat and have a low glycemic index rating. They help to regulate the health of the intestines and in so doing cleanse the body.

potatoes, and hearty stews and broths. You also expend more energy keeping yourself warm, and carbohydrates provide a good slow-release energy source for the body. At warmer times of year, your body no longer needs a covering of body fat to insulate it from the cold, and you don't expend energy simply keeping yourself warm. As a result, you are less likely to crave starchy carbohydrates and heartier meals and less filling foods will satisfy you. This craving can make it more difficult to lose body fat in the cold months than in the warm ones.

the diet for modern living

The modern diet needs to be able to compensate for the effects of stress – emotional and environmental – on the body. It also needs to cope with high levels of oxidation in the body, which occur as a result of poor nutrient intake and low activity levels. My team and I believe that stress, less active lifestyles, changes in the quality of the food people eat, and the faster pace of life all create a more toxic environment in the body.

acid and alkaline foods

To tackle this situation you need to eat foods that can clean up the system, fight against oxidation, and neutralize free radicals. It is also wise to ensure that – at times when stress levels are high – you avoid eating foods that will increase toxin levels in the body. It is logical that different types of food have different levels of digestibility. My team and I believe that foods that are more difficult to digest create more toxic by-products as they are broken down. We call these foods acid-forming because they increase toxin levels in the body after digestion. Foods that are easy for the body to digest, we term alkaline foods.

We believe that eating a diet high in alkaline foods can help to reduce toxin levels in the body. Alkaline foods also put less stress on the digestive system because they are by nature easy to digest and so require less energy from the body.

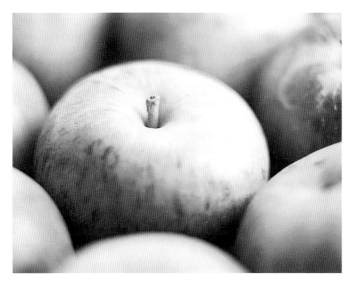

glycemic index of foods

The glycemic index (GI) rates each food according to how quickly it affects a rise in blood glucose levels. The higher a food's GI rating, the more quickly it causes blood glucose levels to rise. Conversely, the lower the GI rating, the more gradual the rise in blood glucose levels. The food guide on pages 34–5 classifies some of the more everyday foods into high, moderate and low glycemic index categories.

The modern Western diet is very high in foods that have a high GI rating. Items such as potatoes, white rice, most refined breads, cereals, cookies, and sugary foods all have high GI ratings. This means that they provide quick-release energy to the body. This sudden rush of energy causes the body to produce high levels of insulin to utilize and transport the sugar within the body. But the energy peak is short-lived, and as soon as it subsides, the appetite is stimulated and the body craves more energy. Quick-release energy is what it will crave, which means reaching for another high glycemic food. This promotes a cycle of energy peaks and troughs fueled by high glycemic snacking.

If your diet is high in high glycemic foods, you'll find it very hard or even impossible to resist your body's temptation to snack. The only way to break the cycle is to eat more foods that have low GI ratings, which provide slow-release energy and do not produce energy peaks and troughs in the body. Foods such as oats, pulses, wholemeal bread, and fresh and dried fruits, for example, all have low GI ratings.

Another negative effect of a high glycemic diet is that it causes excessive insulin production. My team and I believe that having high levels of insulin makes it harder for the body to utilize fat as an energy source, and so prevent effective fat burning. This makes it more difficult to lose excess body fat.

Extensive experience with our clients has shown us that a diet consisting mainly of low to medium glycemic alkaline foods doesn't just help to keep energy levels up, fine though that is. It also promotes good health and is easy to live with.

◀ **apples**
There is common sense in the old saying that an apple a day keeps the doctor away. Apples have a low glycemic index rating and are alkaline-forming; they are rich in vitamin C and high in soluble fiber.

food guide

This easy-reference food guide classifies everyday foods according to their glycemic index rating (*see page 33*) and their acid/alkaline effect on the body.

low-glycemic alkaline foods

These foods should make up 40% of your diet.

fruit

Apples
Apricots (fresh)
Berries (except blueberries)
Breadfruit
Cherries
Dates (fresh)
Figs (fresh)
Gooseberries
Grapes
Kiwis
Limes
Mangoes
Melons (all varieties)
Papaya
Passion fruit
Pears

vegetables

Asparagus
Broccoli
Brussels sprouts
Cabbage
Carrots
Cauliflower
Celery
Cucumber
Eggplant
Endive
Ginger (fresh)
Kale
Leeks
Peppers

Rhubarb
Sweet potato
Squash
Spinach
Turnips
Zucchini

grains

Amaranth
Millet
Quinoa
Wild rice

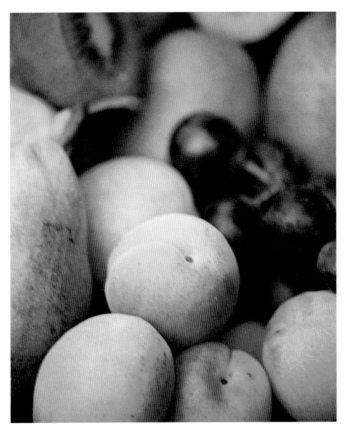

beans

Butter beans
Chick peas
Haricot beans
Kidney beans
Lentils
Peas
Soybeans (all soybean
   products, including tofu)

nuts and seeds

Almonds
Brazil nuts
Chestnuts
Sesame seeds

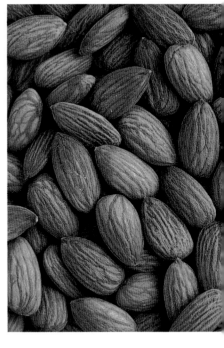

oils

Almond oil
Avocado oil
Fish oils (from oily fish)
Olive oil
Safflower oil
Sesame oil

medium-glycemic alkaline foods

These foods should make up 30% of your diet.

fruit

Pineapple
Strawberries

dairy

Milk (skimmed)
Dairy-free milk such as soy
   or rice milk

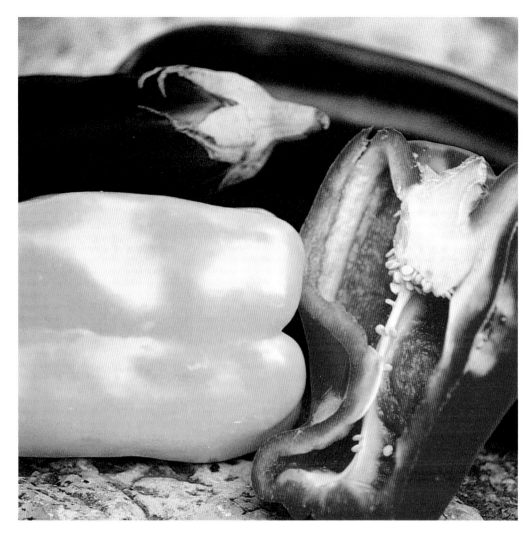

White pasta
Basmati rice
Popcorn
Pastries, cookies, cake

fruit
Citrus fruit
Cranberries
Plums
Prunes
Tomatoes

nuts
Cashews
Pistachios
Macadamias
Peanuts
Pecans
Walnuts

other occasional foods and drinks
Processed foods
Red meat
Chocolate
Tea, coffee
Alcohol

grains
Wholemeal bread
Wholemeal pasta
Brown rice
Couscous
Oats
Puffed rice
Puffed millet

seeds
Sunflower seeds
Pumpkin seeds

vegetables
Sweet corn

high-glycemic alkaline foods
These foods should make up less than 10% of your diet.

sugars
Honey
Syrup

vegetables
White potatoes
Parsnips

fruit
Bananas
Dried fruit

acid-forming foods
These foods should make up no more than 20% of your diet.

dairy
Butter
Cheese
Cream
Custard
Full-fat milk
Full-fat sweetened yogurt

grains
Wheat flakes
White bread

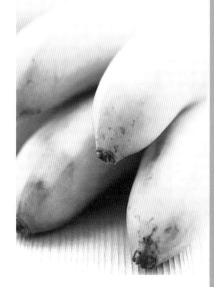

healthy eating

meal suggestions

A healthy diet should optimize your nutritional intake without compromising your enjoyment of the food. I recommend that you eat from the low-glycemic, low-alkaline-forming food groups (*see pages 33–5*). Where possible, eat fruit and vegetables in their fresh, raw state; and experiment with new ingredients. Here are some suggestions for meals that are enjoyable as well as nutritious. Most are quick to prepare and require little skill in the kitchen.

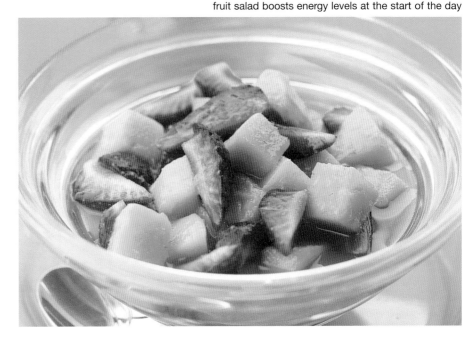

fruit salad boosts energy levels at the start of the day

breakfast

Breakfast really is the most important meal of the day. It should be substantial enough to last you through to lunch without the need for snacks. Vary your breakfast options.

Wheat-free breakfast cereal with skimmed or semiskimmed milk

Fruit salad with low-fat yogurt, or combine in a blender for a smoothie

Wholemeal toast with a little jam or marmalade

Oatmeal made without cream

Poached free-range eggs on wholemeal toast

Egg white omelette with mushrooms and peppers

lunch

Your body needs nutrients and energy-giving food by lunchtime. Eat a meal that consists of about 70 percent starch.

Wild rice salad with beans and asparagus

Bean salad with smoked salmon

Wheat-free pasta salad with pesto dressing

Wholemeal pasta with sun dried tomatoes

Sushi made with fish or vegetables

Avocado and salad sandwich on wholemeal bread (no mayonnaise)

Couscous salad with chicken or tofu

Marinated bean salad with olive oil, lemon, and chile

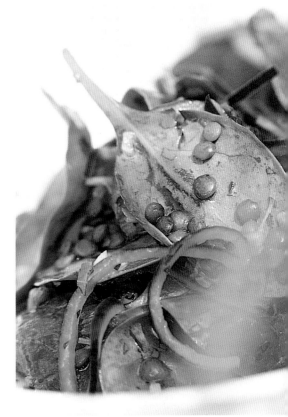

raw vegetables are full of vitamins and minerals

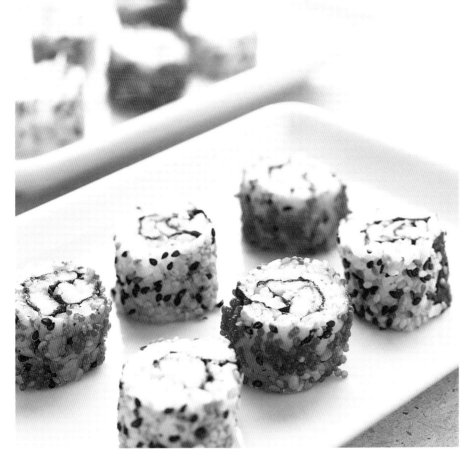

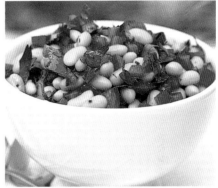

sushi makes a good low-fat lunch

a bean salad is delicious as well as filling

dinner

The later you eat, the more alkaline and vegetable-based your meal should be. Such foods are easier for the body to digest. Rather than adding oil or butter for flavor, experiment with rubs, marinades, spices, and fresh herbs.

Steamed vegetables with grilled or baked fish

Curried lentils with grilled vegetables

Seafood kebabs with grilled vegetables

Stir-fried vegetables such as bean sprouts, broccoli, zucchini, carrots, peppers, and mushrooms

Grilled chicken with celeriac and celery salad

Spinach and lentil salad

snacks

Snacking is important, but avoid foods that are high in processed sugar. Your main meals should sustain you through the day, but strategic snacking can keep your body satisfied in between meals.

Fresh fruit such as pears, bananas, apples, grapes, papaya, berries, mango, and kiwis

Almonds or brazil nuts

Small handfuls of dried fruits such as raisins, apricots, or prunes

Sunflower seeds

Pumpkin seeds

eating out

Eating out can be a challenge if you are watching your diet. Follow the few simple guidelines below to ensure that it's still a pleasurable experience and a treat.

Ask for food to be steamed, baked, or grilled rather than fried or cooked in a rich sauce

Avoid creamy or buttery sauces

Ask for food to be cooked without butter

Avoid the bread basket

Eat heavy dishes that contain red meat only very occasionally

Choose fruit compote, fruit salad, or sorbet for dessert

healthy eating

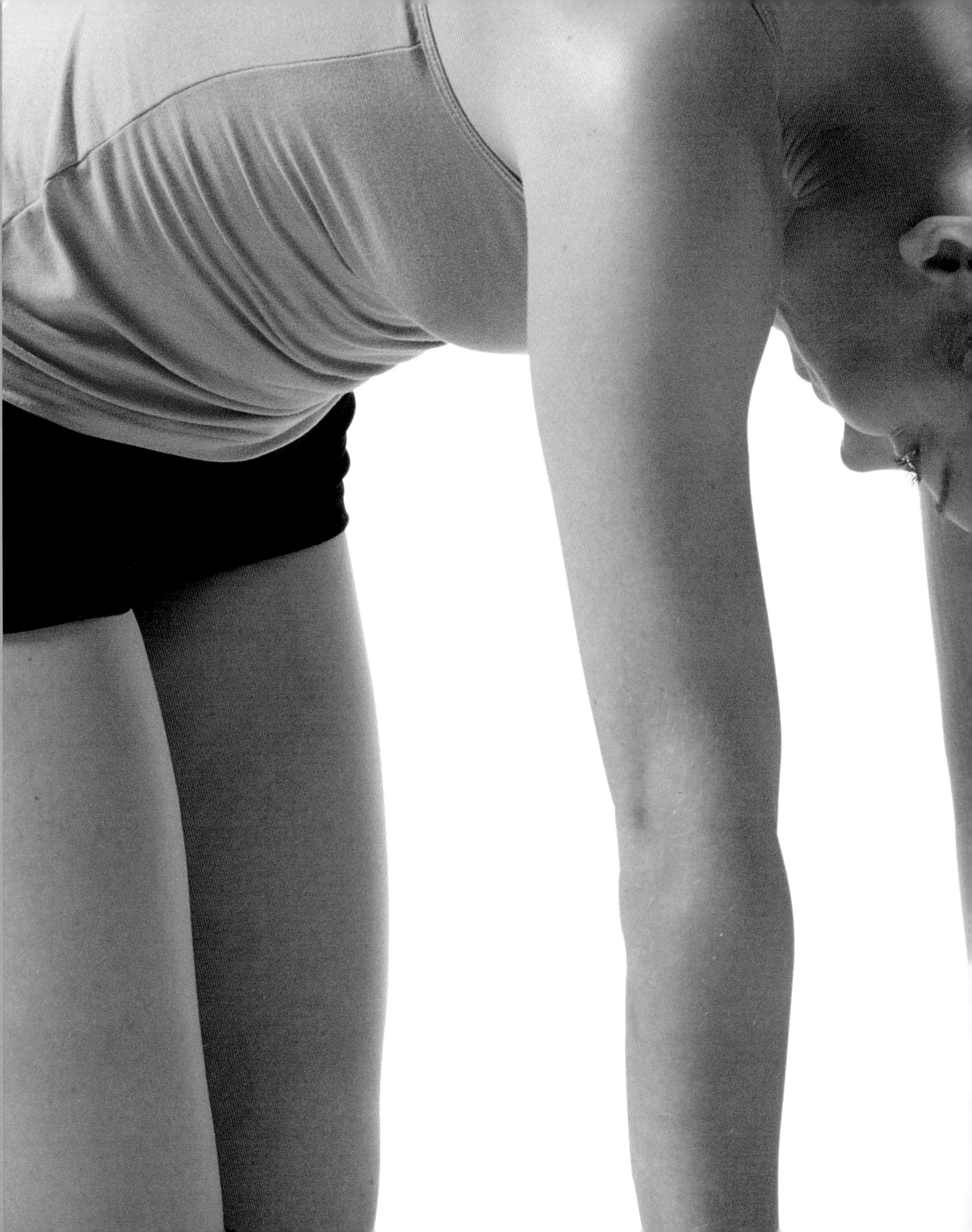

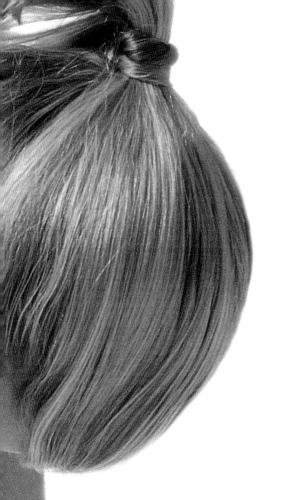

flexibility

It's normal to experience some muscle stiffness as you get older, but that doesn't have to spell an end to exercise and activity. Regular stretching can help to maintain – and even improve – flexibility and mobility, giving you a spring in your step and feelings of renewed vitality. For people who enjoy sports, good flexibility can be the difference between winning and losing. For anyone who is active, it can be the difference between injury and well-being.

flexibility

what does flexibility mean?

Good flexibility means you can enjoy improved mobility in your joints and muscles. Muscles enable joints to move, but the older they get the less elastic they can become. However, regular stretching can help to delay or slow down this process.

know how to stretch

Part of flexibility training is examining the daily demands you place on your body as well as considering any physical requirements unique to you. Maintaining flexibility is equally important whether you're deskbound or lead an active life.

Anyone who has spent years working at a desk without correcting their posture will probably have noticed some stiffness in the back and legs. The effect of the "desk posture" is to shorten the hip flexors, the muscles in the front of the body while lengthening the muscles in the back, which causes the spine to curve forward. In addition, sitting down for long periods can cause the muscles at the back of the legs, the hamstrings, to shorten, which can put pressure on the pelvic area when you are standing. Regular stretching in problem areas such as the back, knees, and ankles elongates the muscles and helps them to maintain a wide range of motion.

However, it is also possible to overstretch your muscles. Your muscles support your skeleton and protect your joints; when you overstretch a muscle, your joints become hypermobile – capable of flexing or extending beyond their normal limits. There is therefore a greater risk of injury because your muscles are less effective at protecting your joints. This is when you might harm the intervertebral discs and surrounding nerves in your back or damage cartilage or ligaments in a hypermobile knee joint. Women are more flexible when pregnant because the body produces the hormone relaxin to help it through childbirth. Therefore, pregnant women should not push the body beyond its usual limits as this may cause harm. The best way to improve your flexibility is through regular and gentle stretching that gradually increases a joint's range of motion.

when should you stretch?

Ideally, do some gentle stretching every day. A simple routine is enough to maintain good flexibility and doesn't require more than 10 minutes – time well spent to insure yourself against future problems. Postexercise stretching is essential. Exercise causes your muscles to contract and shorten, actually reducing flexibility. Stretching after exercise, when muscles are warmed up and as a result more responsive, reduces the shortening and helps to disperse lactic acid that builds up during a workout. You also significantly reduce your risk of injury.

Pretraining flexibility work is important but not essential. A good, slow, progressive warmup that simulates the movements in the main part of your workout or activity will ensure that your joints are sufficiently prepared for exercise.

▼ **new lease on life**
Being flexible increases your range of movement, making any activity more enjoyable, whether it's a challenging sport or a game of Frisbee.

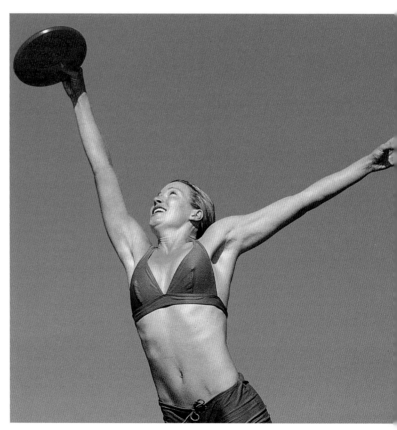

flexibility test

The five exercises below test the flexibility in different parts of your body and will help you to isolate any area that might need work. See pages 42–9 for stretches.

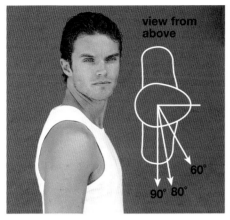

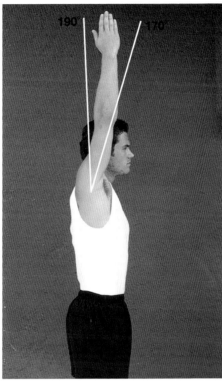

▲ **neck flexion** Stand with arms by your sides and head and neck relaxed. Turn your head toward your shoulder, as far as is comfortable. Measure the degree of motion in your neck.
less than 75° poor; **75–80°** good; **80–90°** very flexible

◀ **arms and shoulders**
Stand or sit with back straight, shoulders relaxed, and arms by your sides. Raise one arm up by the side of your head. Hold your abdominals tight and keep your elbow straight and your hand facing inward. Measure the degree of motion.
up to 170° poor; **170–180°** good; **over 180°** very flexible

▼ **hip flexor and hamstring** Lie flat on your back with both legs straight. Raise one leg up into the air and measure the degree of motion at your hip.
up to 75° poor; **75–90°** good; **over 90°** very flexible

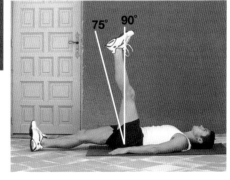

▼ **lower back** Lie flat on your back with your shoulders on the floor and arms out at right angles to keep you in position. Keeping your left leg straight, bend your right leg at 90°, and cross it over your body. Aim to get your right knee to touch the floor, but stop at the point where your shoulder begins to lift off the floor.
less than 45° poor; **45–75°** good; **over 75°** very flexible

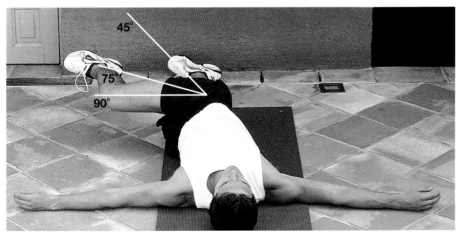

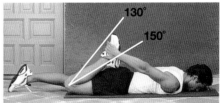

▲ **knee and quads** Lie flat on your stomach with your arms by your sides. Reach back and grasp your right foot with your right hand, and pull your foot toward your butt. **up to 130°** poor; **130–150°** good; **over 150°** very flexible

flexibility

neck and shoulder stretches

The neck and shoulder muscles have to work tirelessly, and bear particular strain if you work in a static position such as at a computer or hunched over a desk. This is where most people store tension, so it's important to maintain good flexibility here.

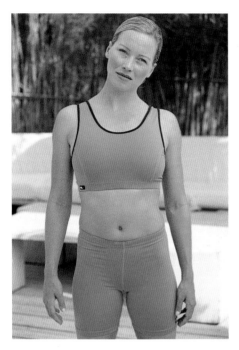

◄ **neck stretch** Stand with feet hip-width apart, shoulders relaxed, and arms by your sides. Gently tilt the head to one side so you feel the stretch in the other side of the neck. Hold for 10–12 seconds, taking care not to push the stretch to the point where it becomes uncomfortable.

▶ **head forward stretch** Stand with feet hip-width apart, shoulders relaxed, and arms by your sides. Keeping your back straight, gently drop your head forward until you feel the stretch in the back of the neck and the upper back. Hold for 10–15 seconds.

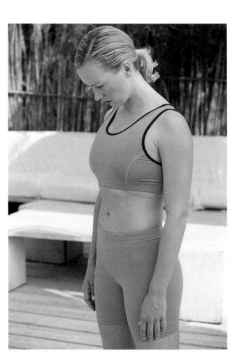

▶ **shoulder stretch** Stand with feet hip-width apart, legs slightly bent. Bend your left arm a little, and bring it across your body so your hand is by your right shoulder. Place your right hand on your upper arm to push the stretch a little further. You should feel the stretch in the back of the shoulder. Hold for about 10 seconds on each side.

▶▶ **anterior deltoid stretch** Stand with feet hip-width apart and back straight. Take one arm behind you and, grasping it by the wrist, gently ease it behind your back. Take care to keep your shoulders straight. Hold for about 10 seconds, until you feel the stretch at the front of the shoulder. Repeat for the other arm.

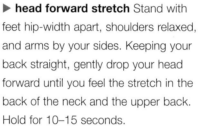

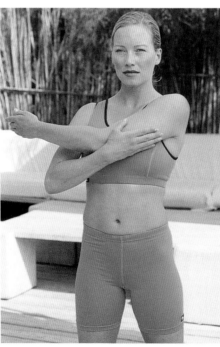

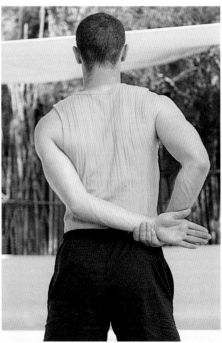

chest and arm stretches

The chest is also a common area for tension to be stored, and as a result the muscles here can become tight and inflexible, which can cause postural problems. Strong and flexible triceps and biceps can prevent muscle tension in the chest and upper back.

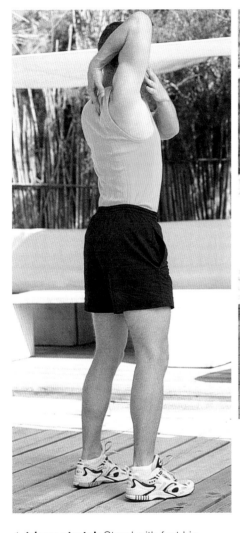

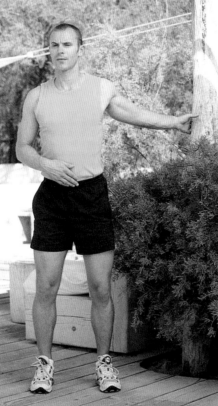

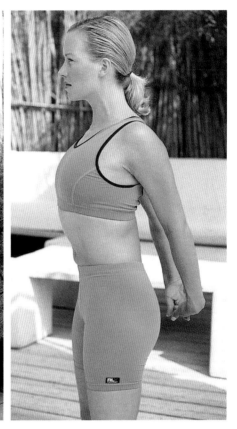

▲ **tricep stretch** Stand with feet hip-width apart, legs slightly bent. Raise your right arm and place your right hand over your back as if you were reaching down your spine. Use your left hand to gently push your right arm back and increase the stretch. You should feel this stretch down the back of the arm. Hold for 10 seconds on each side.

▲ **bicep and chest stretch** Stand an arm's length away from a wall or pole, and place the palm of your hand against it. Keeping your arm straight, gently rotate the body forward, away from your hand, so you feel a stretch in the chest and arm. Hold for 15 seconds. Repeat the stretch using your other arm.

▲ **chest stretch** Stand with feet hip-width apart and legs slightly bent. Hold your abdominals tight and keep your head, neck, and shoulders relaxed. Clasp your hands behind your back and, keeping your back straight, lift your arms behind you until you feel the stretch across your chest. Hold for 10–14 seconds.

flexibility

43

back stretches

The back holds tension more than any other area of the body. It is particularly important to stretch the back properly after exercise because, during a workout, the back muscles contract, increasing the tension even further.

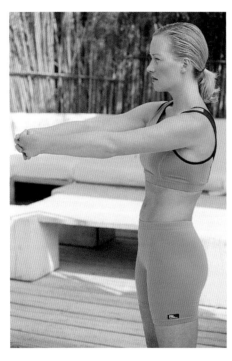

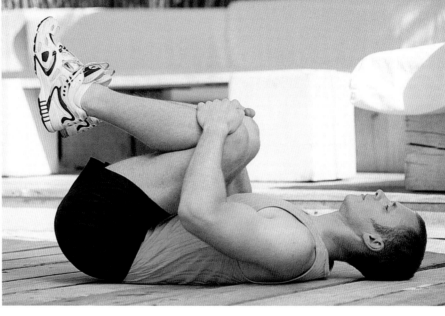

▲ **upper back stretch** Stand with feet hip-width apart and legs slightly bent. Straighten your arms and clasp your fingers together in front of you. Gently push your hands away from you, keeping your lower back firm and your body upright. You should feel this stretch across the upper back and at the back of the shoulders. Hold for about 10 seconds.

▲ **lower back stretch** Lie on your back. Holding the tops of your shins, bring both knees in toward your body. Gently pull your knees in closer until you feel the stretch in your lower back. Hold for 10 seconds.

▶ **hyperextension of back** Lie down flat on your front on the floor. Tuck your elbows in close to your body. Keeping your hips on the floor, push your torso up until you are supporting your body weight on your elbows. Take care to keep your neck relaxed. Hold for 15 seconds.

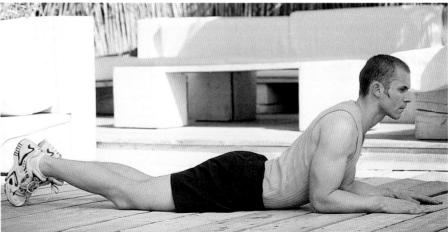

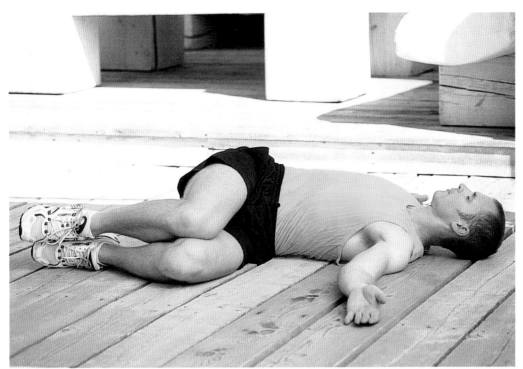

◀ **spine rotation** Lie on your back, arms outstretched at shoulder level. Bend both legs at about 90° and slowly drop your knees to the left until the left knee is touching the floor. Keep your shoulder blades flat on the floor. Don't force the stretch. Hold for 10 seconds.

▼ **cat stretch** Go down on your hands and knees, keeping your back straight. Push your spine upward to create a curve in the middle of your back. Hold the position for 5 seconds, then release the stretch and return to the start position.

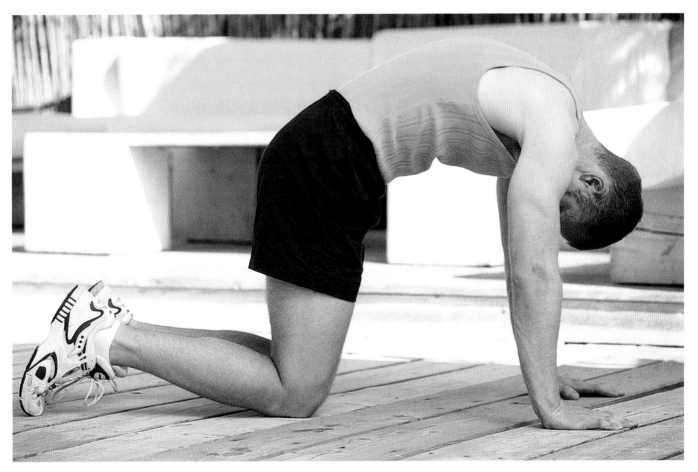

flexibility

leg stretches

These stretches target the major muscles in the legs. It's important to stretch muscles such as the hip flexor because they are often neglected or forgotten. The hamstring stretches are great after a long walk or a jog.

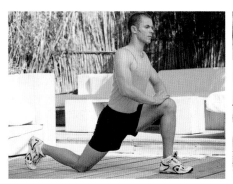

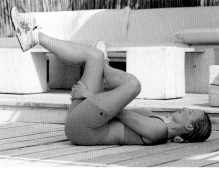

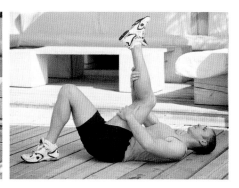

▲ **hip flexor** Kneel on both knees. Step forward with your left foot keeping your right knee on the floor. Place your hands on each side of your front foot. Slide your back leg out behind you until you feel the stretch in the front of the hip. Push your hip forward, straighten your body and place your hands on your front knee to intensify the stretch. Hold for 10-12 seconds.

▲ **glute stretch** Lie on your back on the floor. Bend your right knee, keeping your foot on the floor, and cross your left leg over it, so your left ankle rests just above your right knee. Hold behind the right thigh with both hands and gently pull your leg toward you. You should feel the stretch in your butt and outer thigh. Hold for 10 seconds then repeat for the other leg.

▲ **prone hamstring stretch** Lie on your back on the floor with your right leg bent. Hold your left leg with one hand behind the thigh and one hand behind the calf muscle. Keeping your left leg as straight as possible, gently pull it toward you until you feel the stretch down the back of the thigh. Hold for about 10 seconds, allowing the muscle to relax into the stretch.

▶ **standing hamstring stretch** Stand facing a bench or rail. Place your right foot on the bench or rail and straighten your right leg. Keep your left, supporting leg slightly bent. Slowly bend forward from the hips until you feel the stretch in the back of the thigh, top of calf, and into the back of the knee. Hold for about 8 seconds, without bouncing, then slowly lean in a little further to intensify the stretch. Raise the height of the bench as you become more flexible. Repeat for the other leg.

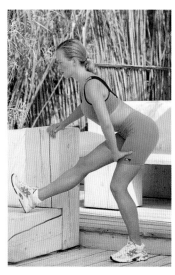

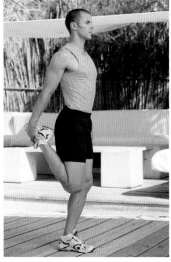

◀ **standing quadricep stretch** You may want to stand against a wall or rail for support. Stand up straight, keeping your left, supporting leg slightly bent. Bend your right leg and, holding the front of your foot, pull your foot up toward your butt. Keep your knees together, your hips pointing forward, and your back as straight as possible. Push the knee of the stretching leg slightly further back to intensify the stretch. Hold for about 10 seconds, then repeat for the right leg.

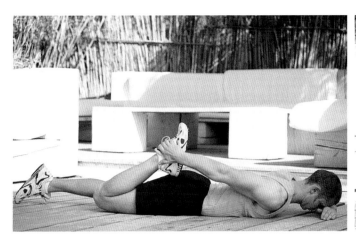

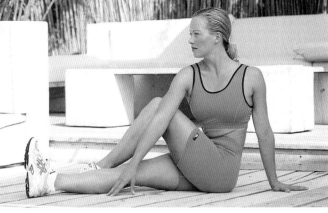

▲ **prone quadricep stretch** Lie face down on the floor. Keeping your hips on the floor, bring your right leg up behind you and hold the front of your foot. Keep your head down and your neck relaxed. Hold for about 10-12 seconds, then repeat for the left leg.

▲ **outer thigh (abductor muscles)** Sit up with your right leg extended straight out in front of you and your left leg crossed over it, so that the foot is on the outside of the knee. With your left arm for support, use your right arm to ease the knee across the body. You should feel the stretch in the outer thigh. Hold for 12 seconds.

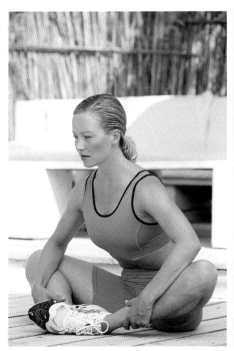

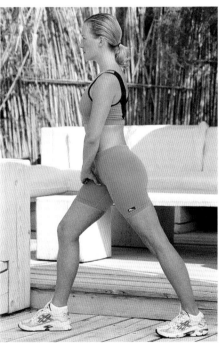

◀ **calf stretch** You may want to use a wall for support, in which case stand at arm's length away from it and place hands on the wall at chest level. Stand with feet together, then step back with your left foot, pushing into the heel and bending your right leg slightly. Keep your back straight. Keep both feet parallel and facing forward and both heels on the floor. Imagine a straight line running from your back heel to your head. Intensify the stretch by stepping further back with your rear leg. Hold for about 8 seconds. As you relax into the stretch, move the rear foot slightly further back, pushing into the heel, and hold for a further 4 seconds. Repeat about 3 times, then stretch the right calf.

▲ **inner thigh (adductor muscles)** Sit up with your back straight. Place the soles of your feet together and, holding your ankles, pull your feet in toward you. Hold the stretch, feeling it in your inner thighs, as your legs relax down toward the floor. Intensify the stretch by placing your hands on your ankles and your elbows on your knees and, keeping your back straight, gently easing the body forward from the hips. If you are very flexible, use your elbows to apply gentle pressure on the top of the inner thigh until you feel the stretch. Hold for 10–12 seconds, then gently ease the stretch a stage further.

flexibility

stretching sequences

Our bodies take a great deal of battering in our every-day life, and it can feel wonderful to release all of that tension with a really good stretching session. Don't forget that stretching after exercise helps your muscles to relax and to reduce muscle soreness or stiffness. The hold times indicated for each stretch are the minimum amount of time that the muscle needs to really relax. There is nothing wrong with holding the stretches for longer, and allowing the muscles to get more out of each stretch. If you do choose to stretch for longer, keep feeling for the point at which the muscle relaxes. Then, ease the stretch a bit further so that the muscle length is constantly developed.

total body stretch sequence

This sequence can leave you feeling like a new person. Take your time, and keep your breathing slow and controlled throughout. You might want to put on some relaxing music.

lower body stretch sequence

If you've done an intense lower body toning routine, or been out walking or running and have plenty of time to stretch, this sequence gives you the ultimate lower body stretch.

short standing stretch sequence

This short sequence is ideal as a cooldown after a run, fast walk or game of golf, softball, or tennis. If you don't have time for a total body stretch, it gives you all the standing exercises that can be done quickly and stretches all the major muscles.

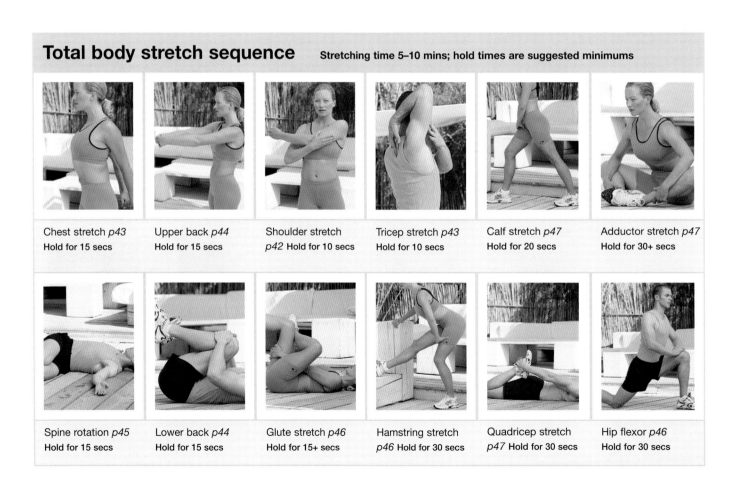

Total body stretch sequence Stretching time 5–10 mins; hold times are suggested minimums

Chest stretch *p43* Hold for 15 secs	Upper back *p44* Hold for 15 secs	Shoulder stretch *p42* Hold for 10 secs	Tricep stretch *p43* Hold for 10 secs	Calf stretch *p47* Hold for 20 secs	Adductor stretch *p47* Hold for 30+ secs
Spine rotation *p45* Hold for 15 secs	Lower back *p44* Hold for 15 secs	Glute stretch *p46* Hold for 15+ secs	Hamstring stretch *p46* Hold for 30 secs	Quadricep stretch *p47* Hold for 30 secs	Hip flexor *p46* Hold for 30 secs

Lower body stretch sequence

Stretching time 5 mins; hold times are suggested minimums

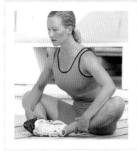
Adductor stretch *p47*
Hold for 30+ secs

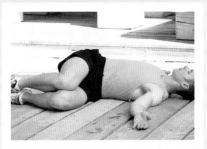
Spine rotation *p45*
Hold for 15 secs

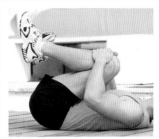
Lower back stretch *p45*
Hold for 15 secs

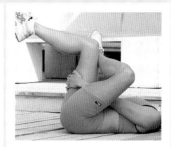
Glute stretch *p46*
Hold for 15+ secs

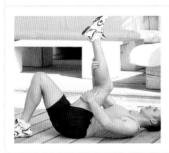
Prone hamstring stretch
p46 Hold for 30 secs

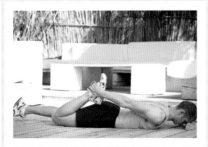
Prone quadricep stretch *p47*
Hold for 30 secs

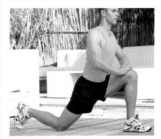
Hip flexor *p46*
Hold for 30 secs

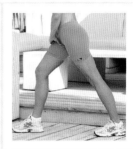
Calf stretch *p47*
Hold for 20 secs

Short standing stretch sequence

Stretching time 5 mins; hold times are suggested minimums

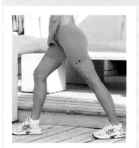
Calf stretch *p47*
Hold for 20 secs

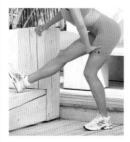
Hamstring stretch *p46*
Hold for 20 secs

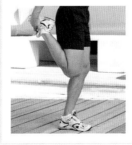
Standing quadricep
stretch *p46*
Hold for 20 secs

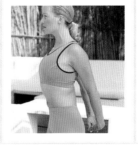
Chest stretch *p43*
Hold for 15 secs

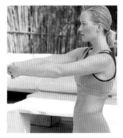
Upper back stretch *p44*
Hold for 15 secs

flexibility

49

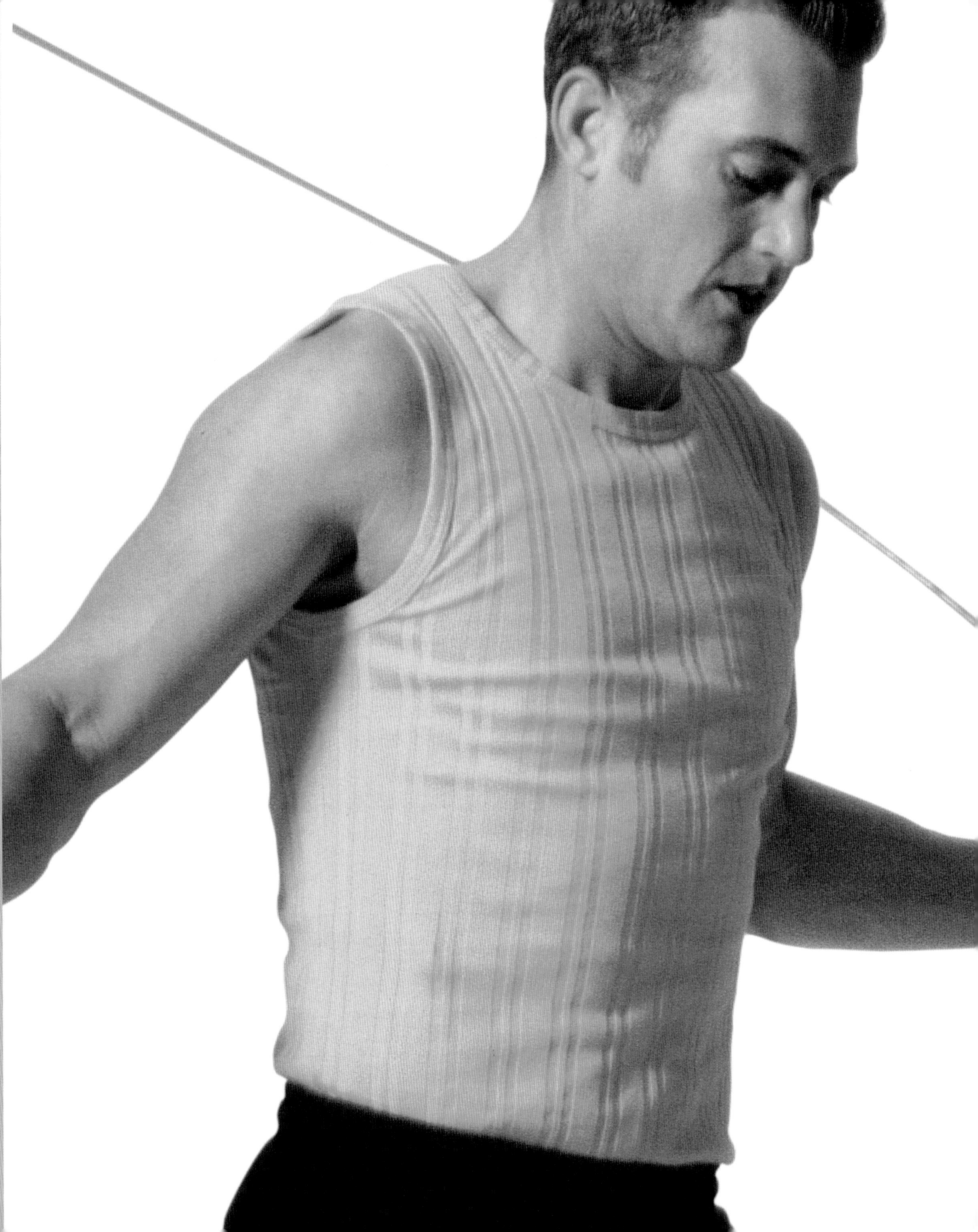

aerobic training

Aerobic training – exercise that raises the heart rate, conditions the heart and lungs, and burns fat – is an important part of health and fitness. I am often asked which aerobic exercise is best for burning fat and building aerobic strength. I always say that the best aerobic exercise is the one that you are most likely to do – and keep on doing. This chapter tells you how to get the most out of whatever aerobic exercise you choose, whether it be running, walking, cycling, or swimming, and whether you do it at the gym or outdoors.

what is aerobic training?

Aerobic training, or "cardio" as it is often referred to, is fundamental to any good fitness program. It works your heart and lungs and helps to improve your physical fitness, but it also has countless other benefits, from boosting energy levels and improving your ability to concentrate, to reducing your risk of heart disease. As you read this book, your body is working aerobically, or "with air." Your lungs extract oxygen from the air that you breathe. When you exercise, you increase your body's demand for oxygen in the same way that the demand for fuel is increased when you drive a car faster. Any activity that gets your heart working harder and raises your heart rate – running, fast walking, rowing, cycling, skiing, swimming, or skating for example – is a form of aerobic exercise.

how does it work?

The oxygen that your lungs take from the air that you breathe acts like a fuel for your body. When you train aerobically, you increase the rate at which your body uses oxygen, and you aim to work within an objective "zone" where you burn energy most efficiently. Your body uses oxygen when you sit or stand or walk down the street. When you push yourself too hard, you begin to exercise anaerobically, or "without air." Your body can't keep up with your muscles' demand for oxygen and you burn out quickly from exhaustion. As you get in better shape, your body becomes more efficient at supplying your muscles with oxygen and you can train harder and for longer periods of time.

why is it so important?

The heart is a muscle and it responds to exercise in the same way as any other muscle in the body: it adapts. As it is pushed to new levels of exertion, it responds by growing stronger. A strong heart has a higher stroke volume – it can pump more blood out of the heart with each beat – and therefore doesn't

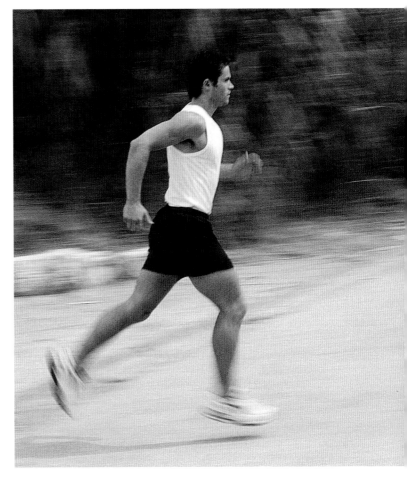

▲ break into a sweat
Aerobic exercise works the heart and lungs, but it can also help you combat stress and sleep more soundly.

need to work as hard to meet the body's increased demand for oxygenated blood as it exerts itself. Your body can cope with higher levels of physical exertion, and your heart rate at rest decreases as well, which means less strain is put on your cardiovascular system. In short, you are in better shape.

When you exercise, your arteries and capillaries dilate, which boosts circulation. If you exercise regularly, the long-term benefits can be reduced blood pressure and lower risk of heart attack; circulatory problems such as cold hands and feet may also be improved. As your aerobic fitness level rises, the intercostal muscles, the muscles that surround the ribcage, become stronger, increasing lung efficiency. You use a very small percentage of your lung capacity when you breathe, but regular aerobic exercise helps to increase this percentage. The effect of this is that the alvioli – the small balloonlike sacs in your lungs that transfer oxygen to the blood – are able to absorb oxygen more efficiently. These small transfer systems can be damaged by smoking, for example, which damages the alvioli and makes them less efficient at transferring oxygen. As a result you experience breathlessness.

Aerobic exercise burns calories, and therefore fat. The body burns fat and sugar reserves as energy sources even while resting. When you exercise aerobically, it draws on its most readily available sources of energy – sugar reserves in the blood and muscles (glycogen) and fat reserves. It uses fats at a lower rate than sugars. Although you burn more sugars than fats when you exercise, you increase the rate at which you burn them, so you still burn more fats than you would in a resting state. If you want to burn fat, you have to work aerobically.

Along with the many physical benefits of aerobic exercise come numerous psychological ones. Apart from boosting your immune system, strengthening your bones, and improving your posture, regular aerobic exercise also boosts confidence, improves concentration, helps you to cope better with stress and helps you to sleep more soundly.

Exercise, and aerobic exercise in particular, awakens a natural instinct to go farther and faster – to work yourself that bit harder and to improve on previous performances. It is the reason that people respond to working toward goals such as running a marathon, for example. Physically, it improves body awareness, but the effects can be more far reaching. It's not unusual for clients of mine to tell me about professional successes or career promotions after having embarked on a fitness program. Exercise will even make you feel more contented. Your body releases adrenaline and serotonin, a chemical that makes you feel happy. Together with increased levels of oxygen in the blood, these produce the general sense of wellbeing that follows aerobic exercise; this is also known as "runner's high." Many regular exercisers use their workout sessions as a release and as a way of setting aside problems and stresses. Research has shown that regular exercise can even help in the treatment of clinical depression.

▶ **exercise to lift your spirits**
Regular aerobic exercise can enhance your mood and lift your spirits. It's a healthy form of stress relief.

when not to exercise

There are times when you shouldn't exercise. If you're feeling exhausted, run down, or as if you may be about to succumb to a cold or flu, take a break from your exercise routine. You can't sweat a cold or flu out of your system. When you are ill, your immune system has to work hard to fight off the infection. Vigorous exercise will deplete the body of the reserve energy it needs to do this, and may make symptoms more severe, the illness more prolonged, and recovery slower.

You should stop exercising immediately if you feel faint or dizzy. You are pushing your body too hard and it just can't cope. This is why it's important to monitor your heart rate when exercising and to work within your optimum training zone (*see pages 54–5*). Go through the physical questionnaire (*see pages 22–3*) before you embark on a program, and always work at the percentage of MHR specified.

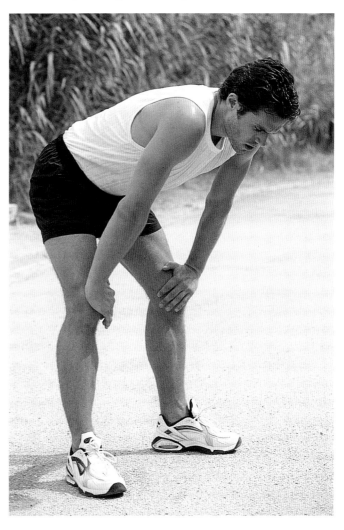

aerobic training

heart rate training zones

Being aware of your working heart rate – your heart rate while exercising – is a little like knowing how to cook. Just as you need to be aware of the correct oven temperature to get a successful result, you need to aim to work out at an optimum heart rate that will work your heart and lungs most efficiently. Whatever your ultimate goal – to lose weight, run a marathon, or improve your performance in a particular sport – being aware of your heart rate training zone is crucial to your success. It allows you to check and monitor your body's response to different levels of exertion, and to maximize the effectiveness of your workouts.

optimum training zone

To work your heart and lungs most efficiently and to burn fat, you need to aim to work at between 65 and 85 percent of your maximum heart rate (MHR) – this is known as your optimum training zone. To calculate your MHR, assume that your MHR when you are born is 220, reducing by one for every year of life. So your MHR = 220 minus your age. If you are 35, your MHR is 185 beats per minute (bpm). Sixty-five percent of 185 (0.65 x 185) is 120, and 85 percent of 185 (0.85 x 85) is 157. When you train, aim to keep your heart rate above 120 bpm but below 157 bpm. If you train above your optimum training zone, you begin to work anaerobically and your body can't keep up with the demand for oxygen. You won't be able to sustain a workout at such high intensity, and will quickly become exhausted. You need to work within your optimum training zone to ensure you get the most from your workouts.

The best way to monitor your heart rate is by using a heart rate monitor (*see right*), or by taking your pulse manually. As you learn more about how your body responds to exertion, you'll find you can recognize what heart rate you are working at by how you feel; you won't have to stop to measure your heart rate. Try using the rate of perceived exertion scale (*see right*), which gives a numerical rating that corresponds to physical symptoms at different levels of exertion.

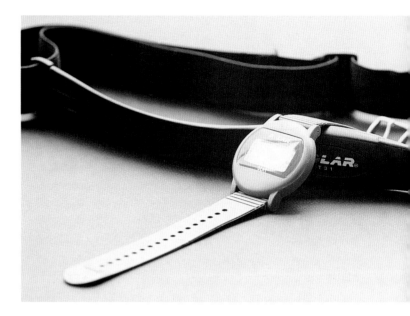

▲ **essential equipment** Take the guess work out of measuring your heart rate, and ensure you get the most out of your workouts by investing in a heart rate monitor. These simple devices vary in price, and some are very affordable.

The chart below shows the percentage of MHR for different age groups in average bpm. Use it to find your optimum training zone.

age	65%MHR	70%MHR	75%MHR	80%MHR	85%MHR
18–25	130	139	149	159	169
26–30	127	134	144	153	163
31–36	124	130	140	149	158
37–42	120	126	135	144	153
43–50	116	121	129	138	147
51–58	112	116	124	133	141
59–65	108	110	118	126	134
65+	104	106	114	121	129

monitoring your heart rate

The most reliable methods for monitoring your heart rate are to take your pulse manually or to use a heart rate monitor. You can also use the rate of perceived exertion (rpe) scale, when you are more familiar with how your body responds to exercise.

taking your pulse manually

You can take your pulse at your wrist or neck. Find your pulse at your wrist by following the line of your thumb and placing two fingers approximately 1in (2cm) below your wrist joint. The pulse at the side of your neck is just below the jawbone. Always use two fingers (not your thumb) to take your pulse. Count for 15 seconds, then multiply by 4 to get a bpm figure.

using a heart rate monitor

This is the easiest and most accurate way to measure heart rate. You wear a strap around your chest, which monitors your heart rate and transmits a signal to a watchlike device on your wrist. It gives you a continuous reading. See page 213 for more information on choosing a heart rate monitor.

using the rate of perceived exertion (rpe) scale

If you don't have a heart rate monitor, or don't want to stop to take your pulse, the rpe scale is a convenient way of monitoring how hard you are working. The scale gives a physical symptom for each level of exertion that corresponds to a number from one to 10: at number one you are at rest, and at 10 you are working at your hardest. Each number on the scale also corresponds to a percentage of MHR. In the chart below, MHR estimates start at 6 because everyone has different heart rates at rest. Look at the descriptions of how you can expect to feel at different levels of exertion, and once you are used to the system, you should be able to monitor how hard you are working and adjust the intensity of your workout accordingly.

Many people prefer this method of monitoring their performance when working out. It can give you a better understanding of how your body responds to exercise. The scale does not change as your fitness level improves. From time to time, check your heart rate against the scale to ensure that your perception of the intensity of your exercise is accurate.

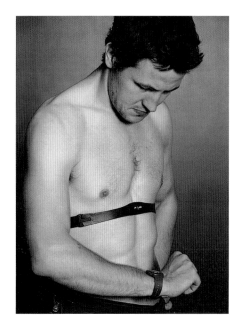

▲ accurate and convenient
The strap around your chest monitors electrical activity in your heart and transmits signals to a watchlike receiver on your wrist. With a heart rate monitor, there's no need to interrupt your workout to check your heart rate – you simply glance at your wrist.

rate of perceived exertion

at rest	**1**	nonexercise heart rates
low level activity, sitting working	**2**	nonexercise heart rates
light exertion such as gentle walking	**3**	nonexercise heart rates
purposeful walking	**4**	nonexercise heart rates
brisk walking	**5**	nonexercise heart rates
medium- to fast-paced walking	**6**	60% MHR
breathing becomes more difficult	**7**	65–75% MHR
breathing heavily, conversation just possible	**8**	80% MHR
sweating, difficult to hold conversation	**9**	85% MHR
maximum effort, hard to maintain for long	**10**	maximum heart rate

aerobic training

55

aerobic training techniques

Different training techniques work the heart and lungs – and therefore build aerobic strength – in different ways. There are two principal training techniques: constant pace training, which builds endurance – the strength you need for a long run; and interval training, which builds stamina – the strength you need to play team sports where you often stop and start or regularly change intensity.

constant pace training

Working for extended periods at a steady pace, or at least keeping your heart rate within a small working zone, is called constant pace training. It is a training technique that builds endurance and helps the body to use oxygen more efficiently. It increases lung capacity and local muscle endurance.

While you will burn marginally more fat with interval training, constant pace training is crucial for building a good base level of fitness. This will improve your performance in any field of sport or exercise.

interval training

This is where you work for a short period at a high intensity, recover by working for a short period at a low intensity, and then repeat the cycle. Interval training builds aerobic strength and stamina because it enables you to work the respiratory and cardiovascular system at a very intense level. The effect of this is to overload the heart and lungs – they have to become stronger to meet the physical challenge, and, as a result, you become fitter. Interval training places high energy demands on your body. It's a more effective method of burning fat than constant pace training because it raises your base metabolic rate (bmr), the rate at which you burn calories when at rest. Interval training also has an "afterburn effect," which means that it raises your metabolic rate for as long as 18 hours after your exercise session.

peripheral heart action (pha)

This is a form of interval training. It is in fact a resistance training technique, but it also conditions the heart. It alternates exercises between the upper and then the lower body, so the heart has to work hard to supply blood to the muscles at each end of the body. This has the same effect as interval training since the heart rate increases in response to large shifts of blood from one part of the body to the other. When you weight train normally, it might feel as though the heart is pounding, but this is more as a result of the increase in blood pressure that results from high exertion than from an increased heart rate. Circuit training uses pha training; because you rest between exercises you maintain obvious heart rate peaks and troughs.

training techniques and heart rate

The charts below illustrate the effects that constant pace and interval training have on the heart rate. Both charts clearly show the effect of the warmup and cool-down periods. When constant pace training, you might need to lower the intensity of your workout to maintain a steady heart rate toward the end of the 20 minutes. Most people would find the interval training heart rate pattern difficult to maintain for the entire session. As your fitness level improves, it becomes easier to control your heart rate and you need less time to recover.

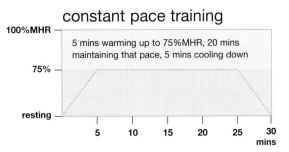

constant pace training

5 mins warming up to 75%MHR, 20 mins maintaining that pace, 5 mins cooling down

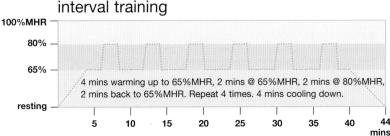

interval training

4 mins warming up to 65%MHR, 2 mins @ 65%MHR, 2 mins @ 80%MHR, 2 mins back to 65%MHR. Repeat 4 times. 4 mins cooling down.

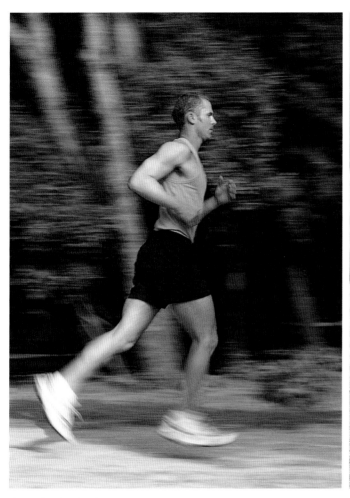

▲ run to stay in shape
Running is a form of constant pace training. It's a good aerobic exercise that will help you to burn calories, but try introducing interval training techniques to get the most out of a session.

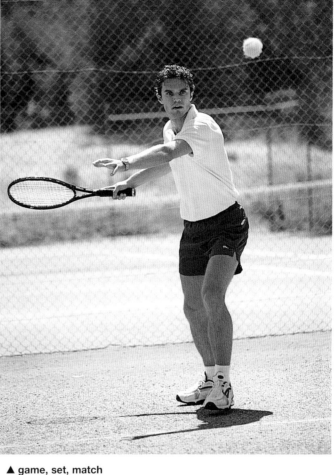

▲ game, set, match
Reduce rest time between points to ensure that a game of tennis provides a good interval training session. Professional players often rush their opponents between shots if they suspect they are less fit.

training techniques and sports

Just as training techniques work your body in different ways, most sports and aerobic activities make different demands on your body and fall into either the constant pace or interval training category. You can concentrate on either endurance or stamina building, depending on the demands your sport makes of you. For example, soccer involves short bursts of energy when you attack for possession of the ball or run to tackle someone, so a player should work at interval training.

Running, assuming you run on flat terrain and at a steady pace, is generally performed at a constant heart rate, so this is a form of constant pace training. The heart rate rises as the body gets tired, not because you are pushing yourself to work at a higher intensity. The total calorie burn is high because the heart rate is constantly at a moderate to high level. For a more effective workout that will burn a greater number of calories, try introducing interval training into your jogging program because this will push your body that bit further, and help you to achieve overload.

Tennis, on the other hand, is a form of interval training, but the periods of high intensity are generally quite short. The average tennis game allows reasonably long rest periods between points and rallies, during which the heart rate is allowed to fall. If you play tennis as a significant part of your fitness routine, reduce the time between points played and at the end of each game. This way you keep your heart rate at a higher level and burn more calories as a result.

aerobic training

swimming

Performed with good technique, swimming is a fantastic exercise. Not only does it improve your fitness level and burn calories more effectively than many other forms of aerobic exercise, it has a dual effect of building cardiovascular strength while also toning and strengthening the body's major muscles. To get the most benefit from a swimming workout, a good program is essential. Think of the swimming pool as another piece of gym equipment, and use swimming as the aerobic element of your workout.

the importance of the front crawl

A few lengths of gentle breast stroke are certainly better than doing nothing at all and have some benefit as a warmup, but for a really effective workout it's best to use stronger strokes such as the front crawl. Push yourself and concentrate on good technique and on working your body as intensively as possible. This is one of the most difficult strokes to master, and you will last longer in the water and get more from your workout if your technique is correct.

▼ breathe in
The most common problem with front crawl is the breathing. Turn your head to the side to breathe in, bringing your ear closer to your shoulder rather than lifting your head out of the water.

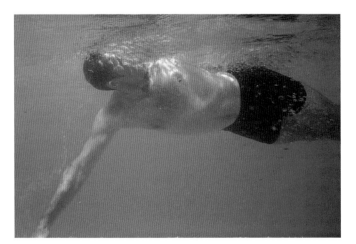

breathing

The problem that most people have with front crawl is getting the breathing right. Often people attempt to breathe both in and out while their head is out of the water. This means that they can't take in enough air, resulting either in rapid fatigue or in an interrupted, irregular stroke pattern that is not only exhausting but prevents any momentum from being built up.

The key is simple: to breathe out under the water. From mid-stroke to the end of stroke you should be exhaling into the water. When you turn your head to the side, breathe in. Practice by using a float. Put one arm on the float, holding it close to the body, and use the other arm to pull through the stroke. Kick gently and practice breathing out into the water. When you breathe in, turn your head away from the float, bringing your ear toward the shoulder rather than trying to lift your head out of the water.

Start off by breathing every other stroke; then once you feel confident, discard the float and practice breathing with both arms performing the stroke. At this stage keep breathing with every other stroke and breathe on the same side of the body that you practiced with the float. Progress to breathing every three strokes so that your head turn alternates. Once you've mastered the breathing, the rest will come more easily and you won't feel as if you are rushing for breath.

▼ breathe out
Try to keep your breathing as regular as possible. The key is to exhale while underwater as you pull through in the middle to end phase of the stroke. Start by breathing with every other stroke.

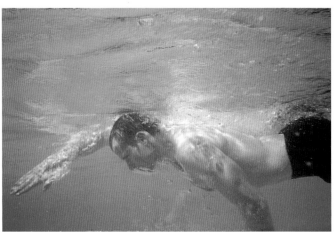

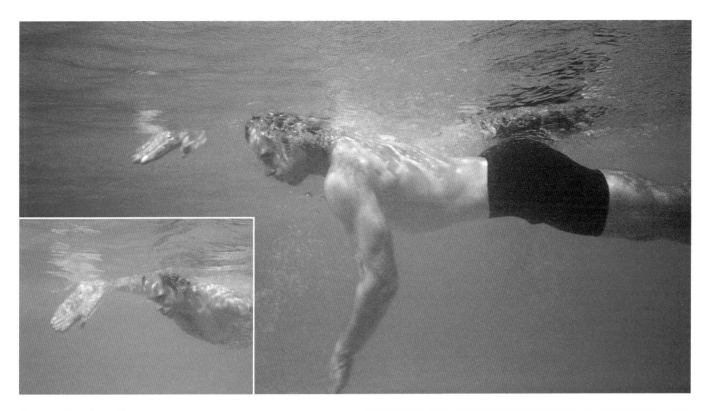

▲ **correct hand position**
Reach directly in front of you. Keep the hand in a slightly cupped
position as you pull through the stroke; this helps to move you
forward through the water.

arm stroke

Concentrate on keeping each stroke long, steady, and strong.
• Reach directly in front of you, but without overstretching
the shoulder. The hand should enter the water in a slightly
cupped position, with fingers together.
• As the arm enters the water, pull through the central line
of the body, keeping the arm slightly bent. Straighten the arm
a little at the end of the action to propel the body forward.

kicking

Often, people tire themselves out by kicking too hard.
• Aim to minimize splashing and movement above the water.
• Kick from the hip, using the entire leg, not just the bottom
half. This works the abdominals and can help to create a trim
and toned stomach area.
• Start with long, slow kicks to get used to the movement
coming from the hip, then gradually speed up the kick once
you feel comfortable with it.
• Keep your feet pointed, but relaxed.

the front crawl program

Once you've mastered the stroke, this program
will provide a challenging workout.

6 lengths of front crawl a comfortable pace. Keep the
strokes long; try to use fewer strokes for each length.

30 seconds rest

6 lengths with a float between the legs so that you
are using just your arms at 80% of maximum effort.

30 seconds rest

6 lengths full stroke working at 90% of maximum effort.

30 seconds rest

6 lengths holding a float with front crawl kicking action.

30 seconds rest

4 lengths full stroke at 100% effort.

30 seconds rest

6 lengths comfortable full stroke at 70% of maximum
effort, using as few strokes for each length as possible.

fast walking

Walking is one of the best, and certainly one of the most versatile, ways to keep fit, and is suitable for all fitness levels. It is a low impact exercise that works the glutes and all the muscles in the leg, in particular the quadriceps and hamstrings. You can walk outside, but you will get just as much from a walk indoors on the treadmill when time is short or the weather poor. Because it is easy to monitor and control how hard you work, walking is a good way to learn about how your heart rate responds to different exertion levels.

good technique

I see many fast walkers who are hindered by poor technique. Some are unable to walk fast enough, and so don't get a good workout; others push themselves to walk faster, but put the body under unnecessary strain as a result. Check your posture and aim to keep the body aligned at all times.

neck and shoulders

One of the most common mistakes when walking is tensing the neck and shoulders.

• Before your walk, relax the neck and shoulder muscles by gently dropping the head from side to side; this helps lengthen and relax the muscles in the neck and upper shoulders.

• While walking, extend the neck, but keep the muscles as relaxed as possible. Keep you walking posture tall and elegant, not tense and hunched.

• Walk with your chin up and look forward rather than down. Keep a good gap between you chin and neck, and don't "squeeze" or tense the neck and shoulder muscles. This will also make breathing easier.

• Relax your shoulder muscles by pulling your shoulders down, then letting them bounce back up to their natural position. Try to maintain this natural position throughout the walk.

▼ take it in stride
The longer the stride, the more effort you need to put into it, but the more you slow yourself down. Concentrate power in your back leg as you push off the ground.

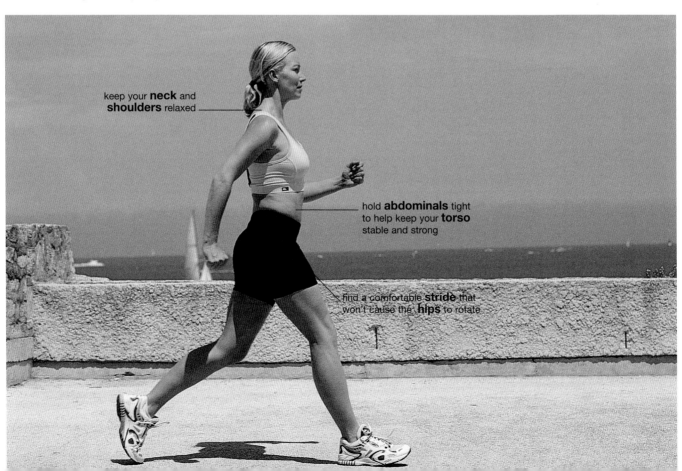

keep your **neck** and **shoulders** relaxed

hold **abdominals** tight to help keep your **torso** stable and strong

find a comfortable **stride** that won't cause the **hips** to rotate

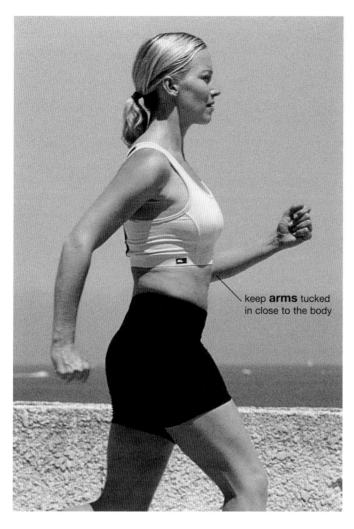

keep **arms** tucked in close to the body

◄ **stepping out**
On the forward step, the heel should plant down on the ground with the body weight on the front foot as it rolls through the step. When the weight is transferred, the back leg can push through into the stride.

• Try not to lean too far backward or forward as you walk because this puts extra pressure on the hips and spine.
• Breathe deeply. Try to breathe from the stomach to increase the percentage of lung capacity used so that you can draw more oxygen into the body with each breath. It's common for people to breathe from the chest when they exercise which means that the intercostal muscles in the ribs do all the work. When you breathe more deeply, the diaphragm contracts, and this helps you to suck more air into your lungs.

hips and butt

The hips act as stabilizers, but the glutes, the muscles of the butt, are the real workhorses of fast walking because they provide the power as you walk.
• Keep the hips square and facing forward; imagine they are like car headlights. This enables the legs to work hard and prevents you from twisting your lower back.
• The most important phase of the walk is the backward push, which is powered by the glutes. If you have good technique, you should be able to feel the glutes and the hamstrings at the back of the thighs working.

legs and feet

Don't put all your efforts into increasing your stride length; ultimately, this will only slow you down.
• Keep your stride length short so the body is not forced to rotate through the hips.
• As you step forward, the heel should plant down on the ground first and the body weight should then roll through. Once the weight is transferred, push through with the glutes. Roll through the back foot, keeping your toes on the ground until the very end of the stride.
• The push through phase is longer and more powerful than the step forward.
• Keep your hips, knees and feet aligned and pointing directly forward. If your feet don't naturally point forward, this may feel awkward, but persevere and make an effort to maintain the alignment.
• Keep your feet as relaxed as possible as you walk. This helps to prevent tightness developing in the shins.

arms

Your arm movements balance your leg movements.
• Hold the arms at a relaxed 90° angle as you walk, with forearms relaxed and hands cupped, not tensed into fists.
• For the arms, the important phase in the stride is the strong backward motion as you pull your arm back at the same time as pushing the back leg out to gain power.
• The forward motion should be a shorter movement with the hand coming up to chest height so that the elbow comes only slightly further forward than the body. Big arm movements will do nothing but waste your energy and exhaust you.

the torso

The torso provides the strong base for the legs to work fast; it moves very little as you walk.
• Keep the abdominals tight and the body upright or angled just slightly forward.

common problems

Fast walking carries a lower risk of injury than running, but painful shins or sore ankles are familiar complaints.

painful shins

One of the more common problems when people first start fast walking is pain in their shins; sometimes it can be painful enough to discourage them from fast walking altogether. The muscles in the shins – the tibialis anterior – have to work hard to constantly pick up the toes as you walk. In most people who aren't practiced fast walkers, the shins are very weak while the muscles in the calves are much stronger. There are simple exercises you can do to strengthen the shins and prevent this from happening. Try standing up and continually lifting your toes off the ground so that you feel the muscles in the shins working. Similarly, sometimes people experience tightness in their calves after fast walking. Remedy this with a simple calf stretch after your walk (*see page 47*).

Try walking on grass where possible: it acts as a shock absorber and lessens the impact on the shins. Treadmills are another option because they are bouncy and more shock absorbent than roads or other hard paved surfaces.

sore ankles

Any pain experienced in the ankles is more than likely to come from wearing incorrect or unsuitable footwear. If you have feet that pronate (roll inward) or supinate (roll outward) when you walk, it is important to wear shoes that provide the correct support and prevent this from happening. Any good sporting goods store should employ trained staff to advise you on the footwear that is most suitable for your needs.

choosing the correct footwear

When you walk your feet are in constant contact with the ground. Therefore, it is essential that the feet have a solid landing base, are properly supported, and are adequately protected at every point in your stride.

This is especially important if you pronate or supinate. The best way to work out if you have a tendency toward either of these is to look at an old pair of shoes. If you tend always to wear out the inside sole of your shoes, then you are almost certainly a pronator – your foot rolls inward when you walk. Choose a pair of shoes that support the inner side of the foot and prevent this rolling effect.

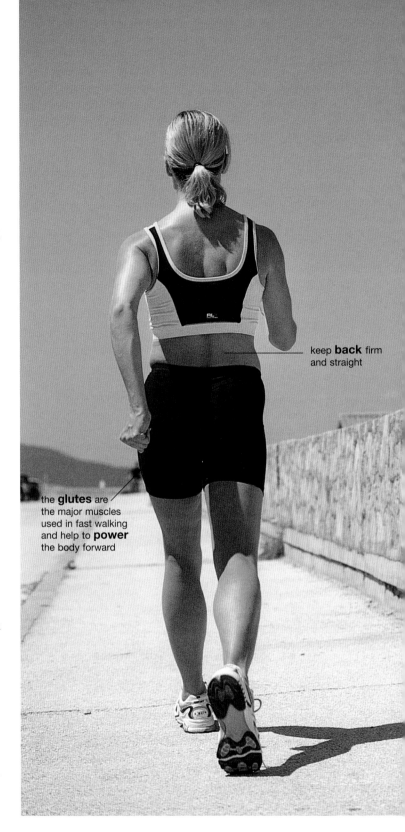

keep **back** firm and straight

the **glutes** are the major muscles used in fast walking and help to **power** the body forward

▲ **walk on**
The glutes are the real workhorses of fast walking and provide the power. Fast walking helps to tone the glutes and keep your bottom looking lean and trim.

If, on the other hand, you find that you always wear out the outer side of the soles of your shoes, you are more likely to be a supinator. This means that your foot has a tendency to roll outward when you walk. Choose shoes that provide good support on the outer side of the foot, and also make sure that the soles are quite wide so that there is less chance of general roll through the foot. As well as these considerations, look for shoes that have the following features:

• Good cushioning on the heel to support the heel on landing.

• Flexibility that accommodates the natural bend of the foot, so that movement through the walking action is easy.

• A wide base to the shoe to prevent foot roll.

• Good height around the ankle to support it.

• Light so that the legs do not bear too much extra weight, which can cause calf or other muscle pain when you walk.

important stretches

After a walking session, take time to stretch out all the major muscles that have been worked: the glutes, hamstrings, calves, quadriceps, shins, hip flexors, and lower back. This can help to prevent subsequent uncomfortable muscle ache. For leg and back stretches, see pages 44–7.

walking programs

To achieve the best results from fast walking, try to vary the pace and intensity of your walk. Alternating training techniques will give you a good aerobic workout and will also tone and strengthen your leg muscles.

• **To build endurance**, practice walking at a steady pace for an extended period of time. This is known as constant pace training (*see page 56*). So, for example, you might warm up by walking for 4 minutes until your heart rate is at 75%MHR, maintain that pace for 20 minutes, then cool down by slowing your pace for 4 minutes.

• **To build stamina**, you should walk for short periods at a high intensity and alternate these with short periods of low intensity work that allow you to recover. This is known as interval training (*see page 56*). A possible program might be to take 4 minutes to warm up to 65%MHR and walk at that pace for 2 minutes, then work up to 80%MHR and walk at that pace for 2 minutes. Alternate between the two heart rates, and repeat the sequence five times.

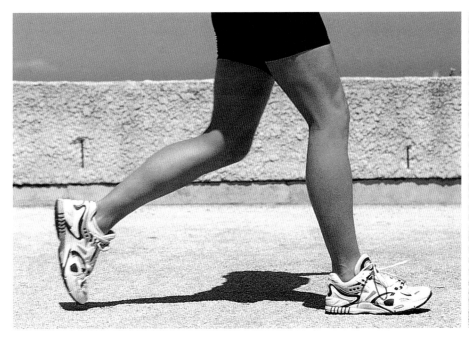

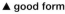 **▲ good form**
Toes point forward and hips, knees, and feet are aligned. Maintain a purposeful pace and a comfortable, easy stride. Experiment with different training techniques and programs to get the most out of your walks.

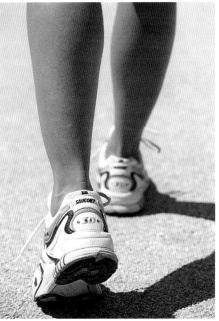

▲ foot fall
Your toes stay on the ground until the very end of your stride. You push forward with the ball of your foot and your toes.

aerobic training

running

Marathons such as those run in London, New York, and Berlin grow in size every year, a good indication of how popular running has become. This adaptable sport can take you outdoors, although many people don't get farther than the treadmill at the gym. It's important for beginners to start slowly, concentrate first on good technique, and then build up the length and intensity of runs. The only equipment you need to invest in is a good pair of shoes. Because it is a high-impact sport, running is not suitable for anyone with knee problems.

good technique

Running is a high-intensity, high-impact exercise, so good technique is important; it will ensure that you get the most from a run – that you get a good aerobic workout, but also that you don't sustain any unnecessary injuries. Running with poor technique can cause pain in the lower back and hips.

neck and shoulders

One of the more common problems when walking is tension in the neck, shoulders, and upper back. The temptation to pull the shoulders up and, as a result, create tension in the neck is even stronger when running.

• Try to keep the neck extended and the shoulders down in a relaxed, comfortable position.

• At the beginning of a run, pull your shoulders down; after some time, you'll find you do this naturally. During longer runs, keep checking your shoulders and correct them if you feel yourself starting to pull them up. While you are running, the neck and shoulders should feel relaxed and easy to move, not stiff or rigid.

• If you begin to suffer from stiffness in the neck, try a simple neck stretch (*see page 42*).

▶ **powerful exercise**
Running requires more power than walking; at one point in the running action both feet are off the ground at the same time. The feet hit the ground with more force, which makes running a high-impact exercise.

arms

Your arm movements help you to power yourself forward and maintain your pace.

• Aim to keep your arms and hands loose and tension-free.

• Once your shoulders are relaxed, open the angle at your elbows and straighten your arms a little.

• Relax your hands rather than tensing them into tight fists.

• As you run, use your arms to help your momentum. Swing them forward and backward, but be sure not to exaggerate the action; if you bring them up too high, you'll create tension in the arms, hands, and shoulders.

• On easier sections of your run, such as when going downhill, drop the hands and allow the arms to straighten a little – this can help to ease tension in the neck.

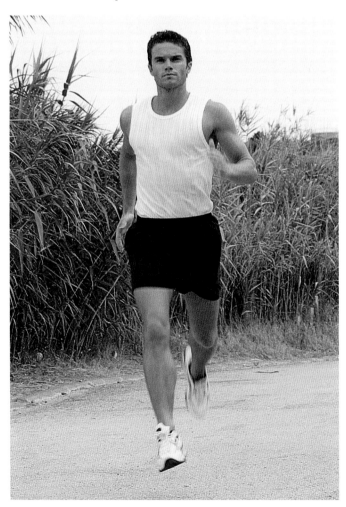

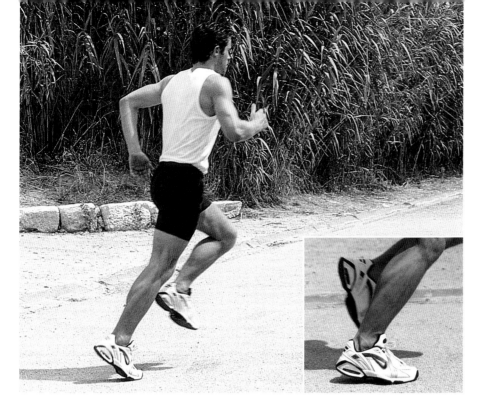

Maintain a good, strong posture, and keep your back as straight as possible. Keep your feet close to the ground and be sure not to "bounce" as you run. Land on your heels, and use the power in your glutes and hamstrings to take off from your toes.

torso

Running requires a great deal of effort from the muscles of the lower back and stomach. As a result, you not only strengthen this area, you also work off any excess body fat there.

• When you run, keep the torso upright and straight, and hold the abdominals tight; like for fast walking, this provides a solid base for the legs to power from. It's common to experience some muscle tightness in the stomach after running; this is generally as a result of tensing your abdominals to hold you in the correct position as you run.

• Do exercises to strengthen the abdominal muscles (*see pages 102–5*) and the back muscles (*see pages 90–5*). The stronger the torso, the easier you'll find running, and the less strain you'll put on your body.

• Keep your back straight and tall to prevent the upper body and shoulders from hunching forward. A straight back will help to diffuse tension in the upper body, and means you can maintain a relaxed running position more easily.

hips and glutes

With the stomach muscles and the lower back muscles held firm, the hips can also provide stability. The glutes – the muscles of the butt – are integral to the running action because they provide the power.

• When you run, the glutes work hard to push power through the legs and propel the body forward. A common fault is to underutilize the glutes and to rely instead on the hamstrings, the muscles at the backs of the thighs. This can often lead to hamstring strain and pain in the lower back.

• When you run you should feel the glutes powering the leg at the end of the running action. If you cannot feel the glutes working, your technique is incorrect.

legs and feet

My advice to new runners is often "don't try so hard." When people first take up running as a sport, the temptation is to emulate a character from the movie *Chariots of Fire* and run with exaggerated high-knee lifts, long strides, and big bouncy steps. Running in this fashion will tire you out, but it will also put unnecessary strain on the ankle and knee joints. Once you have mastered fast walking, running is the natural progression because the technique is so similar. But unlike the walk, where one foot is always in contact with the ground, when you run, both feet come off the ground for a brief moment.

• Keep the feet close to the ground and maintain a good, strong body posture.

• Try not to bounce too much when you run.

• Land on your heels and roll through the whole foot, then take off from your toes. Use the glutes and hamstrings (the muscles at the backs of the thighs) for power.

• Short, fast strides are better than long ones that tend to require a lot of effort.

aerobic training

common problems

Poor technique, doing too much running, or running for too long at a time may cause problems. Here are some of the more common running-related complaints I have encountered and advice on how to treat them or – even better – prevent them in the first place.

knee pain

This is one of the more familiar running injuries. It's often caused by wearing unsuitable shoes. Running is a high-impact exercise where the body has to absorb shock as you pound along. Choose shoes that cushion the body and ease the pressure on the knees as you run. For more advice on footwear, see pages 62–3.

Excess pressure on the knees can be another cause of knee pain. If you are carrying a little more weight than you should be, pressure on the knee joints can be dramatically increased when you run, and this can damage the knees. In this case it is better to try an exercise such as fast walking that doesn't put so much pressure on the knees. Once you've lost the extra pounds you can go back to running as your way of keeping the weight off.

Muscle weakness or imbalance can also cause knee pain. Weak quadriceps, for example, can concentrate movement on the knee joint and put extra pressure on it. You might feel the pain in the center or at the sides of the knee. This can occur, even in advanced, seasoned runners, when one side of the body is weaker than the other. Similarly, muscle imbalance where, for example, there are strong quadriceps but weak hamstrings, can cause knee pain. The advice is usually to stop running and work on balancing the strength in the muscles. To prevent running-related knee problems, keep all the muscles in the legs strong.

shin pain

Runners, like fast walkers, often suffer from shin pain, or shin splints. Sometimes your footwear may be to blame. Shin pain can be the signal that your shoes are worn out and are no longer supporting your feet – or body – correctly. People who run regularly should buy new shoes every six months. If you have just bought new shoes or have just started running, it may be that your footwear is unsuitable.

You might also experience shin pain if you push yourself too hard when you run. The shins absorb much of the impact when you run and can be the first part of the body to complain. Listen to your body, and try to vary your running programs as much as possible.

calf tightness

Running can put strain on the calf muscles. As most runners don't stretch after running, that tightness is often left in the calf muscles. Always stretch after a run (*see pages 46–7*).

▶ **running indoors**
Running on the treadmill is a great way to reduce pressure on the knees. However, because your feet are moved backward by the belt, the glutes and hamstrings do not have to work as hard as when you run outside.

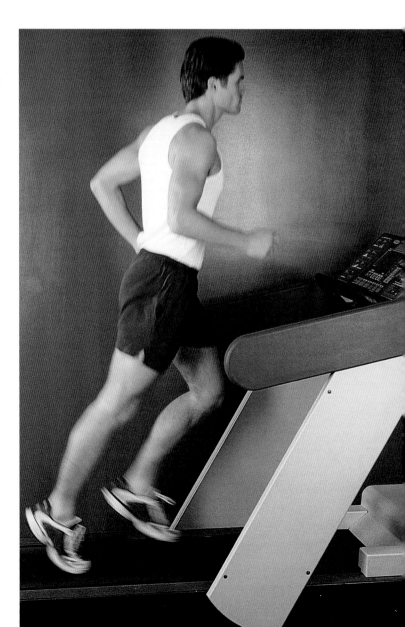

running programs

New runners should begin by interval training where you run for short periods, then fast walk until you recover, then run again and continue to repeat the pattern. Make sure that you have mastered fast walking first and progress to running only when you feel confident with fast walking, or even begin to find it too easy. Don't push yourself to move on to running too quickly. Fast pace walking is a great exercise and I include it in programs for even my healthiest clients. Always start by warming up; try fast walking for five minutes to gently raise the heart rate.

beginner and intermediate programs

Once you have mastered fast pace walking, introduce short bursts of running into your walk to increase the intensity of the workout slightly. So, for example, you might walk for three minutes, run for one minute, then go back to fast walking for three minutes. You could repeat this cycle five times to build an effective 20-minute workout.

As your skill level develops, gradually extend the running period. You might do two minutes of walking followed by two minutes of running. You could progress to one minute of walking followed by three minutes of running. Monitor your heart rate at all times: a good program (*see right*) should always give you percentage of maximum heart rate (MHR) targets that control the intensity of your workout. Running is a high intensity aerobic workout, so it can cause the heart rate to rise rapidly. Increase the intensity of your workout only when the old routine is becoming too easy for your heart.

Gradually building up the length of your running time will mean that eventually you'll be able to run for long periods without needing to stop and walk in between to recover.

advanced programs

Advanced runners often complain that they run three times a week and yet never really see any improvement in their performance. This is often becaue they've found a route that they like, so they do the same run every time they go out. Introduce some variety: work on stamina, high intensity work in short bursts repeated several times, and endurance, low intensity work over a long period of time. Combine long steady pace runs with short fast runs and interval training. By varying your training techniques, the body is continuously being challenged and continues to improve its performance.

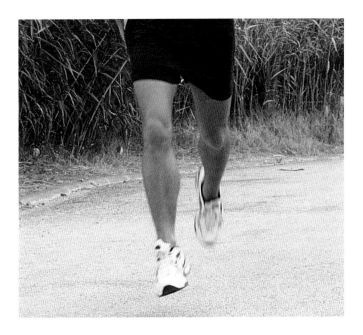

▲ listen to your body
Runners can suffer from problems such as knee and shin pains. Focus on good technique, and wear shoes that cushion and support the feet and ankles. Maintain muscle strength in the legs, and follow a good running program that varies the intensities that you work at and challenges all the muscles in the legs.

the running program

This 2-week program will ensure that your body is continuously challenged when you run.

Day 1 25mins@75–80%MHR (flat terrain)
Day 2 day off
Day 3 40mins@75%MHR
Day 4 day off
Day 5 2mins@85%MHR, 2mins@70%MHR (x5)
Day 6 day off
Day 7 day off
Day 8 60mins@70–75%MHR
Day 9 day off
Day 10 220yd (200m) sprint, 40 secs walk (x6), 4 mins rest, then repeat 1–2 times
Day 11 day off
Day 12 day off
Day 13 20mins@80–85%MHR (flat terrain)
Day 14 day off

aerobic training

cycling

A great low-impact aerobic exercise, cycling works the muscles of the thighs, buttocks, and lower legs, while also toning and strengthening the lower back and stomach muscles. It has the added benefit of being easy to control – because you can change gears and choose between hilly and flat terrains, you can alter the intensity of your workout.

good technique

Be sure to position your body correctly on the bicycle. Feeling comfortable and relaxed will help ensure that you get a good workout, that your muscles are working effectively, and that you don't put unnecessary strain on any part of the body. Good technique is just as important when you are working out on the cycling machine at the gym.

saddle height

The correct saddle height prevents strain on the knees and ensures that the leg muscles can generate as much power as possible. In the downward phase of the cycling action, the leg should be extended, but bent slightly at the knee.

neck and shoulders

When you cycle, your head and shoulders should not move around. It is your legs that should do all the work.
• Keep your neck and shoulders relaxed.
• Don't tense your shoulders. Be sure to keep them down in a comfortable position to prevent straining the neck.

▼ **easy rider**
Once saddle height is correct, maintaining good posture on the bicycle is easy. A slightly bent knee when the leg is extended allows a long downward pedal action. This means you can put more power behind each cycling action.

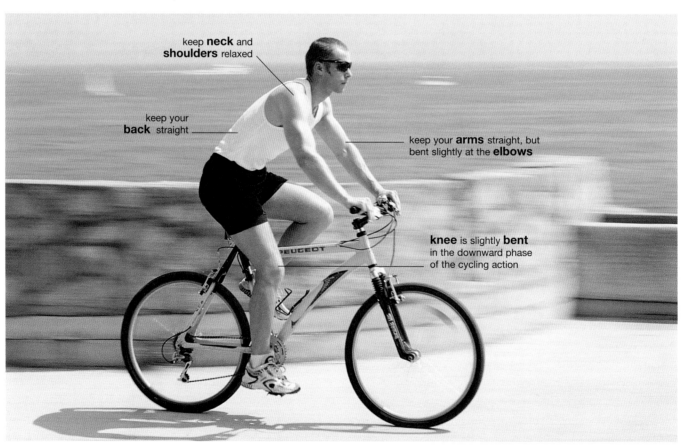

keep **neck** and **shoulders** relaxed

keep your **back** straight

keep your **arms** straight, but bent slightly at the **elbows**

knee is slightly **bent** in the downward phase of the cycling action

▶ an effective workout
When you cycle, you can vary the intensity of your workout. Rise out of the saddle when you sprint, but don't allow the bicycle to sway from side to side. The legs should still do all the work.

arms and hands
The main role of the arms and hands is to stabilize and control.
• Keep your arms relaxed, with a slight bend at the elbows.
• Keep a relaxed but firm grip on the handles. If you grip too tightly, you'll cause muscle tension in the forearms.

torso, back, and hips
The torso provides the stability for the entire cycling motion; it is the base that enables the legs to power through as you pedal. The stronger the mid-section, the less likely you are to move the rest of your body when you cycle.
• Hold the torso muscles – the abdominals, obliques, and erector spinae – tight. This will help to stabilize you.
• Keep your back straight and as upright as possible. Pull your stomach muscles tight to prevent your back from slumping forward.
• Don't allow your shoulders to drop toward the handlebars, because this will put pressure on the upper back.

legs
As long as saddle height is correct (*see opposite*), leg position will be correct too.
• Angle the foot so the toe is pointed slightly downward and the heel is slightly higher in the downward phase of the cycling action. This prevents tension through the calf muscle.
• Use toe clips. When you cycle without toe clips, the cycling action is powered by the muscles at the fronts of the legs, the quadriceps, as you push down to pedal. When you cycle with toe clips, your feet are attached to the pedals and you use the muscles at the fronts and backs of the legs, the hamstrings, glutes, and calf muscles, to power the movement.

tips for off-roading
Leave traffic and busy roads behind and explore some more rugged terrains. The following tips will help to keep you safe and enhance the quality of your workout.
• On corners, keep your inside pedal high so that it doesn't hit any uneven ground and throw you off balance.
• On a hilly route, lower your seat a little. This will enable you to move your body around more easily to maintain balance.

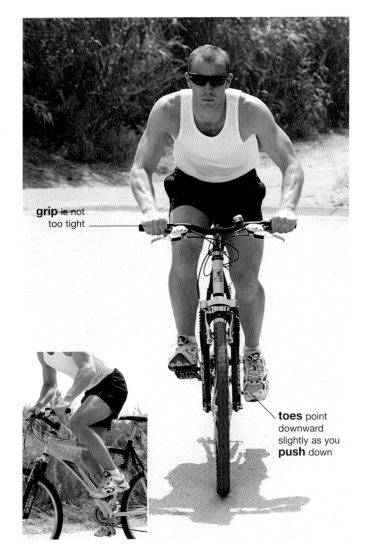

grip is not too tight

toes point downward slightly as you **push** down

• When cycling downhill, move your bodyweight back over the seat to prevent the back of the bike from lifting.
• When cycling up a steep hill, try to stay seated so your bodyweight is evenly distributed over the bike.
• Brake with front and back brakes, otherwise you risk sending yourself flying over the handlebars if you brake suddenly.
• Always wear protective clothing.
• Wear cycling gloves so you can grip the handlebars firmly.

pre-cycle-ride checks
• Check that your tires are inflated to the correct level.
• Make sure the saddle height is correct.
• Check that your brakes are tight and in good working order.
• Carry a flat repair kit with you.
• Make sure your bike has a pump on it.

aerobic training

aerobic gym machines

If it's not possible to exercise outdoors, your best option is the wide variety of aerobic machines at the gym. Vary your workouts, and use as many different machines as you can: don't stick to a single favorite. That way you challenge the body in different ways.

rowing machine

This provides excellent aerobic exercise that works the upper and lower body at the same time. Rowing requires some coordination, and it is easy to perform it incorrectly. To get the maximum benefit, remember to generate most of the stroke power from the legs. Keep a relaxed grip on the handle so that your forearms don't tire prematurely. If your arms tire before your legs, check and correct your technique. Exhale with the effort, as you pull back, and inhale as you return to the start position. Try not to put excessive strain on the back, and take care not to lean too far back at the end of the stroke. Avoid going for speed at the expense of technique by keeping your stroke rate at about 25–35 strokes per minute.

step machine

The step machine, stepper, or Stairmaster after the company that originally produced it, is commonplace in most gyms. The exercise is based on the action of climbing stairs, which, if you climb enough of them, offers a good aerobic workout that also tones the quadriceps, the muscles at the fronts of the thighs, and the calf muscles.

The main difference between step machines is that some have dependent stepping actions, and others have independent stepping actions. On a dependent stepper, the two pedals you stand on cantilever each other; as you step down on one pedal the other one comes up. On independent steppers, the pedals work individually to provide a more demanding workout.

Because the step machine targets the quadriceps, if you work out on this machine exclusively there is a risk of over-developing these muscles. You might want to swap between aerobic machines to give your quadriceps a rest. The step machine is a good machine to use in preskiing training, but not suitable for people with weak knees or knee complaints.

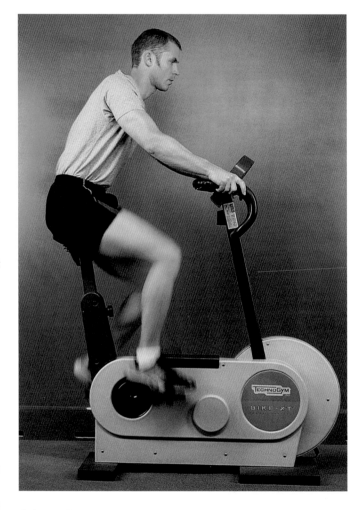

▲ **the cycling machine**
Make sure saddle height is correct before you begin your workout, and try to keep your back straight at all times. For advice on correct body positioning and cycling programs, see pages 68–9.

cross-country skier

Cross-country skiers are renowned for being the healthiest sports people in the world. The cross-country skier takes this great sport indoors. This machine is suitable for those with a good level of fitness. It can also be used as part of a circuit as it can provide a good high-intensity workout that raises the heart rate in a short period of time.

Although the machine helps you to maintain the correct posture as you exercise on it, common areas to experience strain are in the hip muscles and the lower back. To prevent this, try to keep your body weight centerd and distributed evenly over both legs at all times. This machine is not suitable for anyone with lower back problems.

cross-trainer

Also known as the elliptical motion machine, the cross-trainer was devised with multiple purposes: to provide an alternative to running on the treadmill, to target a wider range of muscles than the step machine and to enable you to work for a longer time than possible with the cross-country skier. The resulting machine takes the legs through an elliptical motion that is a cross between running and cross-country skiing and offers the benefits of both of these exercises without any of the downsides.

The cross-trainer takes the impact out of the running action and reduces the risk of knee strain that can result from the cross-country skiing action. It works more leg muscles and lower body muscles than any other aerobic machine in the gym; and because it works them all fairly evenly, there is no risk of any one muscle group becoming more developed than another.

arm ergometer

Probably the least popular of all the aerobic gym machines, the arm ergometer should not be overlooked. It resembles a bicycle, but with the pedals placed up at shoulder height. It works in the same way except that you turn the pedals with your arms instead of your legs.

Arm ergometers offer a good aerobic workout while also having a toning effect; however because they work the smaller muscles of the arms rather than the large muscles of the legs, it is very hard work and raises the heart rate very quickly. My only criticizm is that it is so tiring, it can be difficult to sustain the exercise for long and achieve a true aerobic effect.

Arm ergometers are great as part of a circuit training workout where you want to raise the heart rate quickly for a short period of time. Beginners should start slowly and combine this machine with other aerobic machines to get an effective workout.

the cross-trainer ▼
The increasing popularity of cross-training means that most gyms have this machine. It provides a good low-impact aerobic workout that targets many different muscles.

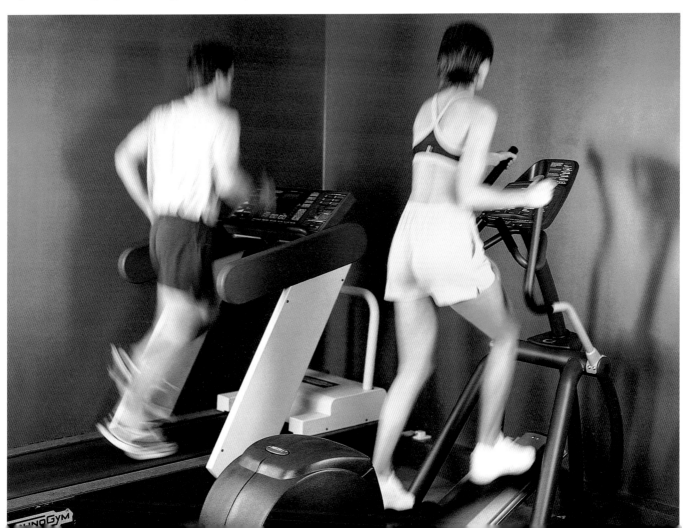

aerobic training

gym circuit aerobic exercises

You can introduce variety into your training routine at the gym by doing some circuit training as part of your usual workout. This involves performing a series of exercises in quick succession with the aim of raising the heart rate and testing the muscles in different ways. Any aerobic workout should aim to keep the heart rate elevated for a minimum of 20 minutes. Try including some of the following exercises in your circuit.

skipping

Boxers skip as part of their training. It provides a great high-intensity aerobic workout that also improves coordination. Because it raises the heart rate quickly, it's difficult to keep it up for more than a few minutes at a time. For this reason it is better performed in short bursts as part of a circuit.

When you skip, aim to keep the body close to the floor at all times, with the skipping rope passing close under the feet as you bring them gently off the floor. Most people start with more of a jumping action, which can put strain on the knees. Aim instead for an easy transfer of body weight from one foot to the other as you skip. The quicker a new skipper can learn this lower impact skipping technique, the better.

Skipping can elevate the heart rate so rapidly that it can take you beyond your optimum training zone (*see page 54*) in no time at all. Unless you have a very high level of fitness, it's best to start by skipping in short bursts and resting for short periods in between. It is a high-impact exercise and is not suitable for anyone with weak knees.

▼ a hop and a skip
Try including skipping in your circuit routine. It provides a good high-intensity aerobic workout and also improves concentration. All you need is a skipping rope.

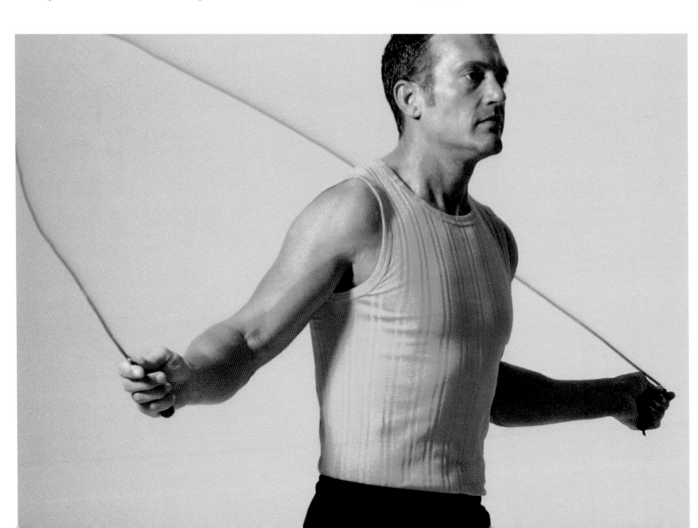

shuttle runs

These are regularly used as part of sports training and are excellent for improving agility. They may bring back dreaded memories of school phys. ed. classes, but they are still a fantastic aerobic exercise to include as part of a circuit.

Mark two points about 32–50ft (10–15m) apart. Sprint between the two markers for either a specified number of sprints or a specified period of time. Keep the markers fairly close together so that the exercise involves plenty of turning.

This is a high-impact exercise because it involves short bursts of high-speed running and turning. Wear shoes with good support and high shock absorbency (*see pages 62–3*).

If you are training for a sport that involves lots of short explosive sprinting, for example tennis, netball, soccer, or basketball, you should definitely include shuttle runs in your circuit routine.

cone runs

An advanced form of shuttle runs, cone runs require more agility and stamina and work more leg muscles than are used in straightforward sprinting.

You need at least six cones or markers. Arrange them in two lines with about 7–10ft (2–3m) distance between the lines and about 7–10ft (2–3m) between each cone. Run in a zig-zagging pattern between the two lines of cones. Cone runs provide an excellent aerobic training, but also improve lateral leg strength, turning ability, and speed. This is good training for field sports such as soccer, football, rugby, and field hockey.

Adjust the length and width of the marked area according to the sport for which you are training and the amount of room available. For example, if you play soccer or basketball, put the markers closer together and move between them as quickly as you would if you tackled or dodged in a real game. If you play tennis, move the markers farther apart.

wall climbing

Climbing walls, as well as ladder and rope climbing facilities, are appearing in more and more gyms. Climbing has a good aerobic effect, but also builds upper body strength, which is a great advantage because most other forms of aerobic exercise tend to build strength in the lower body. Wall climbing is very physically demanding and can only really be sustained for short periods, so it makes a good addition to a circuit.

hurdle jumps

This involves small jumps over a line of between 6 and 10 low hurdles. Place the hurdles about one jump's length apart. Jump the hurdles with just one landing between each one until you reach the end of the row.

This is a high-impact activity that does put some pressure on the bones and joints, in particular in the knees. However as hurdles are performed in short bursts, they won't damage the bones; in fact, they will help to strengthen them.

building your own circuit

Below is a suggested circuit routine that combines these aerobic circuit exercises with resistance exercises (*see pages 74–113*). Perform all of the exercises as part of a circuit. Don't waste time between exercises; move quickly and give yourself no more than 30 seconds to recover before moving on to the next exercise. The aim is to keep your heart rate elevated throughout the whole 20-minute circuit. Work on increasing the number of repetitions you do for each exercise every time you do the circuit.

Circuit training program

Aerobic warmup	7 mins
Chest press	30 secs
Squat	30 secs
Skipping	3 mins
Push-up	30 secs
Bent-over row	30 secs
Shuttle runs	2 mins
Lateral raise	30 secs
Lat pull-down	30 secs
Cone runs	2 mins
Ball squat	30 secs
Dips	30 secs
Hurdle jumps	2 mins
Bicep curl	30 secs
Power lunge	30 secs each leg
Wall climbing	15 climbs
Cool-down walk	5 mins
Stretch	Total body stretch (see page 48)

aerobic training

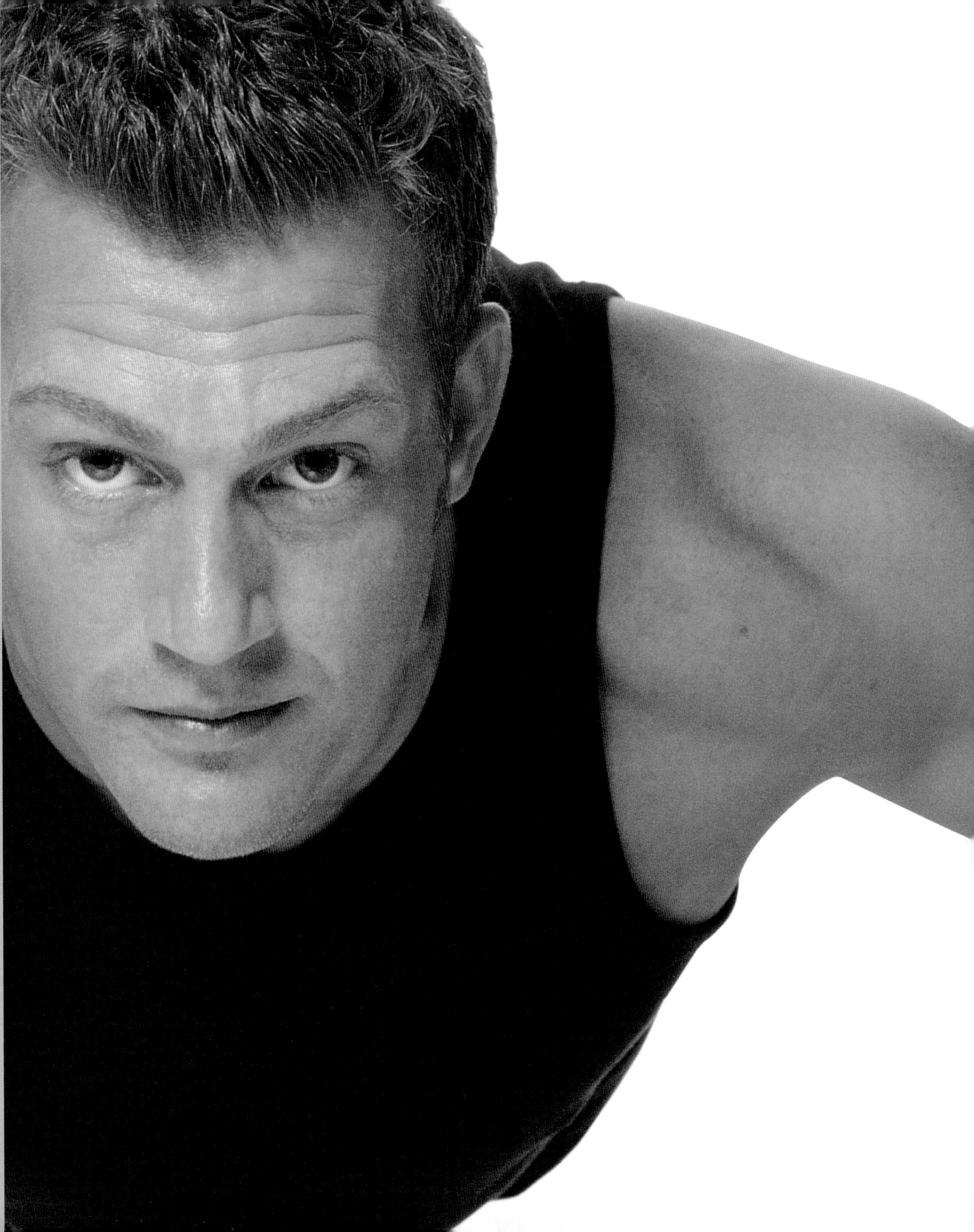

resistance
exercises

Toning and strengthening the muscles of the body is an integral part of any fitness program, whether you are losing body fat, training for a sport, or sculpting your body. This chapter presents a comprehensive range of highly effective toning and strengthening exercises – all organized by the part of the body they target. Vary the exercises you use to work each muscle. That way you challenge the muscles in different ways and will continue to see results.

what is resistance exercise?

Resistance exercise means working, or training, with weights, either free weights, the weights on a gym machine, or your own body weight. By performing simple, often repetitive movements you are able to focus work on a particular muscle or group of muscles. Working with weights, the movement is made harder and requires more physical strength. Resistance work initially damages the muscles, but as they repair themselves they actually become stronger.

muscle fibers

Muscles have two types of muscle fiber that I describe as fast-twitch and slow-twitch. Slow-twitch fibers are used mostly in aerobic activities such as walking, running and cycling and can work for extended periods of time. These fibers utilize energy that is constantly being created by the cardiovascular system.

Fast-twitch fibers are used in explosive actions such as lifting weights or sprinting. These actions require a great deal of energy over a short period of time. Because of the intensity of the activity, they can only use energy that is already stored in the muscles. These muscle fibers can't replace energy stored within them without decreasing the intensity of the action.

Slow-twitch fibers are small, highly efficient fibers. Fast twitch fibers are bigger and therefore require more energy and give a greater size to the overall muscle appearance. We work the fast-twitch fibers when we resistance train, with the aim of toning the muscles or, in some cases, building greater bulk. Improved muscle condition also raises the body's metabolic rate so your body can burn energy more efficiently.

body types and muscle building

People fall into one of three basic body types that respond differently to muscle building. It is as well to understand what your body type can realistically achieve before embarking on a muscle-building program (*see* Building mass, *pages 150–55*).

▶ **pumping iron**
Resistance training, which works the fast-twitch fibers in your muscles, can tone or have a mass-building effect.

Ectomorphs have naturally slim builds. They seem able to eat enormous amounts without ever gaining weight. Ectomorphs will always find it difficult to build body mass and muscle; it's not impossible, but it will take them longer. A mass-building program will help them to achieve a lean and toned body rather than a bulky one. They should pay particular attention to diet and increase their calorie intake to meet the body's increased demand for fuel when training.

Endomorphs have larger builds and tend to gain weight easily. They will find it easier to build muscle than the ectomorph, but often need to burn off excess body fat to reveal the muscle beneath. They should aim to include an aerobic element in their mass-building program otherwise they will just build mass and look bigger, but there will be no muscle definition.

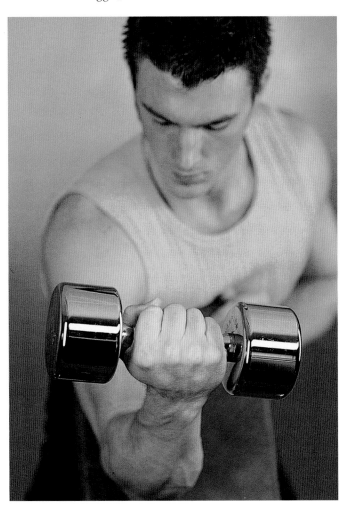

Mesomorphs tend to have athletic builds with lean waists and broad shoulders, a combination that already gives the body a good shape. They will find it easy to build muscle, but, like the endomorph, may need to include some aerobic work to burn fat and emphasize the underlying defined muscle.

resistance training demystified

Some people are reluctant to work with weights. However, resistance training is an indispensable part of any fitness program and, when combined with aerobic training, can help to create a lean, toned body. Below are some of the more common mistakenly held beliefs I have encountered.

lifting weights will give me big muscles

People believe that lifting weights will cause rapid muscle growth in a short period of time. This is not true. Different training techniques will achieve different effects, and building muscle is one of the more difficult ones to achieve, even with a specially tailored program. How easy or difficult you find it to build muscle is dependent on your body type, and even then building up the size of your muscles takes much longer than many other fitness objectives.

If you work your muscles in sets of 14 or more repetitions and stick to a program that works different areas of the body rather than concentrating on just one part as with spot reducing (*see page 78*), you will not build muscle. Instead, you will create lean, toned muscle and a body that burns energy quickly and efficiently.

when I stop training my muscle will turn to fat

Muscle and fat are two completely different tissues – one cannot turn into the other. When you exercise you are not turning fat into muscle. You are burning fat and toning muscle.

When you stop training it is possible to lose muscle and, if you're not careful, you may gain fat. If you stop training, you naturally expend less energy and, as a result, need to reduce your calorie intake. If you eat the same amount as you did when you were training, when your body burned more energy more efficiently, it will store the excess calories as fat.

If you stop training and reduce your calorie intake to account for your lower activity level, you should not gain fat, although you may lose a bit of muscle because you are not exercising. Always be aware of your activity levels and adjust your calorie intake accordingly.

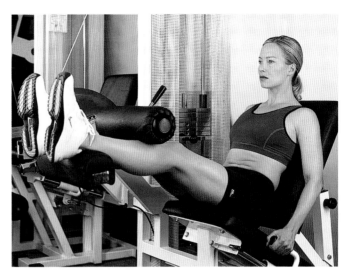

▲ **weight machines**
Resistance training is an essential part of any fitness program. Use the weight machines at the gym, but try to include some free weight work as well, so you challenge your muscles in different ways.

the longer my training sessions, the more effective they'll be

It doesn't take much to work your muscles to the point where they benefit from an exercise and start to become stronger. It does take the right combinations of exercise to achieve specific results, however. The key to successfully attaining your goal is to maximize muscle overload. Once a muscle has reached this point, you should stop working it. There is no need to target the muscles for hours at a time.

Whether your goal is to build muscle size or to tone, it's not how long you spend training the muscles but how you train them. It's the quality of the exercise that you do, and the ability to effectively overload every part of a muscle group that achieves results. The Programs combine different training techniques to achieve different goals, from building mass to toning different parts of the body (*see pages 114–89*).

the heavier the weight I lift, the bigger my muscles will become

For strength gain and muscle building, your long-term aim is to increase the weight you lift – but this should never be at the expense of either technique or precision when performing an exercise. It's just as important to introduce variety into your routine by working with different combinations of rest period and set size. This ensures that your muscles are constantly challenged and that you continue to see results.

resistance exercises

the basics of resistance training

Training with weights, or resistance training, can help to achieve many different effects, from building muscle size and strength to creating definition and tone. It's important to understand how your muscles respond to resistance exercise before starting to work with weights and different training techniques. This will enable you to use the Programs effectively, and help you to achieve your fitness goals with ease.

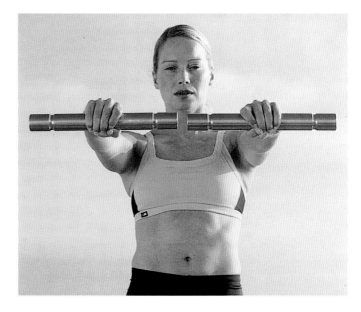

▲ **challenge your muscles**
If you don't continuously challenge your muscles by pushing yourself to work harder and regularly increasing your weights, you will plateau and stop seeing results.

repetition maximums (rm)

This is how you choose the weight that you use when performing an exercise. The rm is the number of repetitions of an exercise that you should perform using a weight that allows you to complete that number of repetitions and no more. For example, if you are told to do 15rm, by the end of the fifteenth repetition you should not be able to perform another repetition without compromising technique. As you perform your 15 repetitions, you should find the last four or five become very difficult and performing a sixteenth would be extrememly difficult. If you find the 15 repetitions easy, you need to choose a heavier weight. If, on the other hand, you find you are unable to complete the 15 repetitions, then the weight is too heavy and you should choose a lighter weight.

Finding the right rm requires some experimentation to begin with, but it means that whenever you perform the exercise you are able to overload the muscles and maximize the effectiveness of the exercise.

The important point to remember about rm is that the effect you feel should never change. As you get stronger, you will need to increase the weights you use so that you still achieve muscle fatigue by the time you have completed the specified number of rm. This will ensure that you continue to challenge the muscles and see ongoing improvement.

overloading

This is the technical term for making a muscle work beyond its comfortable level of exertion. The effect of overloading the muscles is that they are forced to become stronger to cope with the increased demands being made on them. You should always aim to achieve overload when you work out. It means that every time you work out your muscles are working harder than on the previous occasion, and as a result you will see progress constantly.

spot reducing

This is when a person attempts to eliminate weight from a particular part of the body and works on that part to the exclusion of all others. The effect of this to to build muscle whereas in most cases the person needs to lose fat from that area. The end result of fat loss but muscle gain in one area can give the same visual effect – it may even make the area more prominent. Never try to tackle one particular area of your body that bothers you. Always work with the body as a whole.

the plateau effect

Many people give up on exercise routines because they stop seeing results – this usually happens when they reach a plateau. You may be working out, but you may have stopped seeing improvements in your fitness level. This is known as the plateau effect and occurs when the body is no longer being overloaded. The body is not being pushed to new limits and is therefore not being forced to improve itself. It happens most commonly when a person has been following the same workout routine for a long period of time. It is important to vary your workout routines. In many ways it is like playing a game in which you are constantly looking for new ways to challenge the body.

reversibility

This is the next stage on from plateauing. It occurs when a person has been in the plateau stage for a long time and has not been challenging the body. Your fitness level can actually deteriorate even though you are working out. At this stage the body has not experienced overload for some time. This is most likely to occur as a result of not increasing your weights when performing exercises and so not maintaining the rm effect, or as a result of not introducing variety into your exercise routine.

training techniques and their effects

Different training techniques will produce different results depending on factors such as the heaviness of the weight, the number of repetitions and sets you do and the length of your rest periods. Mixing different combinations of rest period and set sizes has the greatest effect. In general, training techniques achieve different effects based on the repetition ranges below:

• Strength gain – very low reps (4–8 reps per set) with long rest periods of two minutes or more between sets
• Building muscle – low to medium reps (6–10 reps per set) with rests of 30 to 90 seconds between sets
• Muscle definition – medium reps (8–14 reps per set) with short rests of between 30 and 60 seconds
• Muscle tone – high reps (15 or more reps per set) with short rests of 30 seconds.

A good tip to remember is that sometimes, using principles from a different training technique can boost the effects of your current one.

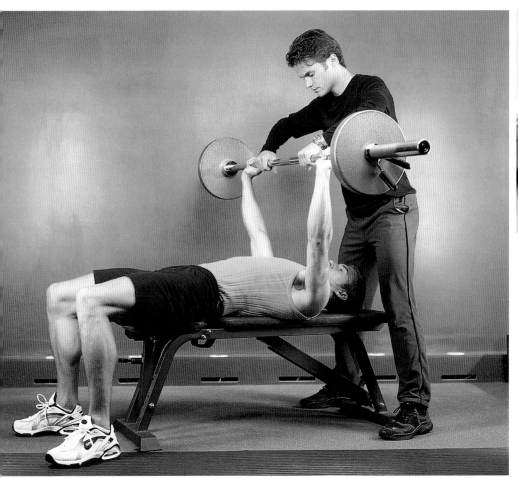

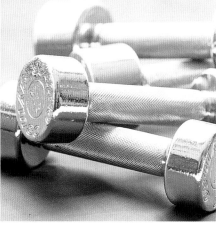

▲ **free weights**
Most gym machine exercises can also be performed with free weights. Exercises with free weights usually require greater muscle control.

◀ **advanced weight lifting**
If you think you might struggle with the last few repetitions, or if you have just increased your weights, your trainer, a member of the gym staff, or a fellow weight lifter might help out – this is known as "spotting."

resistance exercises

resistance training techniques

There is no single technique for muscle gain that can guarantee results. The best training technique for you at this time depends on the technique you've been using up until now, and how long you've been using it. Here I outline the more commonly used resistance training techniques, many of which are part of the Programs (*see pages 114–89*). They are all effective, but experiment and, according to your goal, find the one that works best for you.

drop sets

This is one of the best techniques for achieving muscle overload, whether you are building mass or toning and defining. It is an intensive training technique that delivers results quickly.

Choose your first weight for an exercise with the aim of achieving maximum overload by the end of the set. For example, if you choose 100lb (45kg) on a pec fly with the aim of doing a 12 rep max at 12, by the end of the set you should have completely fatigued the muscle so that you can't perform another repetition. You then change down to a weight that is the equivalent to about 75 percent of the initial weight and perform the same number of repetitions as you did with the first weight – 12 repetitions in this case. This two weight sequence makes up one complete set.

Single drop sets work on the principle that when you overload your muscles you effectively render 25 percent of the muscle unusable without rest. By reducing the weight by 25 percent you account for that loss of power and you can overload the muscle further than when doing a conventional set. Use this principle for any resistance exercise and any muscle group.

pyramid sets

Another high-intensity training technique, pyramid setting is when you perform a series of sets, each one with heavier weights but with lower repetitions, until your muscles reach a point of fatigue where you can't increase the weights, even with lower repetitions. You then decrease the weights, but this still has the effect of overloading the muscles. So a pyramid setting training session might look like this:

Set 1	Set 2	Set 3	Set 4	Set 5
110lb(50kg)	130lb(60kg)	150lb(70kg)	110lb(50kg)	90lb(40kg)
12 reps	8 reps	6 reps	10 reps	12 reps

super setting

Another good technique for achieving effective muscle overload, super setting is also very time efficient as you don't need to stop for rest periods. You work opposing muscles in quick succession so, for example, you might work the tricep and then the bicep. This keeps the intensity of the workout up

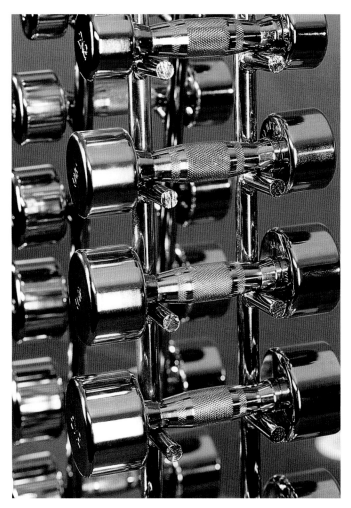

▶ **variety: the spice of life**
Swap between free weights and the weight machines at the gym.

because no rest time is required. As you work one side of the body the other side rests, then you quickly change the side of the body being worked and the other side of the body gets a rest period. An arms super set might look like this:

Set 1	Set 2	Set 3	Set 4
Tricep overhead	Bicep curl	Tricep pushdown	Dips

The most effective combinations for this training technique are: chest and back; fronts and backs of thighs; biceps and triceps.

pre-exhaustion

This training technique is generally used to build muscle. You perform an exercise that works the muscle you want to target as well as other assisting muscles. You perform this first exercise to exhaustion, then choose an exercise that isolates the muscle you want to hit and perform that to exhaustion. By working the muscle along with assisting muscles first, the muscle is overloaded once, then when you ask it to perform the isolation exercise it has to work harder and there is even greater muscle overload. If you were using this technique to work the pectorals, your workout might look like this:

Exercise 1	Chest press	Pectorals assisted by triceps
Exercise 2	Pec flys	Pectorals

compound setting

This works in the opposite way to pre-exhaustion. You perform a number of exercises in a combination that starts by isolating one muscle and you add assisting muscles once this muscle becomes weak. A pectorals compound set might look like this:

Exercise 1	Pec fly	Pectorals
Exercise 2	Chest press	Pectorals assisted by triceps
Exercise 3	Dips	Triceps assisted by pectorals

matrix training

This method of training works on the theory that you are able to target and overload different parts of a muscle at various points in the range of movement as you perform an exercise. So, a full-range bicep curl (*see page 96*) can be divided into two half stages of movement: from the start position to about 90° (halfway to the full position), and from the halfway position to the full position. In theory, you can achieve different effects

by targeting a muscle in each half of the range of motion. You then work the whole range once you have pre-exhausted the two small ranges. This pattern works well using sets of seven repetitions. So working the bicep with the matrix training technique would look like this:

1. 7 repetitions from arms full out to halfway
2. 7 repetitions from halfway to full curl
3. 7 full-range bicep curls

The last seven full-range repetitions should be very hard work and have an extreme overload effect on the muscle, in this case the bicep.

▼ **find the training technique that works for you**
Try a new training technique – it's a good way to introduce variety into your training routine and ensure that you challenge the muscles in different ways. Strive to achieve muscle overload.

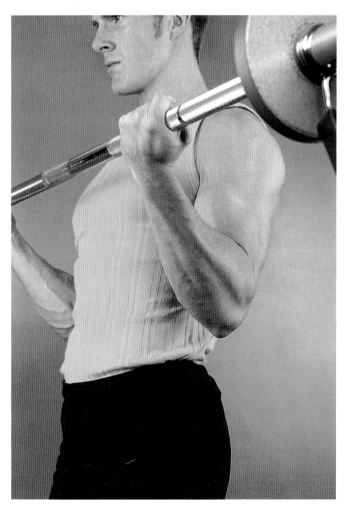

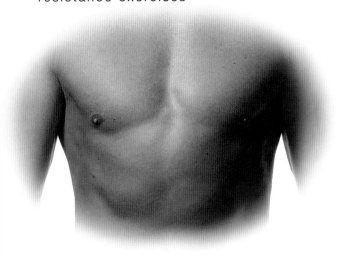

pec fly *pectorals*

This is the definitive exercise for the chest muscles. As always, good technique is crucial.

1 ▼ Lie on your back on a bench with your feet on the floor. Holding a weight in each hand with your palms facing the wall across from you, extend your arms out away from your sides until your hands are at shoulder level.

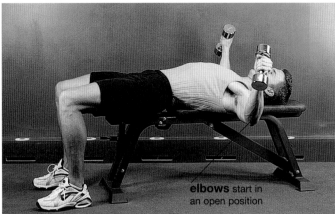

elbows start in an open position

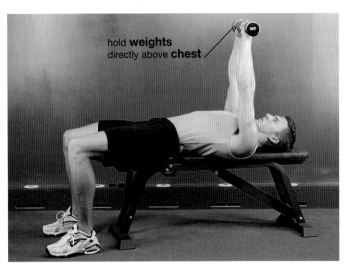

hold **weights** directly above **chest**

2 ◄ While breathing out, use your chest muscles to slowly raise the weights up until your arms are nearly fully extended above your chest. Flex your pectorals, then, breathing in, slowly return to the start position.

machine fly *pectorals*

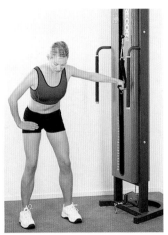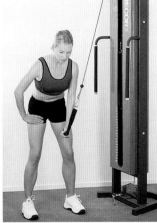

Many gyms have pec fly machines where you perform the exercise seated, but you can also perform it standing using the cable machine.

1 ◄◄ Stand sideways to the cable machine, legs hip-width apart, and knees slightly bent. Grasp the handle, bend forward slightly, and place one hand on your leg for balance.

2 ◄ Keeping your arm almost straight, pull the cable down and across until it is directly in front of you. Return to the start position, keeping the movement slow and controlled.

chest press with dumbbell *pectorals, triceps*

Using free weights for this exercise requires more muscle control than when using the chest-press machine. For best results, keep your abdominals tight.

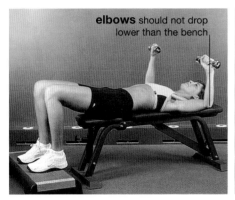

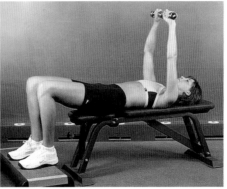

elbows should not drop lower than the bench

take care not to lock **arms** straight

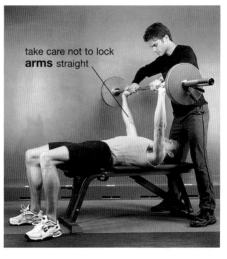

1 ▲ Lie on your back on a bench with your knees bent and feet supported by a step. Holding a weight in each hand, bend your arms so that your elbows are at 90° and your palms face the wall across from you.

2 ▲ Extend your arms upward so that they are nearly straight. Return to the start position, using a pace of about 4 seconds per repetition.

▲ **Barbell alternative** Hold the barbell with hands slightly more than shoulder-width apart; lower it until your arms are bent at 90°. Return to the start position.

machine chest press *pectorals, triceps*

The chest-press machine is standard equipment in many gyms and is great for building strength and shape into the chest area and triceps (back of the upper arm).

1 ▶ Ensure that your lower back is supported by the machine. Start with your arms bent at 90°, making sure your elbows are kept up between chest and shoulder height.

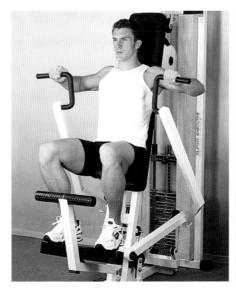

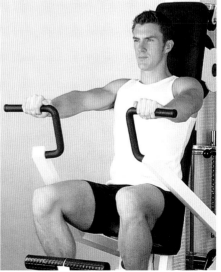

2 ▶▶ Push forward until your arms are almost straight, then bring them back until your elbows are level with your shoulders. Keep the movement slow and controlled, and count 4 seconds per repetition.

resistance exercises

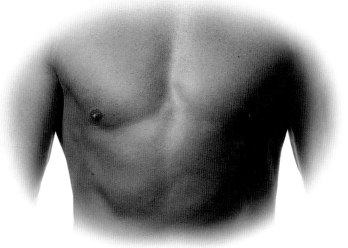

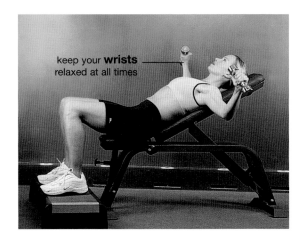

keep your **wrists** relaxed at all times

incline fly *pectorals*

Performing the pec fly with the bench on an incline works the muscles at the top of the chest. Raise the end of the bench so it is at a 40–45° angle. Remember to perform the repetitions in a slow and controlled manner to gain the maximum benefit.

1 ▲ Lie on your back on the bench with knees bent and feet supported by a step. Hold the weights so your hands are level with your shoulders.

2 ▼ Breathe out and extend your arms above you so the weights come together directly above your chest. Slowly return to the start position.

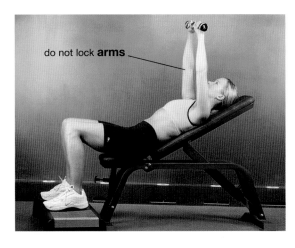

do not lock **arms**

decline fly *pectorals*

Performing the pec fly with the bench on a decline works the pectoris major, the muscles in the lower part of the chest. Position a step under the bench to raise the bottom end by about 30°.

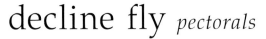

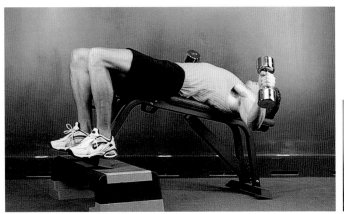

1 ◀ Lie on your back on the bench and hold the weights so your hands are level with your shoulders. Keep your elbows slightly bent and your shoulder blades squeezed back.

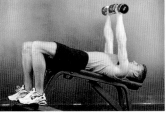

2 ◀ Breathe out, extend your arms above you, and bring the weights together directly above your chest. Take care not to lock your arms straight. Return to the start position.

push-ups *pectorals, deltoids, triceps*

Push-ups use the weight of the body to work the pectorals, deltoids, and triceps (chest, arm, and shoulder muscles). Start with the half push-up and progress to the full push-up once you have built up strength.

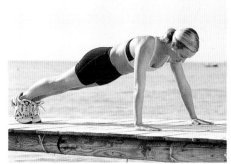
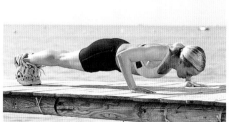
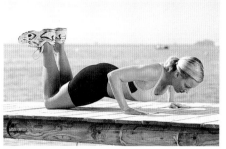

1 ▲ Place your hands directly under your shoulders, or slightly wider if you want to put more emphasis on the chest. Keep your fingers pointing forward and your torso and legs straight.

2 ▲ Bend your arms to about 90° and lower your body, keeping your head in line with your spine. Keep your stomach and thigh muscles tight, which will help to keep your legs straight. Be careful not to point your butt in the air. Push yourself back up to the start position. Remember to breathe in on the way down and out as you push up.

▲ **The half push-up alternative** Keep arms in the same position as for the full push-up, but keep your knees on the mat. Slowly lower the body, then return to the start position.

ball push-ups *pectorals, triceps, abdominals*

Use a stability ball for this more advanced version of a push-up. It works most of the muscles in the chest – in particular the mid-chest area as you squeeze the ball – but also the triceps and abdominals.

1 ▶ Hold your body straight with your toes on the floor. Hold the ball, squeezing it to prevent it from moving, so your hands are positioned just under your shoulders.

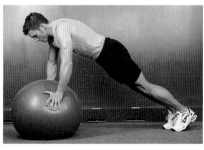
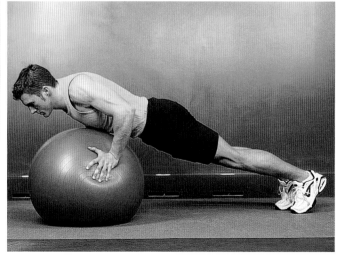

2 ▶ Slowly lower yourself down, keeping your body straight and the movement as slow and controlled as possible. Breathe in on the way down and out on the way up. Count 2 seconds in each direction, longer as you get stronger.

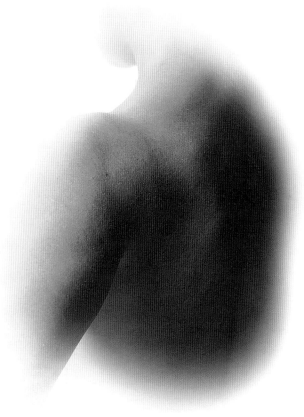

lateral raise *deltoids*

Raise your arms up to parallel with the floor, in the finish position, to ensure that you work all three sections of the deltoids, or shoulder muscles, evenly.

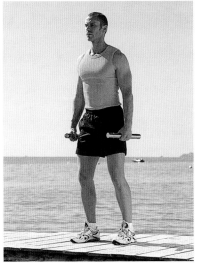 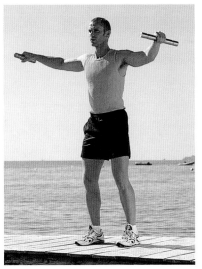

1 ▲ Stand with feet hip-width apart, knees slightly bent. Start with your arms by your sides, holding dumbbells so that your palms face inward. Keep your abdominals tight.

2 ▲ Slowly raise your arms away from your sides, keeping your elbows slightly bent, until your hands are at shoulder level. Keep your palms facing downward; don't allow your hands to twist. Keep your torso still.

bent over lateral raise *deltoids, rhomboids, lats*

You should feel this exercise working the deltoids as well as the muscles across the back. If this is a new exercise for you, you might find that your muscles reach fatigue quickly, so start with lighter weights.

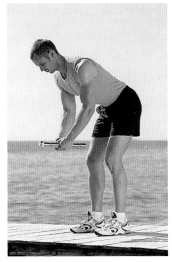 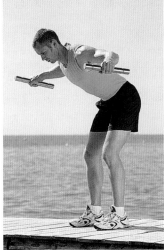

1 ▶ Stand with feet hip-width apart, knees relaxed. Bend forward slightly, holding the weights below your chest with arms slightly bent.

2 ▶▶ Open your arms, and lift the weights until they are level with your shoulders. Hold for 2 seconds, then return to the start position. Take care not to tense the muscles in your neck.

inward thumb lateral raise *posterior deltoids*

Performing the lateral raise with the thumbs turned inward concentrates work on the muscles in the back of the shoulder and the support muscles of the shoulder blade.

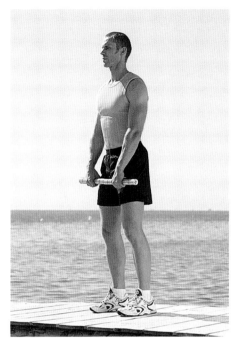

1 ◀ Stand with feet hip-width apart and knees slightly bent. Hold the weights in front of you so your palms face you. Keep your torso straight and hold your abdominals tight.

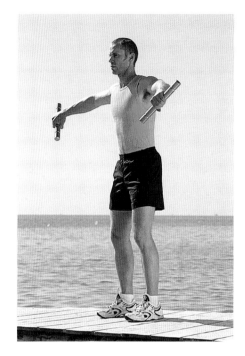

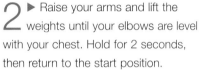

2 ▶ Raise your arms and lift the weights until your elbows are level with your chest. Hold for 2 seconds, then return to the start position.

cable lateral raise
deltoids

Although most gyms will have a lateral raise machine, the exercise can also be performed very effectively on the cable machine. A cable machine has a top and bottom pulley point; use the bottom pulley for this exercise. Some machines may have a variable pulley, in which case position it at its lowest point. Keep your torso still and your shoulders straight at all times.

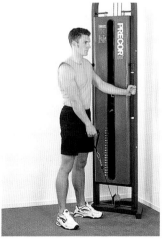

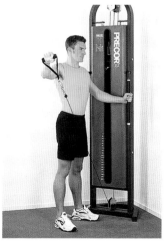

1 ▲ Stand sideways to the cable machine with feet hip-width apart. Hold the cable handle with the outside hand and hold the machine for support with the other.

2 ▲ Raise your hand up to shoulder height, working against the resistance of the cable. Count 2 seconds up and 2 seconds down. Make sure to keep your body steady.

resistance exercises

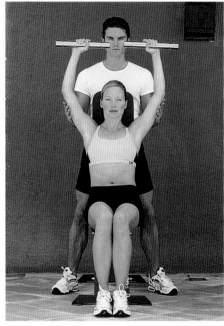

shoulder press *deltoids, triceps*

Performing this exercise while seated concentrates work on the deltoids as the rest of the body is supported by the bench. Stronger exercisers may prefer to do it standing. The pressing action also works the triceps.

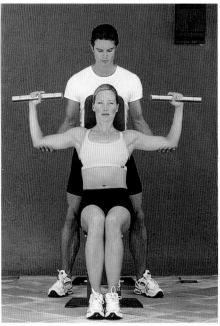

1 ▲ Sit with your back well supported by the bench and legs bent at about 90°. Hold a weight in each hand with your arms bent at 90° and elbows out at shoulder level.

2 ▲ Press the weights upward, raising your arms above your head, but be sure not to lock your arms straight. Your body should not move. Count 1 second up and 1 second down.

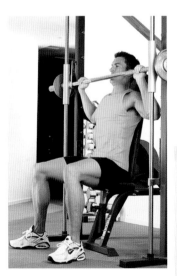

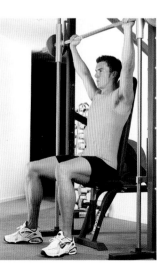

machine press
deltoids, triceps

The shoulder press can be performed on the shoulder press machine, with dumbbells or barbell, or using a bench and the Smith machine, as shown here.

1 ▲ Adjust the bench so that your back is straight and your lower back is supported. Sit with feet hip-width apart and grip the bar with arms bent at about 90°.

2 ◄ Press upward, straightening your arms, but be sure not to lock your arms straight. Keep the movement slow and controlled. Count 1 second up and 1 second down.

upright row *deltoids, trapezius*

This is a good exercise for the deltoids, or shoulder muscles, and the biceps, the muscles at the front of the upper arms. It can be performed using dumbbells or a bar.

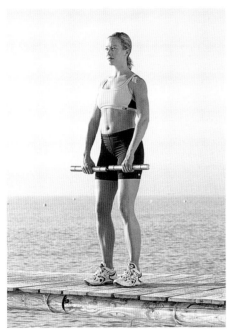

1 ◄ Stand with feet hip-width apart, legs slightly bent, and back straight. Hold the weights in front of you so that your palms face your thighs.

2 ► Pull the weights up to chest height, leading with the elbows. Slowly lower the weights and return to the start position. Count 2 seconds up and 2 seconds down.

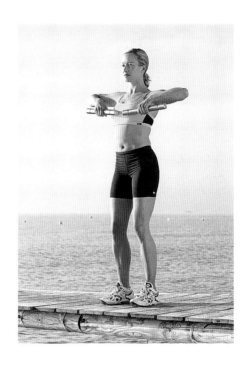

front raise *anterior deltoids*

The front raise tones and improves muscle definition in the front of the shoulder. It can also help to shape the front of the arm.

1 ► Stand with feet hip-width apart, legs slightly bent, and back straight. Hold the weights in front of your thighs.

2 ►► Raise the weights to shoulder height in front of you. Keep your arms straight and maintain a strong upright position. Be sure not to curve your lower back. Count 2 seconds up and 2 seconds down.

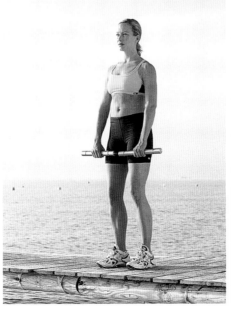

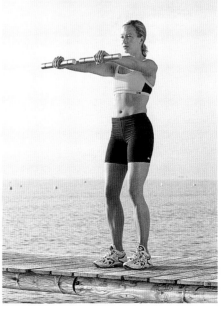

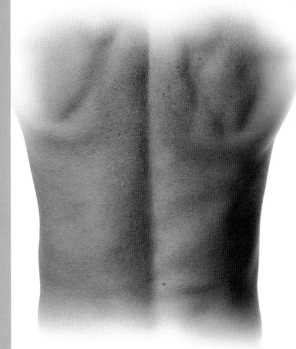

lat pull-down *lats*

This exercise works the large muscles of the back – the latissimus dorsi, or lats, and the rhomboids. Count 2 seconds down and 2 seconds up. Keep your back straight and your abdominals tight at all times

1 ▼ Hold the bar firmly with both hands placed slightly wider than shoulder width. Keep your back straight and your abdominals tight at all times.

2 ▼ Pull down and, as you do so, breathe out. Breathe in as you return to the start position. The whole exercise should take about 4 seconds.

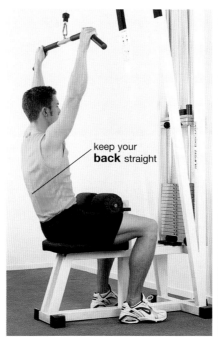

keep your **back** straight

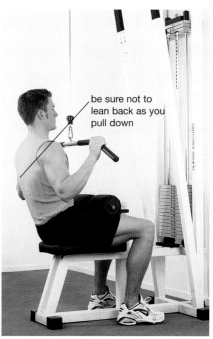

be sure not to lean back as you pull down

reverse fly
posterior deltoids

This is a tough exercise that really targets a specific area – the muscles across the back of the shoulders and in the middle back.

1 ▶ Sit on the end of a bench with knees bent at about 90° and feet hip-width apart. Bend forward, keeping your back straight, and start by holding the weights behind your calves, thumbs facing inward.

2 ▶▶ Lift the weights, keeping your arms slightly bent, until your elbows are level with your shoulders. Hold for 2 seconds, then slowly return to the start position.

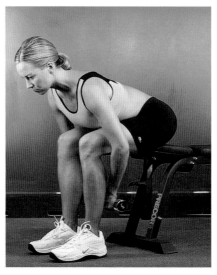

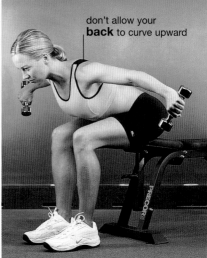

don't allow your **back** to curve upward

single arm row *lats, rhomboids, biceps*

In this exercise you lift a weight toward your body to work the biceps, backs of the shoulders, and upper back. Focus on using the back muscles to pull the elbow through, rather than just relying on your biceps.

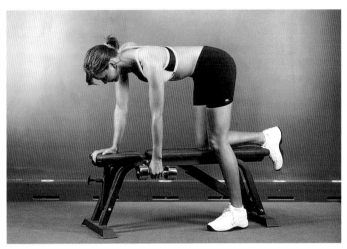

1 ▲ Rest your right hand and knee on a bench, keeping your left foot on the floor. Hold a dumbbell in your left hand so that your arm hangs down toward the floor. Keep your back straight and shoulders parallel to the bench.

2 ▲ Pull the dumbbell up toward your chest, keeping your body stable, your back straight, and your shoulders relaxed. Keep your arm close to your body. Return to the start position, keeping the movement slow and controlled.

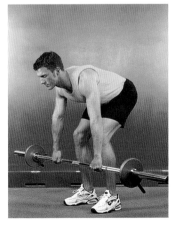
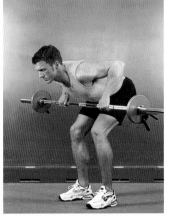

1 ▲ Stand with feet shoulder-width apart, knees slightly bent. Bend forward holding the barbell down in front of your shins.

2 ▲ Pull the barbell up to your chest, hold for 2 seconds, then return to the start position. Keep your back straight at all times.

barbell row *lats*

This is one of the more advanced back exercises. Because it is performed in a bent over position, it requires a greater degree of control, and this concentrates work on the muscles across the back as well as on the general postural muscles in the torso.

resistance exercises

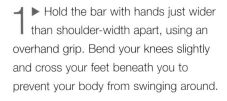

wide pull-up *lats, biceps*

The pull-up can be performed on a pull-up machine, which has a platform that helps support your weight, or on a pull-up bar, as shown here. The wide grip works the lats assisted by the biceps.

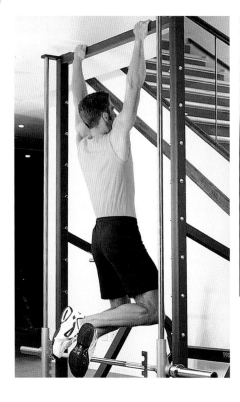

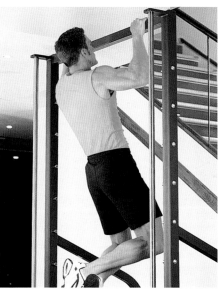

1 ▶ Hold the bar with hands just wider than shoulder-width apart, using an overhand grip. Bend your knees slightly and cross your feet beneath you to prevent your body from swinging around.

2 ▲ Pull your body up until your eyes are level with the bar. Hold for 1 second, then slowly lower yourself back down to the start position.

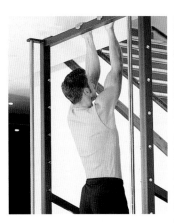

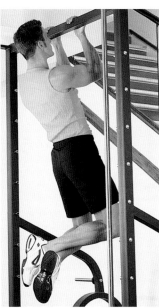

close pull-up
biceps, lats

Performing the pull-up with a close grip works the biceps assisted by the lats. Both types of pull-ups are advanced exercises and should be performed with control rather than momentum.

1 ▲ Hold the bar with your hands slightly closer than shoulder-width apart, using an underhand grip.

2 ◀ Pull your body up until your eyes are level with the bar. Keep your body as straight as possible. Hold for 1 second, then slowly lower yourself back down to the start position.

inward rotator cuff *shoulder stabilizers*

This exercise strengthens the frontal support muscles of the shoulder.
There is a gym machine for this exercise, but it can also be performed
using a bench and a free weight.

1 ▶ Raise one end of the bench to a
45° angle, and sit with your right side
supported by it and your shoulders at
right angles to it. Hold the weight in your
right hand with your knuckles facing the
floor and your arm bent at 90°.

2 ▶▶ Ensure that your right elbow is
supported by the bench, and raise
the weight up to your chest. Hold for
1 second, then slowly lower the weight
and return to the start position.

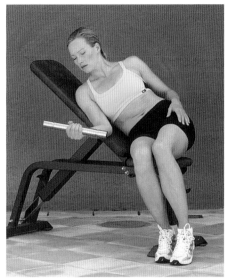
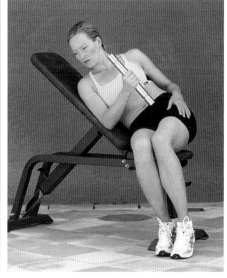

outward rotator cuff *shoulder stabilizers*

This exercise works the minor support muscles of the shoulder. It can be performed
on a gym machine, an adjustable cable machine, or using a bench and free weight.

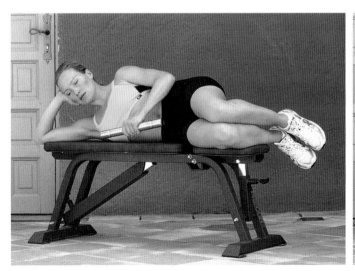
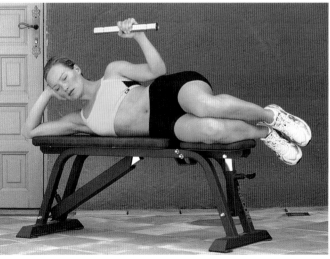

1 ▲ Lie on your right side on a bench with your head supported
by your right arm. Tuck your knees up onto the bench; rest
your left elbow on your hip. Hold the weight in front of you.

2 ▲ Keeping your arm bent at 90° and your elbow supported
by your hip, raise the weight until it is just higher than the line
of your body. Hold for 1 second, then return to the start position.

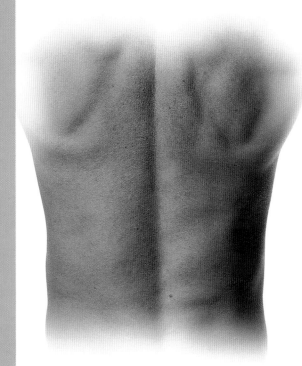

straight arm pull-down
lats, rhomboids, triceps

This works the muscles across the back and also the triceps.
Use the cable machine with a bar attachment.

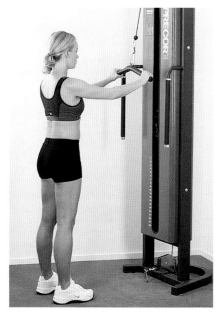 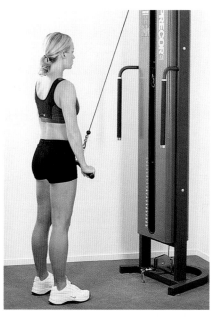

1 ▲ Stand facing the cable machine at arm's length away from it, with feet hip-width apart. Grasp the bar in front of you with both hands.

2 ▲ Keeping your arms straight, pull the bar down until it reaches your thighs. Hold for 1 second, then return to the start position.

seated row
rhomboids, biceps

This exercise tones the muscles of the upper middle back. To get the most from this exercise, keep the torso and legs completely still.

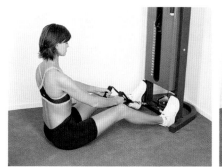 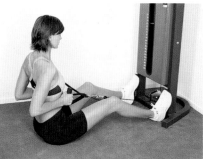

1 ▲ Sit on the floor facing the cable machine, legs out in front of you and knees slightly bent. Hold the bar with both hands; be sure to keep your back straight.

2 ▲ Pull the bar in close to the body, aiming for the lower chest area. Hold for 1 second, then return to the start position. Keep your elbows tucked in close to your body.

dorsal raise *erector spinae*

This is an excellent exercise for the lower back. By strengthening the main muscles that run along the lower part of the spine, the erector spinae, it can help improve posture and also prevent lower back pain.

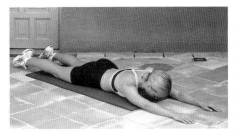

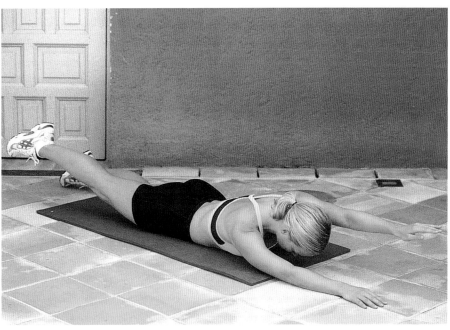

1 ▲ Lie on your front on a mat with your arms outstretched in front of you and legs straight. Make sure not to tense the muscles in your neck.

2 ▶ Raise your left arm and your right leg, keeping them both straight. Hold for 1 second, then slowly lower them. Repeat, raising the opposite arm and leg.

back extension *erector spinae*

This is more demanding than the dorsal raise because here you are using the muscles to control the movement rather than holding them in a static position. Increase the difficulty of this exercise by moving the hands further away from the body – straight out above the head, for example.

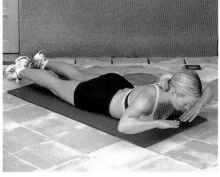

1 ▶ Lie on your front on a mat. Bend your arms and bring your hands up to your chin.

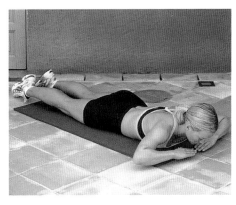

2 ▲ Raise your head and upper torso off the mat, being sure not to tense the muscles in your neck. Hold for 1 second then return to the start position, keeping the movement slow and controlled. Breathe out as you lift and in as you lower yourself down.

resistance exercises

95

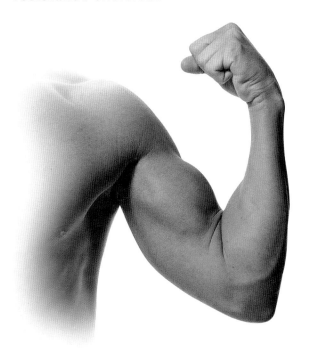

bicep curl *biceps*

A great isolation exercise, the bicep curl gives fantastic definition to the upper arm.

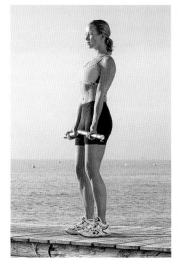
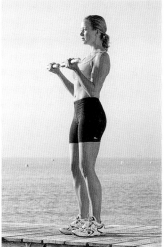

1 ▲ Stand with feet hip-width apart, knees slightly bent, and arms by your sides. Start with your elbows slightly bent; hold the weights so that your palms face outward.

2 ▲ Bend your arms and lift the weights toward your shoulders. Keep your elbows tucked in close to your body. At the top of the movement, flex your biceps to maximize the effectiveness of the exercise. Keep the movement slow and controlled and be sure to keep your back straight as you lift the weights.

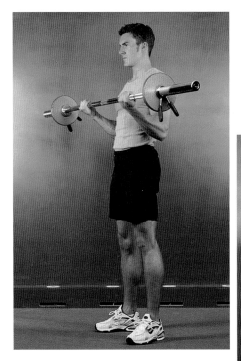

▲ Bicep curl with barbell alternative
Stand with feet hip-width apart and knees relaxed. Slowly raise the barbell to the chest, hold for 1 second, then return to the start position.

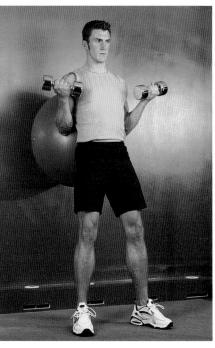

◄ Bicep curl with ball alternative
Position a stability ball between your lower back and the wall. Keep your back straight and your knees relaxed. Raise and lower the weights as for a bicep curl (see above). Leaning on the ball lengthens the biceps because the elbows come slightly further back than usual; this also helps to concentrate work on the biceps.

resistance exercises

hammer curl *biceps*

The hammer curl sculpts and tones the outer sections of the biceps and can actually make your arms appear longer.

1 ▶ Stand with feet hip-width apart, legs slightly bent, and arms by your sides. Start with your arms slightly bent. Hold the weights so that your palms face inward.

2 ▶▶ Lift the weights toward your shoulders, keeping your elbows tucked in close to your body. Flex the biceps at the top of the movement, then return to the start position. Do not allow your body to sway with the movement.

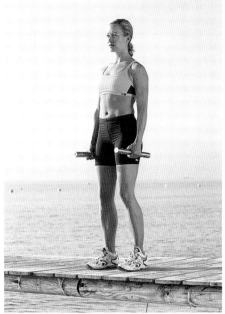

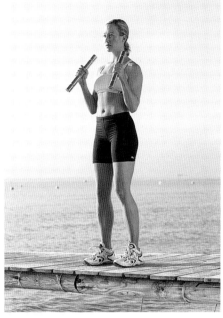

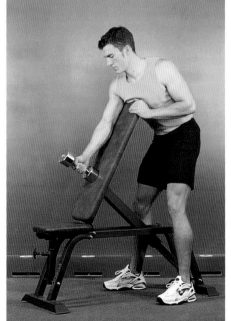

supported hammer curl
biceps

This is an advanced bicep exercise. Because the arm is supported by the bench you cannot move your elbow to help lift the weight, and all the work is done by the bicep.

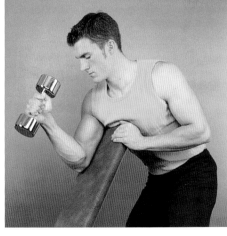

1 ▲ Stand behind a bench that is raised to a 45–55° angle. Keep your back straight, and ensure that your body weight is evenly distributed. Rest the arm with the weight against the elevated bench.

2 ◀ Pull the weight toward your shoulder keeping the upper arm against the bench and maintaining the hammer curl position. Count 2 seconds up and 2 seconds down, keeping the movement slow and controlled. This elongates the bicep rather than giving it a round compact shape.

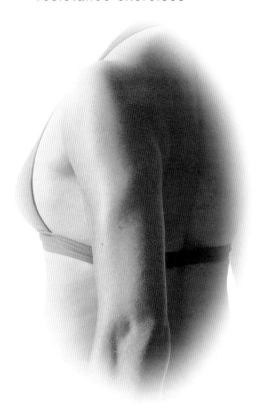

dips *triceps*

This highly effective exercise concentrates work on the triceps. Exercises that involve lifting your own bodyweight help to improve posture and strengthen and protect the skeletal system.

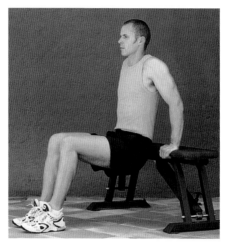

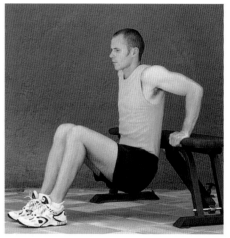

1 ▲ Place feet hip-width apart; keep your back straight and close to the bench and bend your knees at 90°.

2 ▲ Lower yourself down until your arms are bent at 90°, then push back up until arms are straight, but not locked.

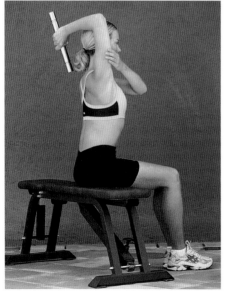

1 ▲ Sit upright on a bench with back straight and feet flat on the floor. Hold the dumbbell behind your head so that your elbow is level with your head.

tricep overhead *triceps*

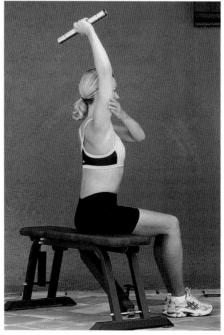

This exercise is an alternative to the tricep extension (*see page 101*). You can perform it standing, but sitting upright on a bench will keep your body steady, which can help to improve technique.

2 ◀ Extend your arm, keeping your elbow close to your head and making sure not to let your elbow "drift" out of position. Keep your abdominal muscles tight to prevent straining the back. Slowly return to the start position.

push-down – thumbs in *triceps*

This is one of the most effective exercises for toning and shaping the upper area of the tricep. The muscle has to work during the upward and downward phases of the exercise. Use a bar attachment on the cable machine.

1 ▶ Stand facing the cable machine with feet hip-width apart. Hold the bar with thumbs pointing in and elbows tucked in.

2 ▶▶ Push the bar down until your arms are straight. Move only the lower part of your arms. Count 2 seconds down and 2 seconds up.

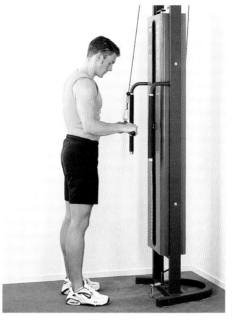
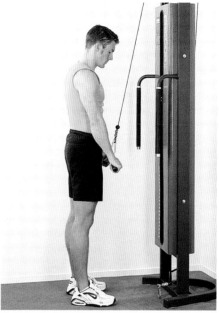

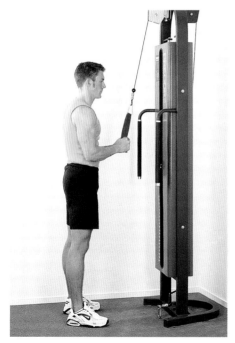

1 ▲ Stand facing the cable machine with feet hip-width apart. Hold the cord with thumbs facing up and elbows tucked in close to the body.

push-down – thumbs up
triceps

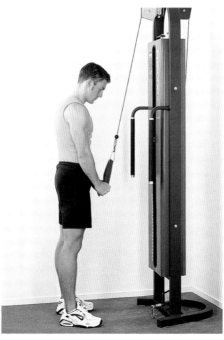

Performing the push-down with thumbs up effectively targets and shapes the outer area of the tricep. Attach a cord or rope to the cable machine so your thumbs are in the correct position.

2 ◀ Bring your lower arms down until your hands are in front of your thighs. Count 2 seconds down and 2 seconds as you return to the start position.

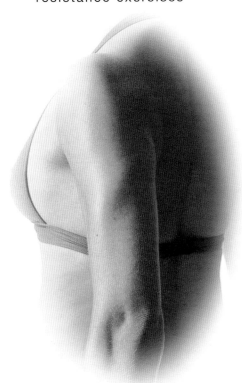

close hand push-up *triceps*

This version of the push-up concentrates work on the triceps. For a less advanced form of the exercise, position your legs as for the half push-up (*see page 85*), with knees on the floor.

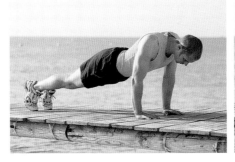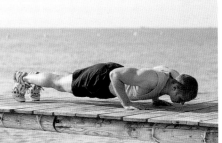

1 ▲ Place your hands slightly closer than shoulder-width apart with your fingers pointing forward. Keep your torso and legs straight.

2 ▲ Bend your arms, and lower your body down, keeping your head in line with your spine and your elbows tucked in. Push yourself back up to the start position.

french press *triceps*

This is one of the most difficult tricep exercises because the muscle is elongated in the start position and is therefore forced to work harder.

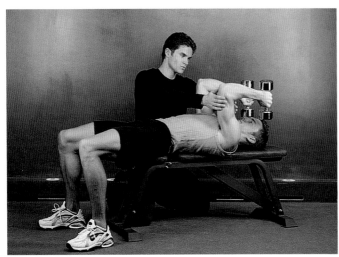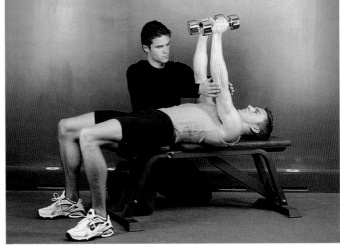

1 ▲ Lie on your back on a bench, feet flat on the floor. Pointing your elbows at the ceiling, bend your arms at 90°, and hold the weights by your head.

2 ▲ Slowly extend your arms until they are nearly straight and the weights are above your head. Move only the lower arms, and be sure not to arch your back.

tricep extension *triceps*

Keep your abdominal muscles tight and your back straight during the tricep extension; this will help you to stay in the correct position and so maximize the effectiveness of the exercise.

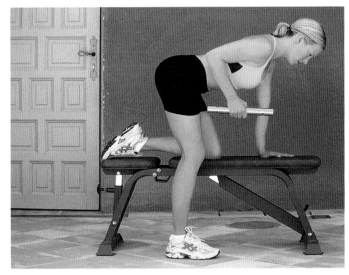

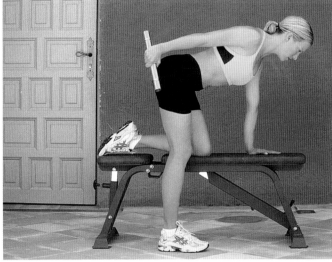

1 ▲ Rest your left hand and knee on a bench, and keep your right foot on the floor. With a weight in your right hand, lift your elbow so that it is at 90° and the upper arm is parallel to the floor.

2 ▲ Hold the elbow position and straighten your arm while flexing the tricep. Slowly return to the start position. Take 4–5 seconds to complete the entire movement.

ball throw *triceps, pectorals*

You need a partner and a medicine ball for this exercise. Stand about 6–10 ft (2–3 meters) apart and use a medicine ball of 7–11 lb (3-5 kg).

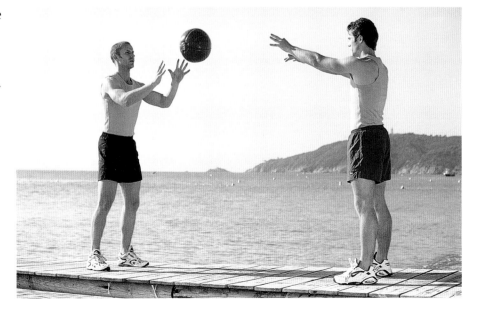

1 ▶ Stand with feet about hip-width apart and legs relaxed. Throw the ball to your partner, following through with your arms as you push it away from your chest. Pull the ball into your chest as you catch it.

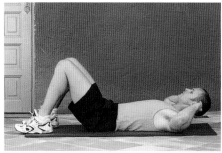

basic crunches *abdominals*

Of all the abdominal exercises, the basic crunch is one of the most effective. The key is to keep the movement slow and to focus on good technique.

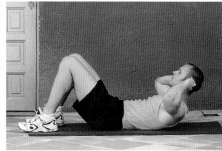

▶ The crunch frame alternative The frame helps to position your body correctly and supports your neck. It also forces you to use your abdominal muscles rather than cheating the exercise.

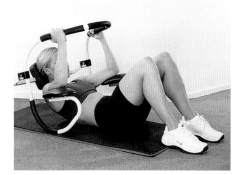

1 ▲ Lie on your back with your knees bent, feet flat on the floor and hands by your ears.

2 ▲ Curl your shoulders forward, keeping your lower back on the floor. Tense the abdominals, breathing out as you lift and in as you lower. Keep a space the size of an apple under your chin, to ensure that your head stays in line with your spine. Each repetition should take about 4–5 seconds in total.

full crunch *abdominals*

The most advanced abdominal exercise, the full crunch combines the movements of the basic crunch (*see above*) and the reverse curl (*see right*) and works the entire stomach area.

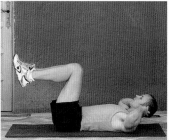

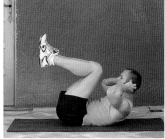

1 ▲ Lie on your back with your legs in the air, knees bent, and hands at each side of your head by your ears.

2 ▲ Curl your legs and pelvis toward your rib cage at the same time curling your shoulders forward. Make sure not to tense the muscles in your neck.

reverse curl *abdominals*

The reverse curl targets the lower part of the abdominal section, putting less strain on the neck area. Used in conjunction with other crunches it can help to give a toned effect to the entire stomach area.

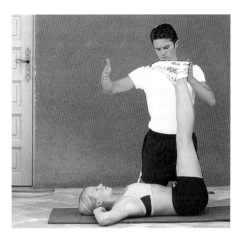

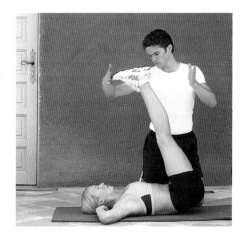

1 ◄ Lie on your back with your hands behind your head, legs straight up in the air. Keep your shoulders and head on the floor at all times. Ensure that your feet never come further back than your head.

2 ► Tighten your lower abdominals and bring your legs and pelvis toward your rib cage. Keep the movement slow and controlled and be careful not to let your legs swing around.

raised reverse curl *rectus abdominalis*

This exercise tones the muscles in the bottom section of the abdomen, the rectus abdominals. The raised angle of the bench adds resistance and makes it more advanced than the standard reverse curl.

1 ► Lie on a bench with the top end raised to an angle of about 10–30°. Hold the top of the bench to keep your body steady and start with your legs straight and your feet in the air.

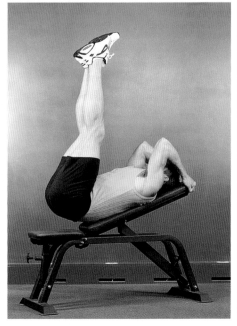

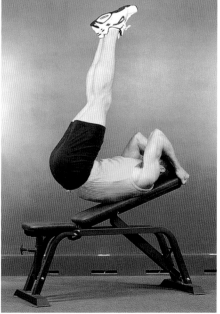

2 ►► Tighten your lower abdominals and curl your legs and pelvis toward your rib cage. Hold for 1 second, then slowly return to the start position.

resistance exercises

103

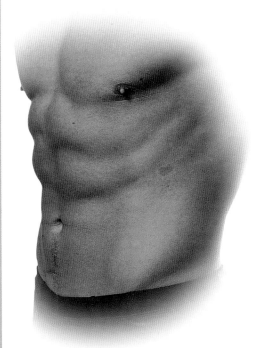

oblique crunch *obliques*

This is the best exercise for the obliques, the muscles at the side of the stomach that run from under the rib cage to the hips.

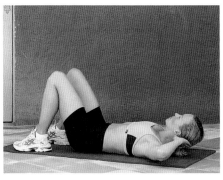

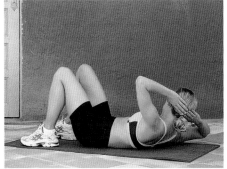

1 ▲ Lie on your back on a mat with your knees bent, feet flat on the floor, and hands by your head.

2 ▲ Slowly raise one shoulder and elbow up toward the outside of the opposite thigh. Change shoulders to work the muscles on the other side.

medicine ball crunch *abdominals*

Performing the crunch with a medicine ball helps to increase the work done by the abdominals and can improve the toning effect of this exercise.

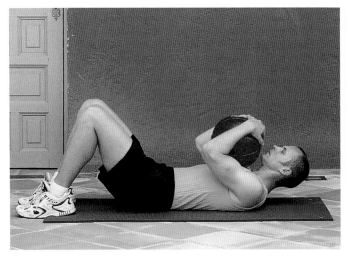

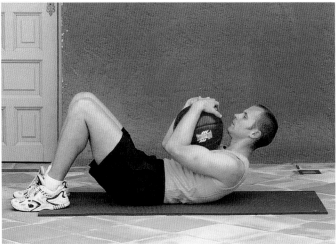

1 ▲ Lie on your back with your knees bent and feet flat on the floor. Hold a medicine ball to your chest with both hands.

2 ▲ Holding on to the medicine ball, curl your shoulders and upper back forward, being sure not to tense the muscles in your neck.

bridge *abdominals, erector spinae*

This is a static exercise that helps to strengthen the muscles in the stomach and lower back. It is an advanced exercise and should only be attempted by stronger exercisers.

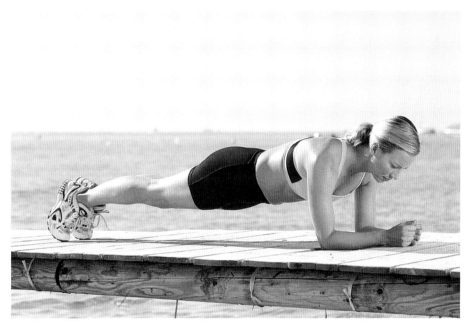

1 ◄ Position yourself so that your toes are on the ground and your elbows are directly below your shoulders. Raise yourself up, keeping a straight line from your shoulders to your ankles, so that your elbows and toes support your body. Use your abdominals to maintain the position, and be sure not to stick your butt in the air.

oblique bridge *abdominals, obliques*

Probably the most difficult of the abdominal exercises, the oblique bridge strengthens the obliques. As with the bridge, it is only suitable for advanced exercisers.

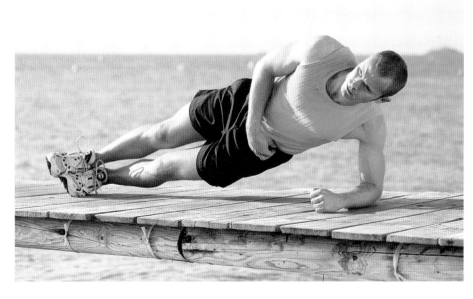

1 ◄ Lie on your side, and position your bottom elbow directly under your shoulder as a support. Place one foot on top of the other, then raise yourself up, keeping a straight line from your head to your toes. Use your obliques to maintain the position.

resistance exercises

lunge *quads, glutes*

A demanding exercise, the lunge can give you wonderfully toned inner thighs and buttocks. Hold hand weights to make it more challenging.

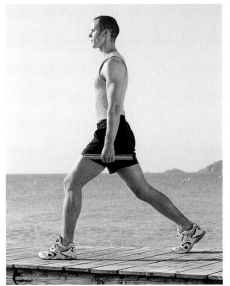

the **knee** should not bend further forward than the toes

1 ▲ Place one foot forward about one stride-length apart from the back leg. Keep your hips facing straight ahead and your arms loose by your sides. Keep your body upright and your abdominals firm.

2 ▲ Bend your knees to bring your front knee directly over your front foot. Put your weight onto the heel of your front foot to work the buttock muscle most effectively. Return to the start position.

power lunge *quads, glutes*

This is a more dynamic version of the lunge (*see above*), but the movement should still be steady and controlled.

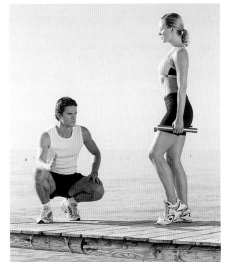

1 ▲ Stand with arms loose by your sides. Holding weights makes the exercise more advanced.

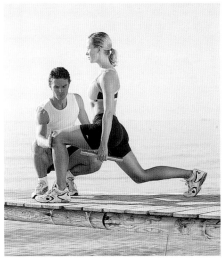

2 ◄ Step forward about 1 stride length from the back foot, making sure that your knee does not bend further forward than your toes. As you do so, lower your body down, then spring back to the starting position, pushing through with the heel of your front foot. Do not allow your body to waver.

walking lunge *quads, hamstrings, glutes*

Unlike repetitive exercises, which often focus on very specific sets of muscles, the continuous forward movement of the walking lunge ensures that all the muscles of the legs and mid section work hard.

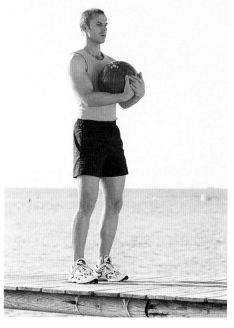

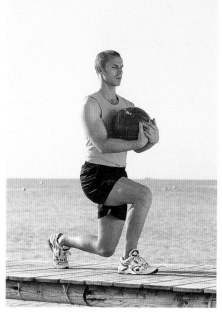

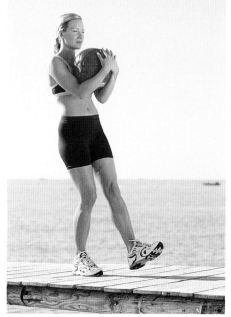

1 ▲ Stand with feet hip-width apart and knees slightly bent. Hold a medicine ball to your chest.

2 ▲ Step forward about 1 stride length from the back foot. In the same movement, lower your body down, hold for 1 second, then raising your body, step forward with the other leg and repeat the lunge. Continue as you move forward.

single leg ball squat *quads*

This is one of the most intensive leg exercises that you can do and really strengthens the stabilizing muscles of the inner and outer thigh. It should only be attempted by regular or advanced exercisers.

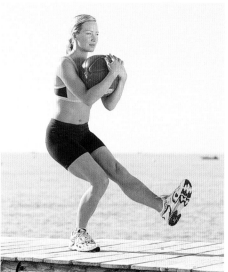

1 ▲ Stand with feet hip-width apart and legs slightly bent. Hold a medicine ball to your chest. Keeping your leg straight, raise it so that your heel is about 3–5 in (8–13 cm) off the ground.

2 ◀ Keeping your back straight, lower yourself down as if sitting in an imaginary chair. Control the movement with your supporting leg which should not be allowed to bend to less than 90° at the back of the knee.

resistance exercises

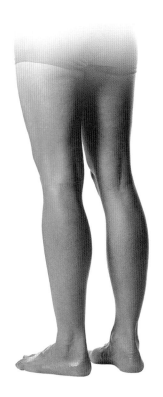

squat *quads, hamstrings, glutes*

Squats work the thighs and buttocks as well as the lower leg muscles, abdominals, and lower back since they are used for balance. Performing the exercise with hand weights increases the intensity and with a barbell over the shoulders builds mass.

1 ▶ Stand with your feet hip-width apart, knees slightly bent. Keep your back straight and place your hands on your hips.

2 ▶▶ Bend your knees to 90° and allow your body to lean forward slightly until it is at right angles to your thighs. Be sure to keep your heels on the floor.

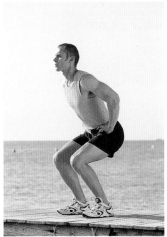
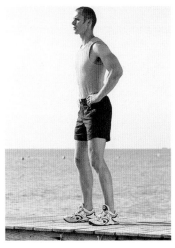

ball squat *quads, glutes*

This exercise simulates the action of the leg press machine and strengthens and shapes the thigh muscles. The stability ball acts as a back support when performing this difficult exercise.

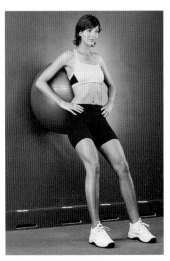
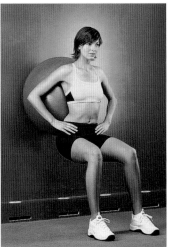
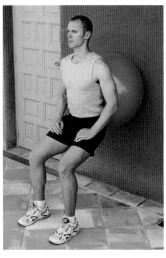

1 ▲ Position a stability ball between your lower and middle back and the wall. Keep your back upright and straight, and place your hands on your hips to steady yourself. Your legs should be almost straight.

2 ▲ Concentrating work on your thigh muscles, slowly lower your body down until your thighs are parallel with the floor. Then, slowly push yourself back up to the starting position.

▲ **Static squat alternative**
Start in the same position as for the ball squat. Lower yourself down until your thighs are parallel with the floor, then hold the position for as long as you can.

step-ups *quads, calves*

Go briskly through this exercise: step-ups work your lower body muscles, but they should also raise your heart rate. Use a step – adjusted so that your knee does not bend to less than 90° when you step onto it – when performing this exercise in the gym.

1 ▶ Stand facing a step or stair. Step up with one foot, placing your whole foot flat on the step. Keep your back straight and your head and neck relaxed but in line with your torso. Step up with your other foot so that both feet are flat on the step. Step down one foot at a time.

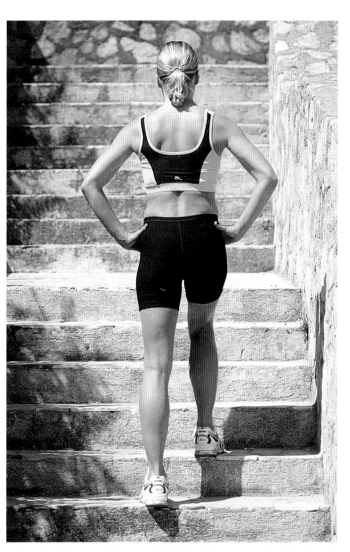

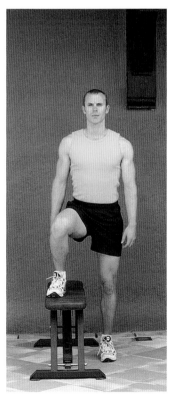 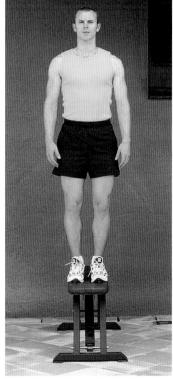

1 ▲ Stand sideways to a bench with arms loose by your sides. Place one foot on the bench. Use that leg to pull yourself onto the bench.

2 ▲ Transfer your body weight onto the other leg, and slowly lower the opposite leg down on to the floor. When that foot touches the floor, pull yourself back onto the bench and repeat.

bench crossover
quads, adductors

This exercise uses the weight of your body as the resistance and builds dynamic strength in the legs. Make sure that your knee does not have to bend to less than 90° when you step onto the bench.

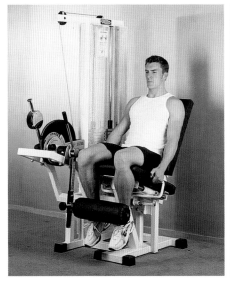

leg extension *quadriceps*

This exercise works the quadriceps, or quads, the powerful muscles at the fronts of the thighs. Take three seconds to lift, then three seconds to return to the start position.

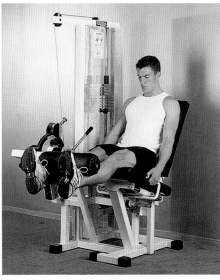

1 ▲ Sit with your ankles hooked behind the roller pad and your legs at 90°. Point your toes forward to ensure that you work the muscles evenly. Pointing the toes to one side can distort leg shape. Keep the lower back well supported.

2 ▲ Slowly extend your legs until they are straight. Hold for half a second, then slowly return to the start position, but don't allow the weights to "touch down." Remember to exhale as you lift the weights and inhale as you lower them.

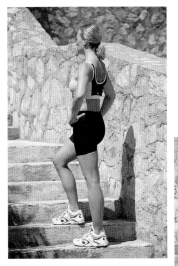

1 ▲ Stand facing a step or stair with one foot on the step and one on the ground. Place your hands on your hips for balance.

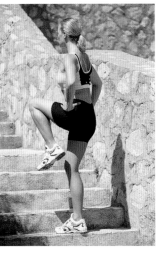

knee raise *glutes, hip flexor*

Another dynamic exercise, the knee raise uses big movements to strengthen and build power in the legs while also raising the heart rate.

2 ◄ Bring your lower leg up, raising your knee as you do so, before bringing it back down onto the ground. Step down with the opposite leg, then repeat on the other side.

leg curl *hamstrings*

The hamstrings are the large muscles at the backs of the thighs. Hamstring work can reward you with longer-looking legs and a slimmer butt. As the muscles develop, they can also increase your body's calorie-burning potential.

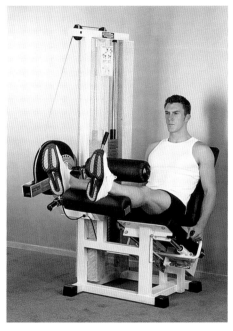

1 ◀ Sit with your legs extended and your ankles on top of the roller pad. Your back should be at right angles to your legs, and your lower back should be supported throughout the exercise. Aim to spread the movement over 6 seconds: 3 seconds to bend the legs and 3 seconds to extend them.

2 ▶ Hold your stomach tight and bend your legs, bringing your heels toward your butt. Hold for half a second, then slowly return to the start position. Exhale as you lift the weights and inhale as you lower them.

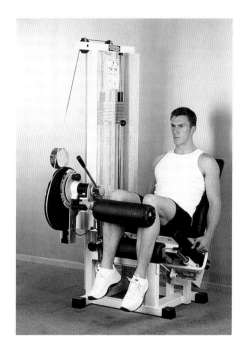

leg press
quads, hamstrings

Many gyms have leg-press machines, but you can also perform this exercise using the Smith machine. When using the leg-press machine, make sure that the lower back is well supported.

1 ▶ Start by positioning yourself under the bar with feet hip-width apart and knees at just more than 90°. Keep the neck relaxed and the back tall and straight.

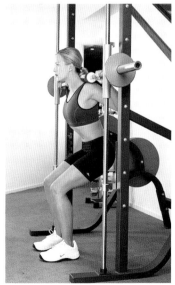

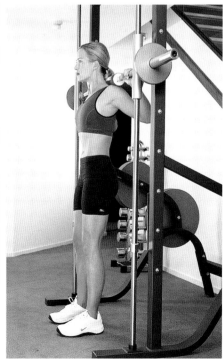

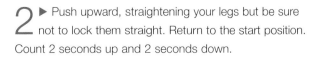

2 ▶ Push upward, straightening your legs but be sure not to lock them straight. Return to the start position. Count 2 seconds up and 2 seconds down.

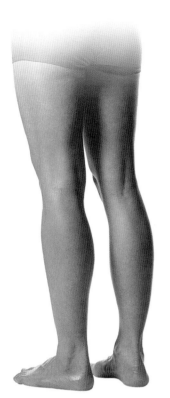

single calf raise *calves*

A good exercise for strengthening and toning calf muscles, the calf raise can also be used for increasing the size of the calves. If you already have large calves, only perform this exercise occasionally.

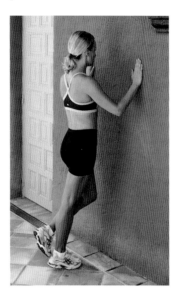

1 ◄ Stand about half an arm's length away from a wall and place your hands on it in front of you. Raise your left foot off the floor.

2 ► Raise your body by going onto tip toe on your right foot. You should feel the contraction in your right calf muscle. Hold for 1 second, and return to the start position.

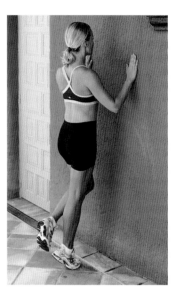

abductor raise *hip abductors*

This exercise targets the muscles of the outer buttocks, the gluteus medius or hip abductor, and is also fantastically effective for toning the outer thighs.

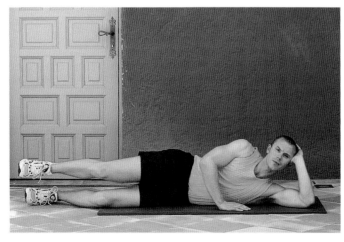

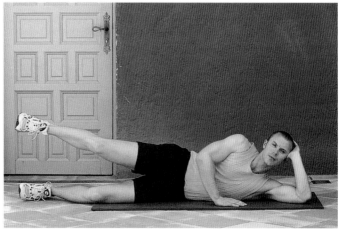

1 ▲ Lie on your left side with your left leg slightly bent. Use your left hand to support your head, and place your right hand in front of you to steady yourself.

2 ▲ Keeping your right leg straight and in line with your body, slowly raise it up with a slow and controlled movement. Hold for 1 second, then return to the start position.

glute raise *glutes, hamstring*

This is an intense exercise that targets the butt, a trouble spot for many people. Performed regularly, you should see results in no time at all.

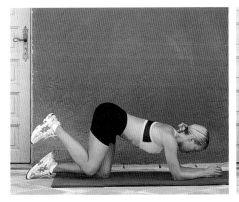

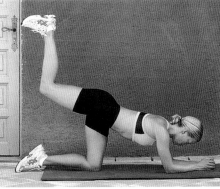

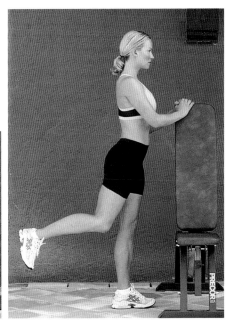

1 ▲ Support yourself on your elbows and knees, with hands together in front of you. Be sure to keep your back straight while performing the exercise.

2 ▲ Keeping your right leg bent, raise it up in the air. Keep your foot flat and press up into the heel. Count 2 seconds up and 2 seconds down.

▲ **Standing glute raise alternative**
Stand straight with abdominals tight. Bend your right leg to 90° and push the sole of your foot away from you. Repeat.

body raise for glutes *glutes, erector spinae*

Make this exercise more effective by pointing your toes away from you in the second step as this intensifies the work on the glutes.

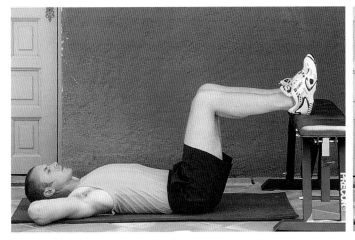

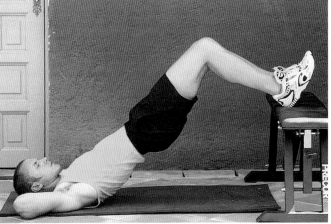

1 ▲ Lie flat on your back with your heels up on a bench, knees bent at 90°, and hands at your head.

2 ▲ Raise your pelvis off the floor until your body is straight from your knees to your chest. Squeeze your buttocks, but don't allow your chest to bow. Count 2 seconds up, 2 seconds down.

resistance exercises

p r

the
grams

The 20 specially tailored programs that I have devised for this section combine different aerobic and resistance training techniques with nutritional advice. They will prepare you for your goal, whether it be to lose weight, maintain your current level of fitness, or run a marathon. There is a program for prenatal fitness as well as one to help recover your fitness after childbirth. As a testament to their effectiveness, five real case studies followed different programs. Each person's progress is charted with a personal training journal and "before," "during," and "after" pictures.

how to use the programs

The programs guide you through workouts that use different training techniques and a variety of aerobic and resistance exercises. The sample program below will help you to understand how to use them. A box at the start of each program tells you whether the program builds strength/tones muscles, burns fat/improves aerobic capacity, or increases flexibility. They are rated as follows: fair ✓ good ✓✓ excellent ✓✓✓.

Workout 2   Workout time 45 mins   (5 mins Warmup + 30 mins Exercise sequence + 10 mins Cool-down)

the exercises

A small "trigger" picture and a page reference will tell you where to find each exercise demonstrated step by step. Sometimes you will see them used in an exercise library, and different charts will tell you how to use the exercises in the workouts.

workout time

This gives the total workout time and will tell you how long each section of the workout takes. So, in this example, the total workout time is 45 minutes: you spend 5 minutes warming up, 30 minutes doing the main body of the workout, the exercise sequence, and 10 minutes cooling down.

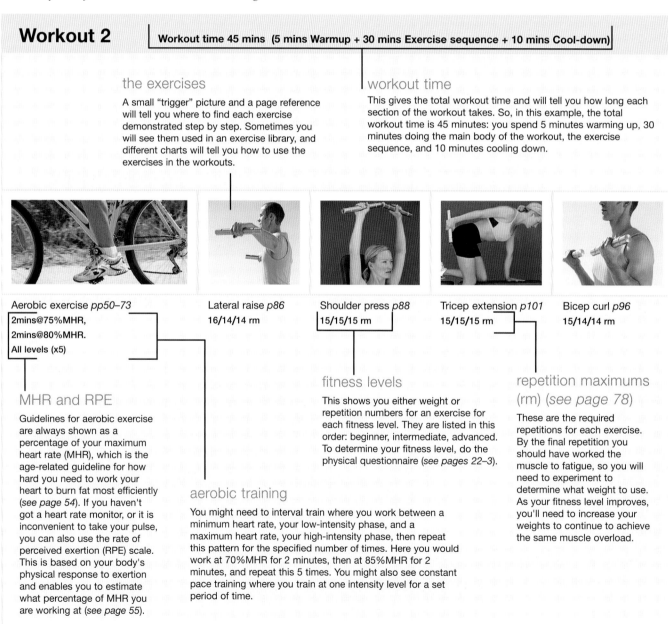

Aerobic exercise *pp50–73*
2mins@75%MHR,
2mins@80%MHR.
All levels (x5)

Lateral raise *p86*
16/14/14 rm

Shoulder press *p88*
15/15/15 rm

Tricep extension *p101*
15/15/15 rm

Bicep curl *p96*
15/14/14 rm

MHR and RPE

Guidelines for aerobic exercise are always shown as a percentage of your maximum heart rate (MHR), which is the age-related guideline for how hard you need to work your heart to burn fat most efficiently (*see page 54*). If you haven't got a heart rate monitor, or it is inconvenient to take your pulse, you can also use the rate of perceived exertion (RPE) scale. This is based on your body's physical response to exertion and enables you to estimate what percentage of MHR you are working at (*see page 55*).

aerobic training

You might need to interval train where you work between a minimum heart rate, your low-intensity phase, and a maximum heart rate, your high-intensity phase, then repeat this pattern for the specified number of times. Here you would work at 70%MHR for 2 minutes, then at 85%MHR for 2 minutes, and repeat this 5 times. You might also see constant pace training where you train at one intensity level for a set period of time.

fitness levels

This shows you either weight or repetition numbers for an exercise for each fitness level. They are listed in this order: beginner, intermediate, advanced. To determine your fitness level, do the physical questionnaire (*see pages 22–3*).

repetition maximums (rm) (*see page 78*)

These are the required repetitions for each exercise. By the final repetition you should have worked the muscle to fatigue, so you will need to experiment to determine what weight to use. As your fitness level improves, you'll need to increase your weights to continue to achieve the same muscle overload.

the case studies

These five people are my case studies. None of them had ever worked out with me before – some had never worked out at all. They each followed a program, and they all achieved their different goals successfully. The most important thing to remember about this group is that they all have normal lives – they all hold down good jobs, and they continued to go out and enjoy themselves while following their programs. They worked out three times a week for 10–12 weeks to achieve the fantastic results that they did.

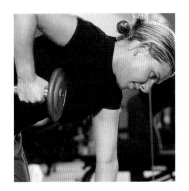

sasha

age **31**

profession **company director**

height **5ft 4in (1.6m)**

weight **152lb (69kg)**

body fat **30%**

dress size **12**

"I wanted to tone up my whole body, and I wanted to enjoy doing it."

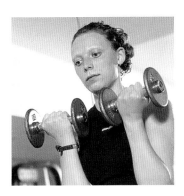

charlotte

age **23**

profession **marketing executive**

height **5ft 6in (1.7m)**

weight **159lb (72kg)**

body fat **32%**

dress size **10/12**

"My ultimate goal was to get down to a size 8, which I have never been."

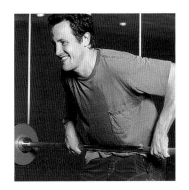

tim

age **26**

profession **journalist**

height **6ft 1in (1.85m)**

weight **178lb (81kg)**

neck **15in (37cm)**

chest **37in(94cm)**

waist **33in (84cm)**

thigh **21in (54cm)**

"My goal was to build muscle on my arms, chest, and shoulders."

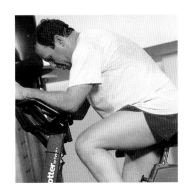

howard

age **40**

profession **cab driver**

height **5ft 8in (1.73m)**

weight **197lb (90kg)**

body fat **36%**

waist measurement **96cm (38in)**

"I felt like I'd really let myself go – I had to dump that extra weight."

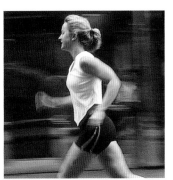

jo

age **31**

profession **magazine comissioning editor**

height **5ft 7in (1.72m)**

weight **140lb (63kg)**

body fat **29%**

dress size **10**

"My goal was to run a marathon, so in the end I could say 'I did it'."

the programs

charlotte

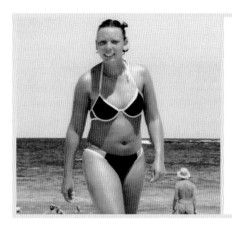

vital statistics

age **23**

profession **marketing executive**

height **5ft 6in (1.7m)**

weight **159lb (72kg)**

body fat **32%**

dress size **10/12**

charlotte's goal

I'd been struggling to lose 15 pounds for over six months. I'd tried lots of different diet and exercise plans, but often they were impractical, and I found I couldn't stick with any of them for longer than a couple of weeks. I also wanted to sculpt my body, but I was scared to work with weights as I build bulky muscle really easily.

matt's assessment

Charlotte gains weight easily, then fluctuates up and down. She wanted to lose weight, but she had just started working and was finding it difficult to balance exercise and a healthy diet with her new lifestyle. The fat loss program provided versatile diet guidelines. The high-intensity aerobic work burns fat, then work with weights helps maintain weight loss and improve muscle tone. This raises the metabolic rate, which helps the body to burn fat more efficiently and results in sustained weight loss.

▼ aerobic and resistance work
Burn fat with aerobic exercise, and tone up by working with weights.

▶ **weeks 1–2**

Just as I started telling people that the exercise wasn't too bad, Matt stepped up the pace and I have to work a lot harder. I feel great after each session except when I am really sweaty and Matt pushes me! I am starting to notice that I sleep a lot better, and my stomach, arms, and thighs are all changing shape. I'm finding the eating plan easy to follow. I feel really good, and it is great not having to weigh and count food. I have my list of foods that I can eat and off I go. I have become a lot more adventurous, and my cooking at home is a lot more tasty as a result of cooking with different, more natural foods. I have not been staying in to avoid the nightclub or having coffee with friends. They know what I am doing and admire my determination (though I did have a little lapse on the weekend). Generally, I just choose alternatives such as herbal teas and juices.

"I feel great after each session, and I sleep a lot better."

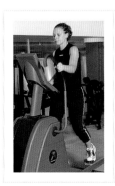
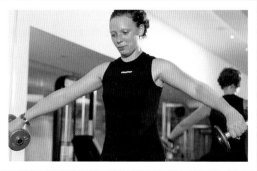
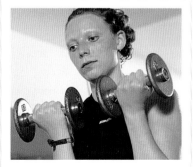
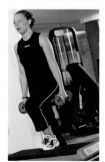

▶ the end of the program
Charlotte achieved her goal by following the fat loss program.

▶ weeks 4–6

I went on vacation for a week, but I went for a run one day and to the gym, which made up for the fact that I was drinking and finding it harder to stick to my eating plan. But I hadn't put on any weight when I got back, and I was really glad that I'd made the effort to do something active. I find that even after a few days, if I don't work out, I get restless and miss it.

▶ week 8

I've found that the occasional time I've eaten or drunk something that I'm not supposed to, such as candy, cake, or wine, I haven't enjoyed them at all. I no longer crave chocolate – the times when I have had it, I haven't been able to finish it and it makes me feel so awful that I don't repeat the performance. My tastes have changed, and I don't have a sweet tooth anymore.

▶ weeks 10–12

I did a 3 mile (5km) run this weekend. I didn't get a cramp and I wasn't even fighting for breath at the end of it. It was a real personal achievement considering that three months ago I had never run. I'm hoping to run the London marathon one day. I was worried at the start of the program that I wouldn't be able to keep up with the exercise, but now I'm quite sad that the program is over.

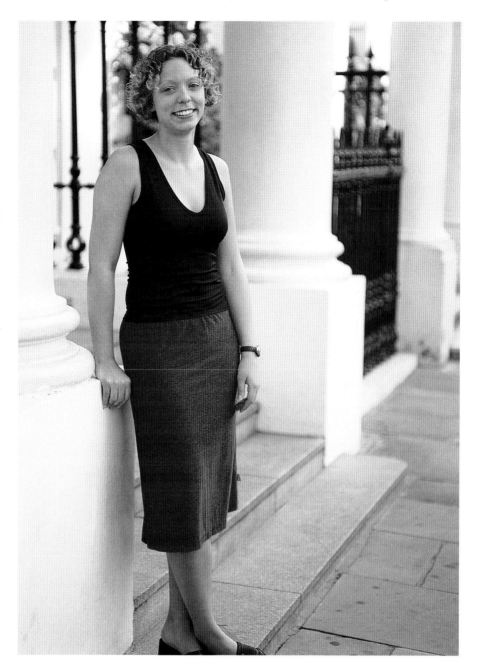

beyond the program

• Charlotte now needs to review her goals and set new ones. It would be great for her to move on to the marathon program or a toning program.

• She should maintain her healthy eating habits and eat a variety of different foods.

vital statistics

weight **145lb (66kg)**
a loss of 14lb (6kg)

dress size **8**
a drop of two dress sizes

body fat **24.5%**
a loss of 7.5%

the programs

howard

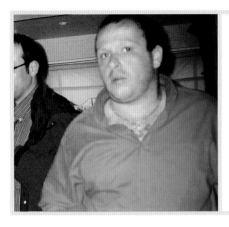

vital statistics

age **37**

profession **cab driver**

height **5ft 8in (1.73m)**

weight **197lb (90kg)**

body fat **36%**

waist measurement **38in (96cm)**

howard's goal

I was much thinner when I was 17, probably because I had a much more active lifestyle then. I've been driving a cab for 12 years, not doing any exercise and snacking a lot in the cab – as a result I've gained a lot of weight. My doctor told me recently that I had very high blood pressure and that I needed to lose weight.

matt's assessment

Because of the nature of his job, Howard had a very inactive lifestyle so he needed a program that would build his aerobic strength and encourage him to be more active. The fat-loss program would increase the rate at which his body burned fat as well as increasing his metabolic rate. A lot of aerobic work at the start of the program encourages fat loss, then resistance work improves muscle tone which helps the body to burn fat – most importantly, it helps it to maintain the weight loss.

▼ **putting howard through his paces**
Aerobic work helps to burn fat and increase the metabolic rate.

▶ weeks 1–2

The biggest shock to the system was the aerobic work. I've never sweated so much in my life. After my first session I couldn't even walk. But I was determined and I started seeing results quite quickly, which was a real motivation. Friends have started to notice changes and comment that I've lost weight, and that's really encouraging. I'm sleeping much better.

▶ weeks 3–4

I had quite good eating habits before I started the program, but now I've really cut down on fat – I've switched to 2% milk and I no longer have mayonnaise on sandwiches. I don't eat as much bread – you can get a salad in most places these days. I don't drink coffee anymore, and I eat a lot more fruit. I'm starting to feel the effects of my improved diet. I have a better idea of how my body copes with food now. Sometimes training is boring, but I know it's good for me, and I'm losing weight. I'm getting used to the gym equipment, and I know how all the machines work now. The best thing about my sessions is the shower when I've finished.

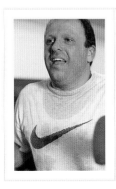 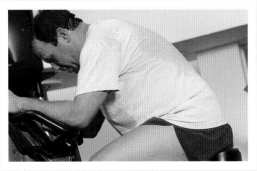 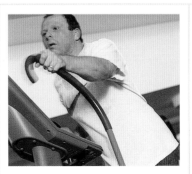 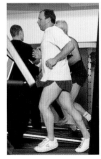

▶ **the end of the program**
Regular exercise can boost energy levels, but also leave you feeling happier and calmer.

▶ **weeks 6–8**

Midpoint, and I thought my resolve would have weakened, but seeing and feeling results is keeping me motivated. My asthma has improved – I'm using my inhaler a lot less than I used to – and my high blood pressure has dropped. Generally, I feel much more energetic, but also calmer and happier than I have in a long time. I'm physically stronger than I used to be – I went cycling with a few friends over the weekend and I was the first one up to the top of the hill. I've lost 14lb (6kg) now. A friend told me that I looked younger. My wife can't believe how much weight I've lost – she wishes she'd started the program with me.

▶ **weeks 9–12**

I used to have a weakness for hamburgers, but I've trained myself not to want them anymore. If I did have one, I know I wouldn't enjoy it. I gave in and had a little creamy dressing with my salad, but I didn't feel too bad about it – I won't make a habit of it, and I'm working it off with my training. I couldn't walk for 3 minutes when I started this program, now I can run for 15 and cycle for 20. I've started doing martial arts classes twice a week – I'm sticking with the program, but it offers a change from the gym. I can't imagine not exercising – it's a part of my life now. My pants are falling off me and I've lost my butt.

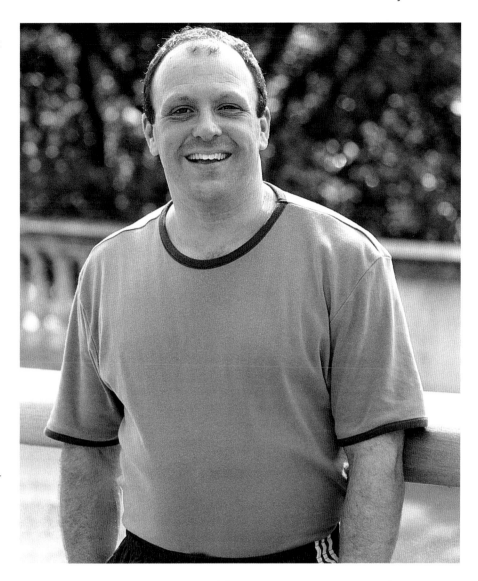

"I'm physically stronger than I used to be"

beyond the program

• Getting fit doesn't have to revolve around the gym. Howard should continue to lead an active life by walking more, or by taking the family cycling on weekends, for example.
• He should continue to challenge his body by varying the exercise he does.

vital statistics

weight **172lb (78kg)**
a loss of 25lb (12kg)

waist measurement **34in (83cm)**
a loss of 4in (13cm)

body fat **26%**
a loss of 10%

the programs

fat-loss program

This three-month program will help you to shed body fat at a safe rate. It combines a diet plan with tailored exercise routines, so it will also shape your body and ensure permanent weight loss. You can lose weight simply through dieting, but this slows your metabolism down: your body shape will fluctuate and you'll find it difficult to maintain the weight loss.

Benefits

builds strength / tones muscles ✓

burns fat / builds aerobic capacity ✓✓

increases flexibility ✓

how the program works

The aim is to burn fat while also increasing your metabolic rate; this is achieved through aerobic work. Constant pace training, where you train at a steady pace for a long period, builds endurance. Interval training, where you train for short periods at high intensity, builds stamina and also boosts the metabolic rate, so you burn fat more quickly for as long as twenty hours after your session.

High repetition resistance training will tone the large muscles of your legs, chest, and back in particular. This boosts your base metabolic rate (*see page 76*) – as your muscle is more active – which helps you to keep the weight off.

Exercise library

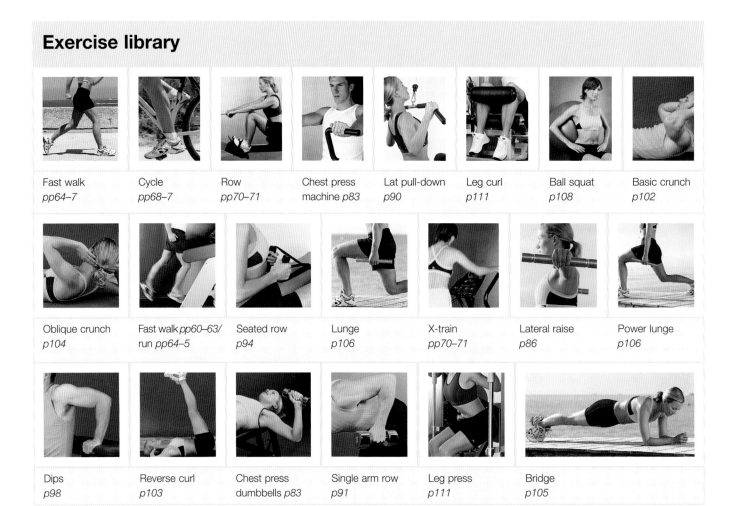

Fast walk *pp64–7*	Cycle *pp68–7*	Row *pp70–71*	Chest press machine *p83*
Lat pull-down *p90*	Leg curl *p111*	Ball squat *p108*	Basic crunch *p102*
Oblique crunch *p104*	Fast walk *pp60–63/* run *pp64–5*	Seated row *p94*	Lunge *p106*
X-train *pp70–71*	Lateral raise *p86*	Power lunge *p106*	
Dips *p98*	Reverse curl *p103*	Chest press dumbbells *p83*	Single arm row *p91*
Leg press *p111*	Bridge *p105*		

Month 1

Work out 3 times a week in month 1: do workouts 1, 2, and 3 once each week.
If you want to train 4 times a week, add another workout 3.
Always try to have at least two days off a week.

Workout 1

Warmup	5 mins aerobic exercise, gradually raising heart rate		

Exercise sequence	beginner	intermediate	advanced
Hill walk (3% incline)	10mins@ 70%MHR	10mins@ 70–75%MHR	10mins@ 70–75%MHR
Cycle	10mins@ 70%MHR	10mins@ 70–75%MHR	10mins@ 75%MHR
Row or X-train	10mins@ 70%MHR	10mins@ 70–75%MHR	10mins@ 75%MHR
Chest press	16rm	16rm	16rm
Lat pull-down	16rm	16rm	16rm
Leg curl	16rm	16rm	16rm
Ball squat	16	20	25
Basic crunch	10 (x2)	15 (x2)	20 (x2)
Oblique crunch	10 (x2)	15 (x2)	20 (x2)

Cool-down	Total body stretch sequence (see page 48)		

Workout 2

Warmup	5 mins aerobic exercise, gradually raising heart rate		

Exercise sequence	beginner	intermediate	advanced
Fast walk/run	2mins@80%MHR 3mins@65%MHR (x2)	2mins@80%MHR 2mins@70%MHR (x3)	3mins@80%MHR 2mins@70%MHR (x3)
Chest press	16rm	16rm	16rm
Leg curl	16rm	16rm	16rm
Seated row	16rm	16rm	16rm
Lunge	14rm each leg	16rm each leg	16rm each leg
Cycle	8mins@75%MHR	10mins@75%MHR	12mins@75%MHR
Repeat the 4 resistance exercises above			
X-train	10mins@70%MHR	10mins@75%MHR	10mins@75%MHR
Basic crunch	10 (x2)	15 (x2)	20 (x2)
Oblique crunch	10 (x2)	15 (x2)	20 (x2)

Cool-down	Total body stretch sequence (see page 48)		

Workout 3

	Perform any 3 aerobic exercises, or walk/run at the heart rates specified		
Warmup	5 mins aerobic exercise, gradually raising heart rate		

	beginner	intermediate	advanced
Aerobic exercise	30mins@70%MHR	40mins@75%MHR	45mins@75%MHR

Cool-down	Lower body stretch sequence (see page 49)		

Diet plan

Follow the general nutrition guidelines (*see pages 24–37*).

get started

- Drink at least 1 quart (1 liter) of water a day.
- Cut out tea, coffee, and sugary drinks.
- Eat breakfast every day: try hot cereals or wheat-free muesli; or fresh, low glycemic fruits such as apples, pears, berries, mango, kiwi with low-fat live yogurt.
- Make sure only one meal a day contains wheat (pasta, bread, couscous, and cereals).
- Reduce the amount of heavy starch (potatoes, bread, pasta) in your diet to two meals a week.
- Reduce red meat to one meal a week.
- Eat at least five portions of fresh fruit a day and three portions of vegetables.
- Eat plenty of oily fish such as salmon, tuna, mackeral, and sardines as they contain healthy oils that provide the body with energy.

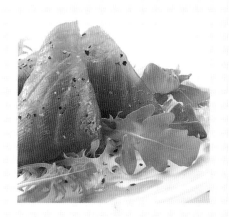

Month 2

Work out 3 times a week in month 2: do workout 1 twice a week and workout 2 once a week. If you want to train 4 times a week, add another workout 2. Always have at least 2 days off a week.

Workout 1

Warmup	5 mins aerobic exercise, gradually raising heart rate		

Exercise sequence	beginner	intermediate	advanced
Hill walk (3% incline)	10mins@ 70%MHR	10mins@ 70–75%MHR	10mins@ 75%MHR
Cycle	10mins@ 70%MHR	10mins@ 70–75%MHR	10mins@ 75%MHR
Row or X-train	10mins@ 70%MHR	10mins@ 70–75%MHR	10mins@ 75%MHR
Chest press	16rm	16rm	16rm
Lat pull-down	16rm	16rm	16rm
Leg curl	16rm	16rm	16rm
Ball squat	16	20	25
Lateral raise	15rm	15rm	15rm `
Power lunge	15 each leg	15 each leg	20 each leg
Dips	15	20	20
Leg press	16rm	16rm	16rm
Repeat the 8 resistance exercises above			
Basic crunch	10 (x2)	15 (x2)	20 (x2)
Oblique crunch	10 (x2)	15 (x2)	20 (x2)
Reverse curl	10	15	20

Cool-down	Total body stretch sequence (*see page 48*)		

Workout 2

Warmup	5 mins aerobic exercise, gradually raising heart rate		

Exercise sequence	beginner	intermediate	advanced
Fast walk/run	2mins@80%MHR 3mins@65%MHR (x2)	2mins@80%MHR 2mins@70%MHR (x3)	3mins@80%MHR 2mins@70%MHR (x3)
Chest press	16rm	16rm	16rm
Leg curl	16rm	16rm	16rm
Seated row	16rm	16rm	16rm
Lunge	14rm each leg	16rm each leg	16rm each leg
Cycle	8mins@75%MHR	10mins@75%MHR	12mins@75%MHR
Repeat the 4 resistance exercises above			
X-train	10mins@70%MHR	12mins@75%MHR	15mins@75%MHR
Basic crunch	10 (x2)	15 (x2)	20 (x2)
Oblique crunch	10 (x2)	15 (x2)	20 (x2)

Cool-down	Total body stretch sequence (*see page 48*)		

Diet plan

Maintain all of the good habits from month 1.

keep up the good work

- Aim to eat your heavier starch meals at lunchtime and light vegetable and protein meals in the evening.
- Try to introduce more beans and pulses into your diet.
- Watch your alcohol intake: men should drink under 12 units a week, women under 8 units a week. (*A unit is a glass of wine, a single measure of spirits, or half a pint of beer*.)
- Don't reduce the amount you eat too drastically; try to fill up with vegetables.
- Snack on handfuls of almonds and Brazil nuts, and pumpkin, sesame, and sunflower seeds.

cross-training

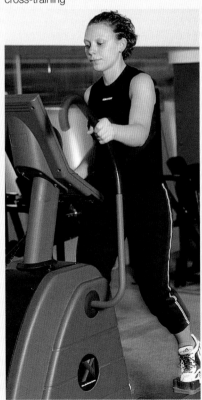

Month 3

Work out 3 times a week in month 3: do workout 1 twice a week and workout 2 once a week. If you want to train 4 times a week, add another workout 2. Always have at least 2 days off a week.

Workout 1

Warmup	5 mins aerobic exercise, gradually raising heart rate

Exercise sequence	beginner	intermediate	advanced
Hill walk (3% incline)	10mins@ 70%MHR	10mins@ 70–75%MHR	10mins@ 75%MHR
Cycle	10mins@ 70%MHR	10mins@ 70–75%MHR	10mins@ 75%MHR
Row or X-train	10mins@ 70%MHR	10mins@ 70–75%MHR	10mins@ 75%MHR
Chest press	16rm	16rm	16rm
Lat pull-down	16rm	16rm	16rm
Leg curl	16rm	16rm	16rm
Ball squat	16	20	25
Dumbbell bench press	16rm	16rm	16rm
Lateral raise	15rm	15rm	15rm
Single arm row	15rm	15rm	15rm
Power lunge	15 each leg	15 each leg	20 each leg
Dips	15	20	20
Leg press	16rm	16rm	16rm
Repeat the 10 resistance exercises above, twice			
Basic crunch	10 (x2)	15 (x2)	20 (x2)
Oblique crunch	10 (x2)	15 (x2)	20 (x2
Reverse curl	10 (x2)	15 (x2	20 (x2)
Bridge	30 secs	45 secs	60 secs

Cool-down	Total body stretch sequence (*see page 48*)

Workout 2

Warmup	5 mins aerobic exercise, gradually raising heart rate

	beginner	intermediate	advanced
Fast walk/run	2mins@80%MHR 3mins@65%MHR (x3)	2mins@80%MHR 2mins@70%MHR (x4)	3mins@80%MHR 2mins@70%MHR (x4)
Chest press	16rm	16rm	16rm
Leg curl	16rm	16rm	16rm
Seated row	16rm	16rm	16rm
Lunge	14rm	16rm	16rm
Cycle	8mins@75%MHR	10mins@75%MHR	12mins@75%MHR
Repeat the 4 resistance exercises above			
X-train	10mins@70%MHR	12mins@75%MHR	15mins@75%MHR
Basic crunch	10 (x2)	15 (x2)	20 (x2)
Oblique crunch	10 (x2)	15 (x2)	20 (x2)

Cool-down	Total body stretch sequence (*see page 48*)

Diet plan

You may be monitoring your diet, but this doesn't mean that you can't eat out.

- Ask for meat and fish in particular to be grilled, steamed, or roasted rather than fried or cooked in a rich sauce.
- Avoid rich, creamy and buttery sauces – they are high in calories and saturated fat.
- Choose boiled new potatoes over fried, gratin, mashed, even baked potatoes, as they have a lower glycemic index rating (*see page 33*).
- Order an appetizer and main course rather than a main course and dessert.

running

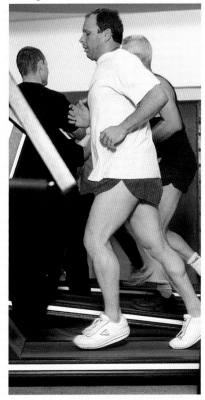

lunchtime workout

If finding the time to get to the gym is your greatest problem, this is the program for you because it aims to achieve maximum results in a minimum length of time. It is a general workout that will build a good base level of aerobic fitness, condition the muscles, and improve and help maintain flexibility in the important structural muscles of the body.

Benefits

builds strength / tones muscles ✓✓

burns fat / builds aerobic capacity ✓

increases flexibility ✓

how the program works

The program consists of two workouts to be alternated over three days a week. Do workout 1 twice a week on day one and day three, and workout 2 on day two. Workout 1 is a high intensity aerobic workout where you work your heart at two levels, or percentages, of your Maximum Heart Rate (MHR). This burns fat and boosts the metabolism for up to 18 hours afterward. The resistance training targets the lower body and then the upper body alternately. This works the heart harder as it has to pump blood to the muscles at both ends of the body and is known as peripheral heart action training. It tones the major muscles of the body while also increasing the body's metabolic rate. The result is a leaner, more athletic-looking body.

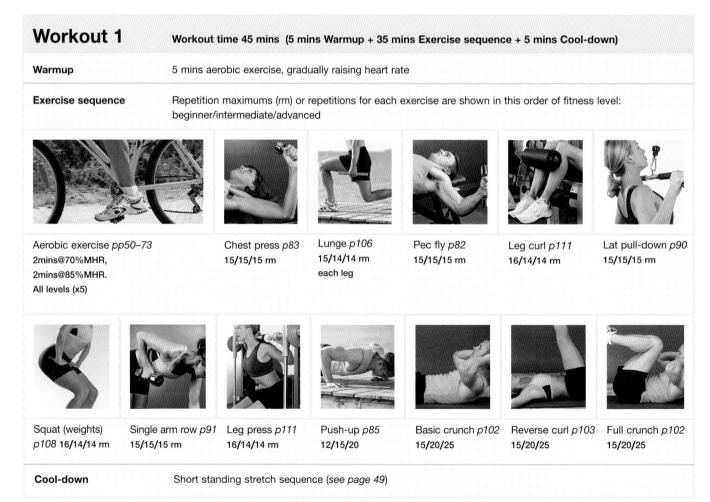

Workout 1	**Workout time 45 mins (5 mins Warmup + 35 mins Exercise sequence + 5 mins Cool-down)**
Warmup	5 mins aerobic exercise, gradually raising heart rate
Exercise sequence	Repetition maximums (rm) or repetitions for each exercise are shown in this order of fitness level: beginner/intermediate/advanced

Aerobic exercise *pp50–73*
2mins@70%MHR,
2mins@85%MHR.
All levels (x5)

Chest press *p83*
15/15/15 rm

Lunge *p106*
15/14/14 rm
each leg

Pec fly *p82*
15/15/15 rm

Leg curl *p111*
16/14/14 rm

Lat pull-down *p90*
15/15/15 rm

Squat (weights)
p108 16/14/14 rm

Single arm row *p91*
15/15/15 rm

Leg press *p111*
16/14/14 rm

Push-up *p85*
12/15/20

Basic crunch *p102*
15/20/25

Reverse curl *p103*
15/20/25

Full crunch *p102*
15/20/25

Cool-down	Short standing stretch sequence (*see page 49*)

try fish for lunch after a workout

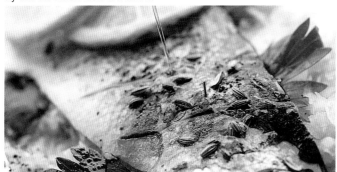

Workout 2 builds aerobic endurance – you work at a constant heart rate during the workout which helps to strengthen the heart and lungs. Choose three different aerobic exercises for this stage of the workout. The resistance work targets the arm and shoulder muscles (biceps, triceps, and deltoids) and will tone flabby upper arms. The crunches and curls will help to tone the abdominals.

Nutrition tips

Don't underestimate the nutrients that your body needs at lunchtime, especially if you are working out. Your postworkout lunch should help your body to replace energy lost while exercising as well as providing enough energy to sustain you through the afternoon.

Preworkout snacks

Half an hour to 45 minutes prior to your workout, snack on easily digestible fruit that is not too high in sugar. Try an apple or a pear.

Postworkout lunches

Eat an energy-rich meal of foods that are high in antioxidants and essential fatty acids. The following suggestions provide the body with slow-release energy and will help prevent mid-afternoon energy dips that can tempt you to snack on sweet things:

- wholemeal pasta salad
- couscous salad
- sushi
- grilled vegetables
- salmon and cottage cheese sandwich on wholemeal bread
- bean and pepper salad
- fresh, raw vegetables with dips such as hummus or tzaziki (but not mayonnaise)
- baked fish such as sea bass
- oily fish such as mackerel, sardines, or herring in a salad or on wholemeal toast.

Workout 2   Workout time 45 mins (5 mins Warmup + 35 mins Exercise sequence + 5 mins Cool-down)

Warmup   5 mins aerobic exercise, gradually raising heart rate

Exercise sequence   Repetition maximums (rm) or repetitions for each exercise are shown in this order of fitness level: beginner/intermediate/advanced

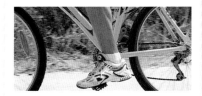

Aerobic exercise *pp50–73*
2mins@75%MHR,
2mins@80%MHR.
All levels (x6)

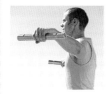

Lateral raise *p86*
16/14/14 rm

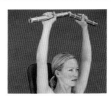

Shoulder press *p88*
15/15/15 rm

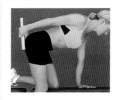

Tricep extension *p101*
15/15/15 rm

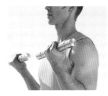

Bicep curl *p96*
15/14/14 rm

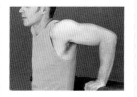

Dips *p98*
10/15/20

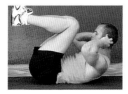

Full crunch *p102*
15/20/25

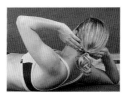

Oblique crunch *p104*
15/20/25

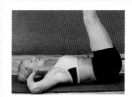

Reverse curl *p103*
15/20/25

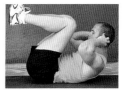

Full crunch *p102*
15/20/25

Cool-down   Short standing stretch sequence (*see page 49*)

the programs

six-week beach body

We all do it; we schedule a vacation months in advance, but only leave getting in shape for it to the last minute. It is not until you try on your swimsuit or beach shorts and experience true horror that the task at hand becomes apparent. This program has all the essential elements for toning and weight loss and will help you to look your best in the shortest time possible.

Benefits

builds strength / tones muscles ✓✓

burns fat / builds aerobic capacity ✓✓

increases flexibility ✓

Exercise library

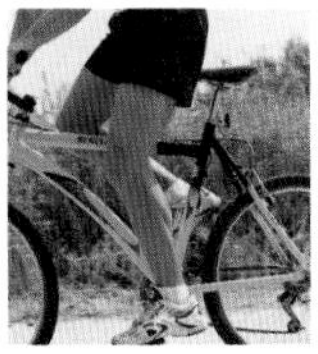

Aerobic exercise pp50–73	Chest press p83	Lunge p106	Lat pull-down p90	Leg curl p111	Push-up p85	Ball squat p108

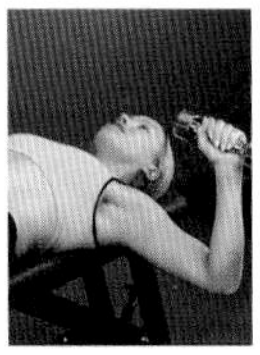

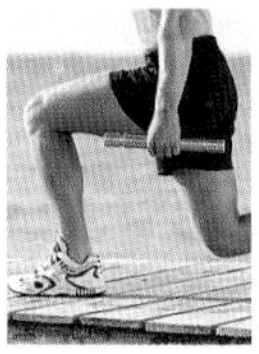

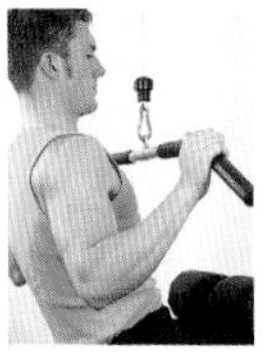

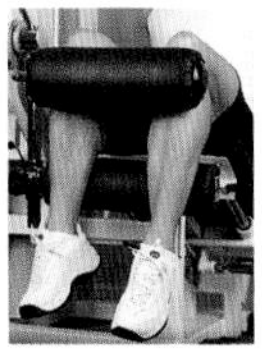

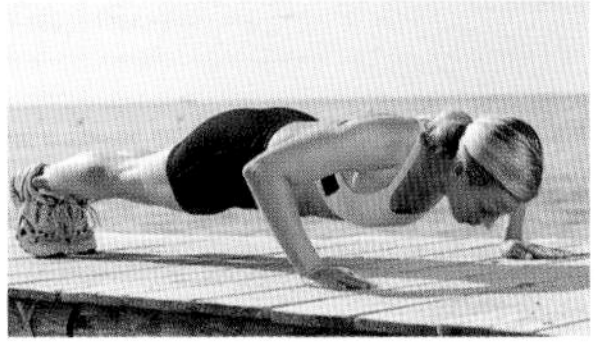

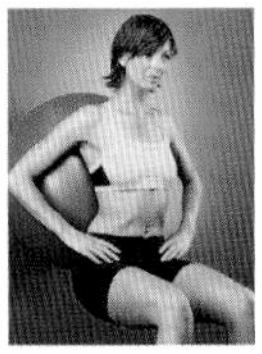

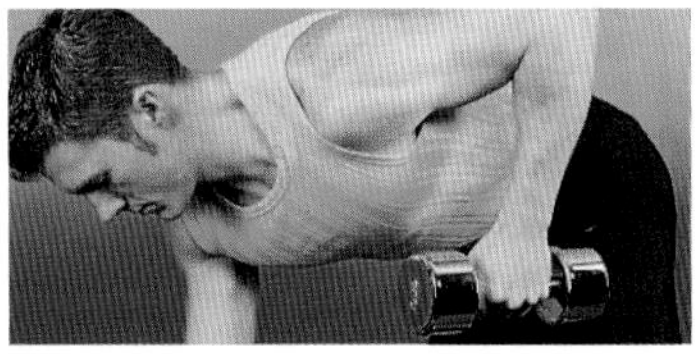

Single arm row p91	Power lunge p106	Dips p98	Reverse fly p90	Glute raise p113	Basic crunch p102

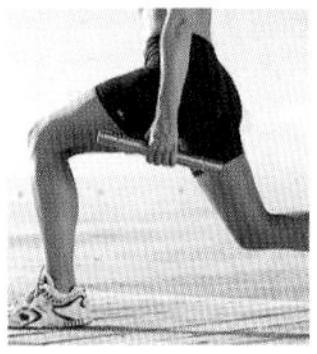

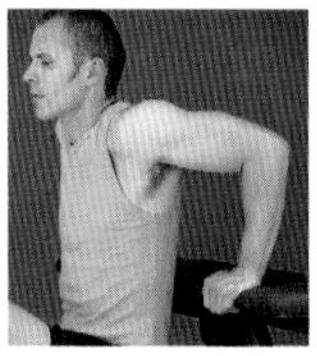

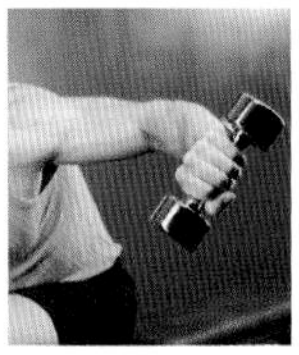

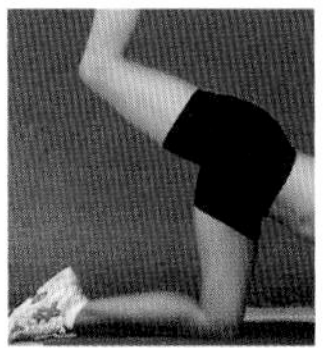

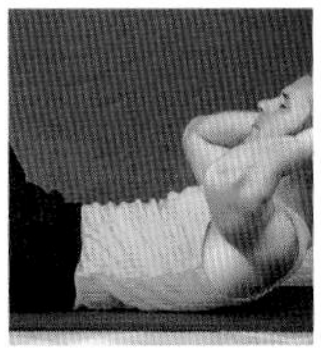

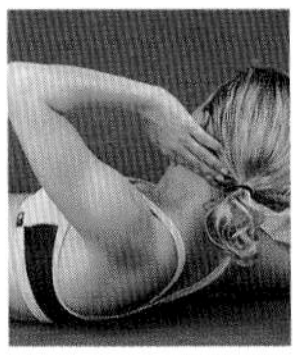

Oblique crunch p104	Bridge p105	Oblique bridge p105	Pec fly p82	Shoulder press p88

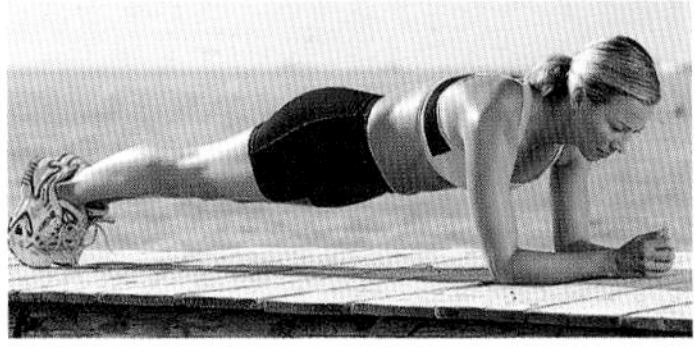

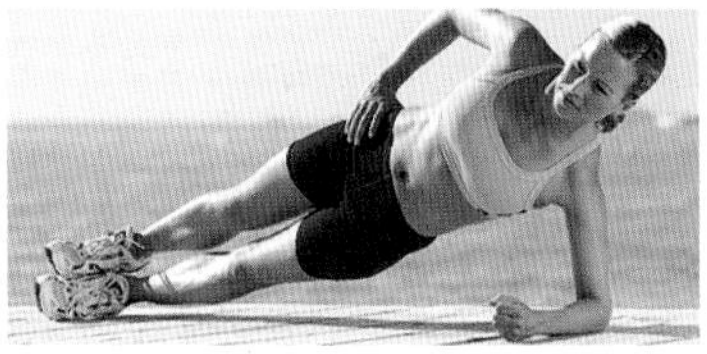

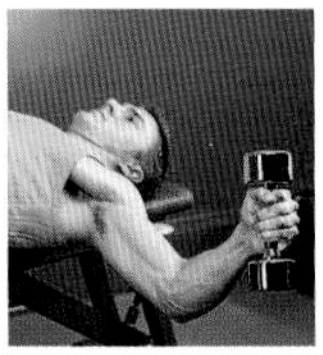

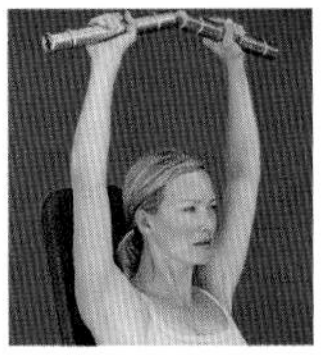

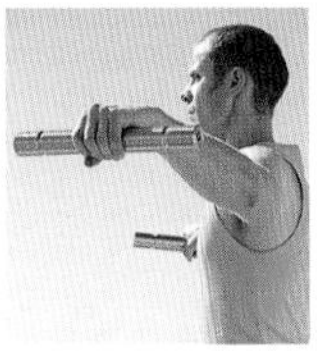

Lateral raise p86	Leg curl p111	Step ups p109	Bicep curl p96	Tricep extension p101	Upright row p89

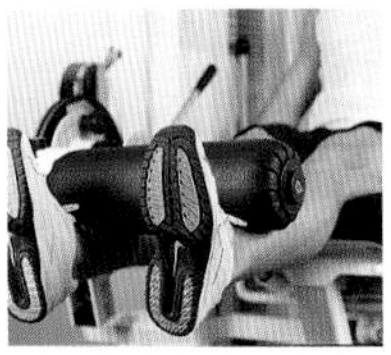

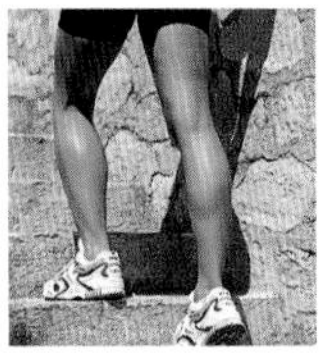

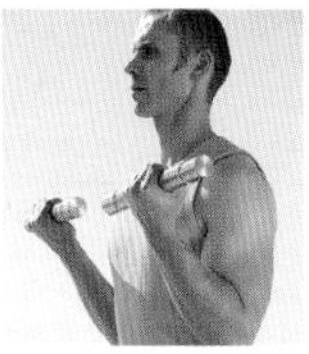

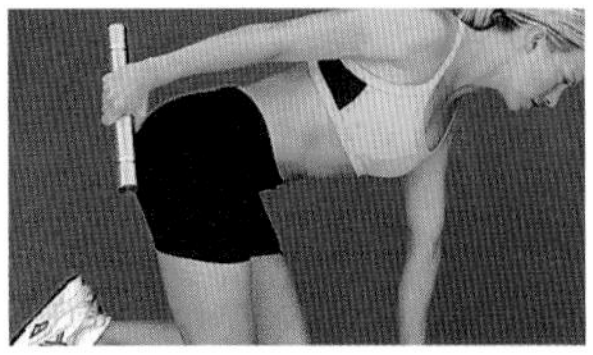

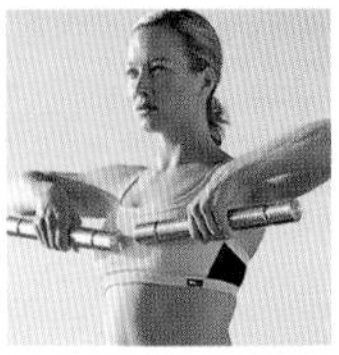

how the program works

The aim is to look thin and lean in your swimsuit or shorts, so the focus in this program is to lose excess body fat. However, six weeks is not long if the task ahead is great. This program includes a lot of high intensity aerobic work, including interval training where you alternate between working at a higher heart rate, then recover working at a lower heart rate. This is one of the most effective methods for burning fat. It also has the advantage of raising your metabolic rate, so that you continue to burn energy quickly and efficiently, even after your workout. Once you have started to lose fat, resistance work targets and tones specific muscles.

General weight loss might be a common goal for both sexes, but men and women have different aims when it comes to shaping and sculpting specific areas of the body.

women's goals

Women need a great waistline. This program helps to shed excess fat from the stomach and create flat, toned abdominals. It will also help to tone the bust area and create a cleavage. Exercises such as the lateral raise and the chest press shape the shoulders, which helps to improve posture and define the female shape. One of the overall effects will also be a reduction in cellulite, if you have any.

men's goals

The main aim in the men's workouts is to get rid of the stomach and define the upper back and shoulders. It will help to tone the shoulders and arms and create strong legs with good muscle definition. Your legs should look powerful – they shouldn't hang out of your shorts like two sticks.

using the program

The programs are broken down into three, two-week long phases. This is a healthy rate at which to lose excess weight and should mean that you can sustain the weight loss. Because goals differ for men and women, in each two-week phase, there are two workouts: the first is for both men and women, then there are two sex specific workouts, one designed to meet the specific needs of women, the other of men.

▶ frolic in the surf
With a lean, toned physique and good muscle definition, you'll want to show off your body on the beach. The programme helps to shape and sculpt the body.

Diet plan

Follow the general nutrition guidelines (*see pages 24–37*).

- Include as many low glycemic, alkaline foods as possible – at least 70 percent of your diet should be made up of these.
- Reduce your intake of tea and coffee to one cup a day.
- Keep your alcohol intake down to 10 units a week for men, and 6 units a week for women. (*A unit is a glass of wine, a single measure of spirits, or half a pint of beer.*)
- Drink 2 quarts (2 liters) of water a day for the entire 6-week period.
- Chew food thoroughly – this makes it easier to digest.
- Graze. Eat 3 small meals, and snack in between to keep hunger at bay and energy levels up. Try fresh or (more occasionally) dried fruit, or a handful of nuts.
- Cut out sugary drinks and foods such as chocolate and snack bars, pastries, candy, and cookies.
- Eat 5 different pieces of fruit a day (not more than one banana).
- Eat brightly colored vegetables like peppers, carrots, and broccoli which are high in antioxidants.
- Try this wheat-free muesli. Mix rolled oats and plain puffed rice in a 2:1 ratio. Add almonds, raisins, and sunflower, pumpkin, and sesame seeds to taste.

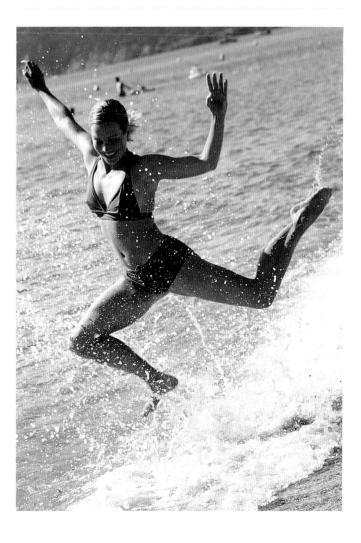

the programs

Weeks 1, 2 & 3 Aim to work out 3 times a week. Do workout 1 twice a week and workout 2 once.

Workout 1 for men and women
Workout time 45 mins (5 mins Warmup + 30 mins Exercise sequence + 10 mins Cool-down)

Warmup	5 mins aerobic exercise, gradually raising heart rate

Exercise sequence	beginner	intermediate	advanced
Aerobic exercise	3mins@80%MHR	3mins 80%MHR	3mins@85%MHR
Chest press	16rm	14rm	14rm
Lunge	16rm	16rm	14rm
Lat pull-down	16rm	14rm	14rm
Leg curl	16rm	16rm	16rm
Aerobic exercise	3mins@80%MHR	4mins@85%MHR	5mins@85%MHR
Push-up	16rm	16rm	20rm
Ball squat	16rm	16rm	16rm
Single arm row	16rm	16rm	16rm
Power lunge	16rm each leg	16rm each leg	16rm each leg
Aerobic exercise	3mins@80%MHR	5mins@85%MHR	6mins@85%MHR
Dips	16	20	25
Leg curl	16rm	16rm	16rm
Reverse fly	14rm	14rm	14rm
Glute raise	16rm each leg	16rm each leg	16rm each leg
Aerobic exercise	3mins@80%MHR	5mins@85%MHR	6mins@85%MHR
Basic crunch	15	20	20
Reverse curl	15	20	20
Oblique crunch	15	20	20

Cool-down	Total body stretch sequence (see page 48)

Workout 2 for men
Workout time 50 mins (5 mins Warmup + 35 mins Exercise sequence + 10 mins Cool-down)

Warmup	5 mins aerobic exercise, gradually raising heart rate

Exercise sequence	beginner	intermediate	advanced
Aerobic exercise	1min@80%MHR 3mins@70%MHR (x5)	2mins@80%MHR 2mins@70%MHR (x6)	2mins@85%MHR 2mins@75%MHR (x6)
Chest press	14rm	12rm	12rm
Chest fly	–	14rm	12rm
Lat pull-down	14rm	14rm	12rm
Single arm row	–	14rm	12rm
Shoulder press	14rm	14rm	12rm
Lateral raise	14rm	12rm	12rm
Leg Curl	16rm	14rm	12rm
Lunge	–	14rm each leg	12rm each leg
Leg extension	16rm	14rm	12rm
Step ups	–	15 each leg	20 each leg
Bicep curl dumbbell	16rm	14rm	12rm
Dips	15	20	25
Repeat the 12 resistance exercises above			
Basic crunch	20	25	30
Reverse curl	5	20	20
Repeat the 2 exercises above			

Cool-down	Total body stretch sequence (see page 48)

Workout 2 for women Workout time 50 mins (5 mins Warmup + 35 mins Exercise sequence + 10 mins Cool-down)

Warmup 5 mins aerobic exercise, gradually raising heart rate

Exercise sequence	beginner	intermediate	advanced	Exercise sequence	beginner	intermediate	advanced
Aerobic exercise	1min@80%MHR, 3mins@70%. (x5)	2mins@80%MHR, 2mins@70%. (x6)	2mins@85%MHR, 2mins@75%. (x6)	Aerobic exercise	3mins@70%MHR, 4mins@80%, 3mins@70%.	3mins@70%MHR, 4mins@80%, 3mins@70%.	4mins@75%MHR, 3mins@80%, 3mins@75%.
Chest press	16rm	16rm	16rm	Reverse curl	15	20	20
Leg curl	16rm	16rm	16rm	Basic crunch	15	20	20
Single arm row	16rm	16rm	16rm	Bridge	20 secs	30 secs	50 secs
Power lunge	16rm each leg	16rm each leg	16rm each leg	Oblique bridge		20 secs	40 secs
Lateral raise	16rm	16rm	16rm	**Repeat the 4 resistance exercises above**			
Ball squat	16rm	16rm	16rm				
Tricep extension	14rm	14rm	14rm	Cool-down	Total body stretch sequence (see page 48)		
Repeat the 7 resistance exercises above							

Weeks 4, 5 & 6 Aim to work out 3 times a week. Do workout 1 twice a week and workout 2 once.

Workout 1 for men and women

Workout time 55 mins (5 mins Warmup + 40 mins Exercise sequence + 10 mins Cool-down)

Warmup	5 mins aerobic exercise, gradually raising heart rate

Exercise sequence	beginner	intermediate	advanced
Aerobic exercise	4mins@ 80%MHR	5mins@ 80%MHR	6mins@ 85%MHR
Chest press	16rm (x2)	14rm (x2)	14rm (x2)
Lunge	16rm each leg	16rm each leg	14rm each leg
Lat pull-down	16rm (x2)	14rm (x2)	14rm (x2)
Leg curl	16rm	16rm	16rm
Aerobic exercise	4mins@ 80%MHR	5mins@ 85%MHR	6mins@ 85%MHR
Push-up	16rm	16rm (x2)	20rm (x2)
Ball squat	16rm	16rm	16rm
Single arm row	16rm	16rm	14rm
Power lunge	16rm	16rm	14rm
Aerobic exercise	4mins@ 80%MHR	6mins@ 85%MHR	7mins@ 85%MHR
Dips	16	20 rest, then 15	25 rest, then 20
Leg curl	16rm	16rm	16rm
Reverse fly	14rm	14rm	14rm
Glute raise	16rm each leg	16rm each leg	16rm each leg
Aerobic exercise	3mins@ 80%MHR	5mins@ 85%MHR	6mins@ 85%MHR
Basic crunch	15	20	20
Reverse curl	15	20	20
Oblique crunch	15	20	20
Bridge	20 secs	30 secs	50 secs
Oblique bridge		20 secs	40 secs

Cool-down	Total body stretch sequence (see page 48)

Workout 2 for men

Workout time 70 mins (5 mins Warmup + 55 mins Exercise sequence + 10 mins Cool-down)

Warmup	5 mins aerobic exercise, gradually raising heart rate

Exercise sequence	beginner	intermediate	advanced
Aerobic exercise	1min@80%MHR 3mins@70% (x5)	2mins@80%MHR 2mins@70% (x6)	2mins@85%MHR 2mins@75% (x6)
Push-up	14rm	12rm	12rm
Chest fly	14rm	14rm	12rm
Chest press	–	14rm	12rm
Lat pull-down	14rm	14rm	12rm
Single arm row	–	14rm	12rm
Reverse fly	16rm	14rm	14rm
Shoulder press	14rm	14rm	12rm
Lateral raise	14rm	12rm	12rm
Upright row	–	14rm	12rm
Leg curl	16rm	14rm	12rm
Lunge	–	14rm each leg	12rm each leg
Leg extension	16rm	14rm	12rm
Step ups	–	15 each leg	20 each leg
Bicep curl dumbbell	16rm	14rm	12rm
Dips	15	20	25
Aerobic exercise	10mins@ 75%MHR	10mins@ 80%MHR	10mins@ 85%MHR
Repeat the 15 resistance exercises above			
Basic crunch	20	25	30
Reverse Curl	15	20	20
Repeat the 2 resistance exercises above			

Cool-down	Total body stretch sequence (see page 48)

Workout 2 for women   Workout time 70 mins (5 mins Warmup + 55 mins Exercise sequence + 10 mins Cool-down)

Warmup 5 mins aerobic exercise, gradually raising heart rate

Exercise sequence	beginner	intermediate	advanced
Aerobic exercise	1mins@80%MHR 3mins@70% (x5)	2mins@80%MHR 2mins@70% (x6)	2mins@85%MHR 2mins@75% (x6)
Push-up	–	16rm	14rm
Chest press	16rm	16rm	14rm
Leg curl	16rm	16rm	16rm
Single arm row	16rm	16rm	14rm
Power lunge	16rm each leg	16rm each leg	16rm each leg
Lat pull-down	16rm	16rm	14rm
Lateral raise	16rm	16rm	16rm
Ball squat	16rm	16rm	16rm
Tricep extension	14rm	14rm	14rm

Exercise sequence	beginner	intermediate	advanced
Dips	15	20	20
Repeat last 10 resistance exercises			
Aerobic exercise	3mins@70%MHR 4mins@80% 3mins@70%	3mins@70%MHR 4mins@80% 4mins@70%	4mins@75%MHR 3mins@80% 5mins@75%
Reverse curl	20	25	25
Basic crunch	20	20	25
Bridge	30 secs	40 secs	60 secs
Reverse curl	15	15	15
Oblique bridge		20 secs	40 secs
Repeat the 5 resistance exercises above			

Cool-down	Total body stretch sequence (see page 48)

three-week detox

If your're feeling under the weather, have endured a long period of stress, continuously suffer from colds or constantly feel sapped of energy, this program can help. Detoxing can help to ease the pressures on your body. It can boost energy levels and help reduce and prevent water retention. It might also help you to fit into that suit or dress that's just a little too tight.

Benefits

builds strength / tones muscles ✓
burns fat / builds aerobic capacity ✓✓✓
increases flexibility ✓

toxins

Our bodies are constantly exposed to toxins – in the environment, in the food that we eat, and in the air that we breathe. They can also build up in the body as a result of stress and hectic modern living. The body has some mechanisms for ridding itself of toxins, but when toxin levels are very high, they can begin to penetrate the cells and prevent the body from functioning efficiently. High toxicity levels can lead to problems such as weight gain, lethargy, pimples, headaches, bad breath, and reduced immune function.

how the program works

The program has three phases, each a week long. It takes at least three weeks to rid the body of toxins. A detox program any shorter than this will not be effective.

In the first week of the program the aim is to begin to clear toxins in the body and help it to become more alkaline by reducing acid levels. In the next week you begin trying to release the toxins from within the body's cells and vital organs into the circulatory and lymphatic systems and eventually out of the body. In the final phase you help the body to reenergize itself and to generate and use energy more efficiently. Before beginning the program, eliminate the following from your diet: coffee, tea, alcohol, sugary drinks, processed foods, convenience foods, and chocolate.

long-term detoxing

This program helps the body to detox in a very short period of time. Ideally you should cleanse the body constantly and minimize your intake of toxins, but this is not always possible. Diet in particular can raise acidity and therefore toxin levels in the body. As much as possible, try to follow my general diet guidelines (*see pages 24–37*); these should help you to keep toxin levels low and energy levels high. Be careful not to let too many of the foods and drinks that you have excluded as part of the detox slip back into your diet. If at any time you feel that you need to spring clean your system and boost energy levels, use the three-week detox as a quick blitz.

a word of caution

It's not uncommon to experience some unpleasant side effects such as headaches, sickness, or lethargy as your body begins to rid itself of toxins. Drink lots of water to help flush out toxins. Symptoms should last no longer than a week.

Exercise library

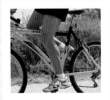

Aerobic exercise
pp50–73

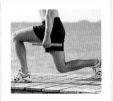

Lunge
p106

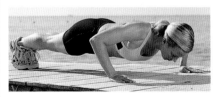

Push-up
p85

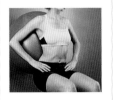

Ball squat
p108

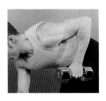

Single arm row
p91

Weeks 1 & 2

In weeks 1 and 2, aim to work out 3 to 4 times a week. Do workout 1 twice and workout 2 once. If you want to train 4 times a week, do each workout twice. Aerobic exercise helps circulation and aids the release of toxins. Choose any aerobic exercise (*see pages 50–73*), but try to alternate between different activities so the body uses different muscles for each workout.

Workout 1 time 40 mins (5 mins Warmup + 30 mins Exercise sequence + 5 mins Cool-down)
Workout 2 time 35 mins (5 mins Warmup + 25 mins Exercise sequence + 5 mins Cool-down)

Warmup	5 mins aerobic exercise, gradually raising heart rate	
Exercise sequence	**beginner**	**intermediate / advanced**
Workout 1		
Any aerobic exercise	30mins@70%MHR	30mins@75%MHR
Workout 2		
Any aerobic exercise	3mins@65%MHR, 2mins@75%MHR. (x5)	2mins@65%MHR, 3mins@80%MHR. (x5)
Cool-down	Short standing stretch sequence (*see page 49*)	

Diet plan

After waking Warm water with fresh lemon juice.
Breakfast Soaked prunes with raw apples, pears, banana, or berries and a tablespoon of low fat live yogurt (add honey if needed).
Mid-morning Fresh fruit such as apple, melon, or banana, and carrot or vegetable juice.
Lunch Brown or wild rice salad, bean salad, raw vegetables such as carrots, cucumbers, and celery with a non-mayonnaise-based dip such as hummus.
Afternoon Low glycemic fruit (*see pages 34–5*); peppermint or ginger tea.
Evening Grilled or steamed oily fish such as salmon, tuna, mackerel, or sardines with steamed vegetables. **Drink** 2.5 quarts (2.5 liters) of water a day.

Week 3

In week 3 you keep up the aerobic work, but add metabolizing resistance exercises that work all the major muscles in the body and raise the metabolic rate. Work out 3 times a week; do workout 1 twice and workout 2 once. If you want to train 4 times a week, add another workout 2.

Workout 1 time 50 mins (5 mins Warmup + 35 mins Exercise sequence + 10 mins Cool-down)
Workout 2 time 45 mins (5 mins Warmup + 30 mins Exercise sequence + 10 mins Cool-down)

Warmup	5 mins aerobic exercise, gradually raising heart rate	
Exercise sequence	**beginner**	**intermediate / advanced**
Workout 1		
Any aerobic exercise	30mins@70%MHR	30mins@75%MHR
Lunge	15 (x2) each leg	20 (x2) each leg
Push-up	15 (x2)	20 (x2)
Ball squat	15 (x2)	20 (x2)
Single arm row	15rm (x2)	15rm (x2)
Workout 2		
Any aerobic exercise	3mins@65%MHR, 2mins@75%MHR. (x6)	2mins@65%MHR, 3mins@80%MHR. (x6)
Cool-down	Total body stretch sequence (*see page 48*)	

Diet plan

After waking Warm water with fresh lemon juice.
Breakfast Hot cereal made with water or skimmed milk; nonwheat muesli (*see page 129*); fresh fruit with low-fat live yogurt, sunflower seeds and sesame seeds (add honey if needed).
Mid-morning Fresh carrot juice, tomato juice, or a fresh fruit smoothie.
Lunch Bean salad; salad niçoise; sushi; rice salad.
Afternoon Handful of almonds and Brazil nuts; peppermint or ginger tea.
Evening Ratatouille and fish; wild rice and grilled chicken; fish and steamed or grilled vegetables; green salad with runner beans, chick peas, butter beans, or kidney beans, or a mixture and olive oil and balsamic vinegar dressing.
Water 2 quarts (2 liters) a day.

the programs

sasha

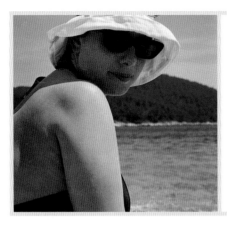

vital statistics

age **31**

profession **company director**

height **5ft 4in (1.6m)**

weight **152lb (69kg)**

body fat **30%**

dress size **12**

sasha's goal

I wanted to tone up all over and to build upper and lower body definition. I did work out regularly, but I concentrated mostly on aerobic training. I'd never really worked with weights, but I was desperate to tone up my flab, especially on my legs and at the tops of my arms. I wanted to get rid of my "grandma's handbags"!

matt's assessment

Sasha had worked out regularly for years, and as a result she had an impressive level of aerobic fitness. She was a very competent runner and able to cope with both stamina and endurance training. The biggest gap in her training was muscle conditioning. The women's upper body tone-up and perfect legs programs have aerobic elements so they assist fat burning; but they also tone, shape, and build muscle strength, without building mass.

▼ tone up with resistance training
The right weight-training program will tone muscles rather than building bulk.

▶ week 1

I had to endure a grueling fitness assessment to begin with. Amazingly, I'm in better shape than I thought I would be – all that time in the gym has paid off. My overall flexibility is extremely good for someone of my age, especially for someone who never stretches before or after any kind of exercise. I have to make some radical changes to my diet – I'm a bit worried about keeping to them since a crucial part of my job entails entertaining clients, which often means eating out and drinking. I thought that giving up caffeine would be extremely difficult as I was a complete caffeine addict, but the headaches stopped after the first three days, and I have actually started to enjoy herbal teas and water.

▶ week 2

By the end of week 2 I've done six training sessions and I'm learning that variety is the key – which is good because I have an extrememly low boredom threshold and I need variety to keep me interested and committed. By doing different exercises – a combination of resistance and aerobic – for different lengths of time and at different intensities, I'm starting to challenge my

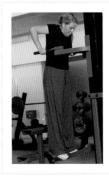

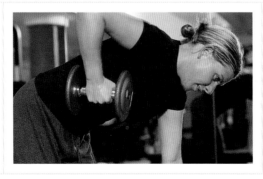

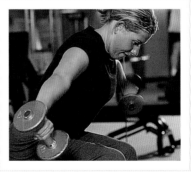

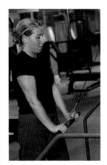

body. I realize that up until now I've had a "Groundhog Day" approach to my workouts; they always started with a long, stable treadmill run of about 30 minutes – always at the same speed – followed by either a short burst on the step machine or the bike, then the same number of abdominal crunches. Now, I've suddenly started seeing results. Short bursts of high intensity running combined with step-ups, squats, leg curls, and lunges have started to define the muscles in my legs. I'm pleasantly surprised and proud to be developing firm, toned thighs.

▶ week 3

My upper body routine is paying off, too – my grandma's handbags have finally started to firm up! I always feel uplifted, positive, and energized after a session. I'm always proud to have successfully completed an exercise that I normally

▶ **toned in all the right places**
Introducing resistance exercises and some variety into Sasha's workout routines made all the difference.

would have given up on or avoided altogether. Even the rowing machine has become an attractive challenge. My general fitness has really improved and my lungs feel noticeably stronger – so do my limbs and bones. I don't experience the same day-to-day aches and pains that I used to – I used to get pains in my arms after a frantic bout of typing, but I don't get them at all now. I've had the occasional lapse on the diet front – sometimes I found it was just too difficult to stick to a totally alkaline diet, especially when entertaining. On the whole I've been good, and I feel that my success with the workouts compensates for any diet slips. When I was faithful to the diet, I did notice that I felt energized, positive, and much less hungry (always a good thing!).

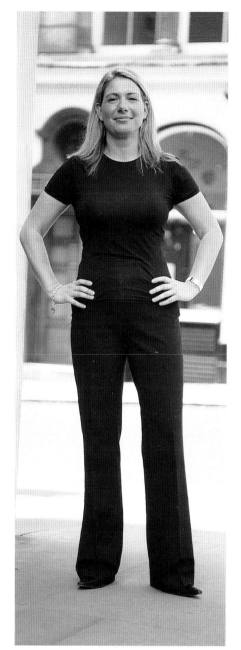

> "I'm pleasantly surprised and proud to be developing firm, toned thighs."

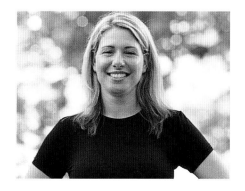

beyond the program

• Sasha has shown that lifting weights doesn't have to build muscle – it actually makes it easier to maintain body shape. Sasha should continue to work on toning, but needs to make sure that she keeps the repetitions high (15+) to prevent bulking.

vital statistics

weight **145lb (66kg)**
a loss of 7lb (3kg)

dress size **10**
a drop of one dress size

body fat **25%**
a loss of 5%

the programs

women's upper body tone-up

The key to sculpting the upper body is to strengthen and tone muscle areas, such as the triceps and pectorals, that may have become weak, either through inactivity or as a result of a poorly designed training program. This gives a more "lifted" appearance to the breasts and tones the upper arms, so you'll look fantastic in anything low cut or backless.

how the program works

The program is structured over three weeks. Each week there are two routines, each to be performed twice a week. The aim is to tone the torso and arms, not to build mass. In the first two weeks of the program, you work with heavier weights and concentrate on high muscular utilization. Initially, this causes the muscles to store more fluid and, as a result, you may feel that your arms are starting to bulk up slightly. Don't worry, this is a temporary effect and fades by week three as you focus more on muscular endurance, which has a toning effect.

Fat burning is also important for muscle definition. Perform the workouts after a warmup or aerobic session; or you could combine this program with the Fat Loss (*see pages 122–25*) or Six-week Beach Body (*see pages 128–31*) programs.

Exercise library

Straight arm pull-down *p94*

Reverse fly *p90*

Lat pull-down *p90*

Seated row *p94*

Single arm row *p91*

Bicep curl *p96*

Upright row *p89*

Basic crunch *p102*

Incline fly *p84*

Chest press *p83*

Tricep overhead *p98*

Push-up *p85*

Back extension *p95*

Tricep extension *p101*

Lateral raise *p86*

Bridge *p105*

Oblique bridge *p105*

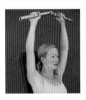
Shoulder press *p88*

Incline fly *p84*

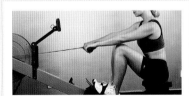
Row *pp70–71*

X-train *pp70–71*

Week 1

In week 1, alternate between workouts 1 and 2, and do each one twice so you work out 4 times a week. Sometimes you will be asked to repeat an exercise or a sequence of exercises within the Exercise sequence.

Workout 1

Workout time 55 mins (5 mins Warmup + 40 mins Exercise sequence + 10 mins Cool-down)

Warmup 5 mins aerobic exercise, gradually raising heart rate

Exercise sequence	beginner	intermediate	advanced
Straight arm pull-down	15rm	15rm	10rm
Reverse fly	15rm	12rm	10rm
Lat pull-down	15rm	15rm	12rm
Seated row	12rm	12rm	10rm
Single arm row	12rm	12rm	10rm
Rest	2 mins	2 mins	2 mins
Repeat the 5 exercises above	**(x2)**	**(x3)**	**(x3–4)**
Bicep curl dumbbells	20rm	20rm	20rm
Upright row	15rm	15rm	12rm
Rest	30 secs	30 secs	30 secs
Repeat the 2 exercises above	**(x2)**	**(x3)**	**(x3–4)**
Basic crunch	25 (x3)	40 (x5)	50 (x5)

Cool-down Total body stretch sequence (*see page 48*)

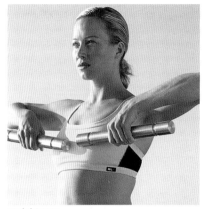
upright row

Workout 2

Workout time 55 mins (5 mins Warmup + 40 mins Exercise sequence + 10 mins Cool-down)

Warmup 5 mins aerobic exercise, gradually raising heart rate

Exercise sequence	beginner	intermediate	advanced
Incline fly	12rm	12rm	12rm
Chest press	15rm	12rm	12rm
Tricep overhead	15	20	to failure
Push-up	to failure	to failure	to failure
Rest	2 mins	90 secs	60 secs
Repeat the 4 exercises above	**(x2)**	**(x3)**	**(x3–4)**
Back extension	15	20	30
Basic crunch	25	40	50
Repeat the 2 exercises above	**(x2)**	**(x4)**	**(x5)**
Tricep extension	15rm	15rm	15rm
Rest	30 secs	30 secs	30 secs
Repeat the exercise above	**(x2)**	**(x4)**	**(x4)**
Shoulder press	20rm	15rm	15rm
Rest	30 secs	30 secs	3 secs
Repeat the exercise above	**(x2)**	**(x3)**	**(x4)**
Lateral raise	15rm	12rm	12rm
Rest	30 secs	30 secs	30 secs
Repeat the exercise above	**(x2)**	**(x3)**	**(x4)**

Cool-down Total body stretch sequence (*see page 48*)

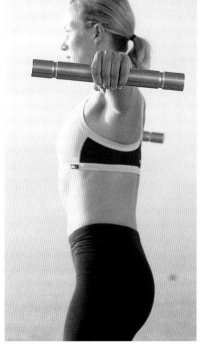
lateral raise

the programs

Week 2

In week 2, alternate between workouts 1 and 2 and do each one twice so you work out 4 times a week. Sometimes you will be asked to repeat an exercise or a sequence of exercises within the Exercise sequence.

Workout 1

Workout time 55 mins (5 mins Warmup + 40 mins Exercise sequence + 10 mins Cool-down)

Warmup — 5 mins aerobic exercise, gradually raising heart rate

Exercise sequence	beginner	intermediate	advanced
Straight arm pull-down	15rm	15rm	10rm
Reverse fly	15rm	12rm	10rm
Lat pull-down	15rm	15rm	12rm
Bicep curl	20rm	20rm	20rm
Upright row	15rm	15rm	12rm
Seated row	12rm	12rm	10rm
Single arm row	12rm	12rm	10rm
Repeat the 7 exercises above	**(x2)**	**(x3)**	**(x3–4)**
Basic crunch	25	40	50
Reverse curl	20	25	30
Rest	30 secs	30 secs	30 secs
Repeat the 2 exercises above	**(x3)**	**(x5)**	**(x5)**
Row	750m (2460ft)	1250m (4104ft)	2000m (6560ft)

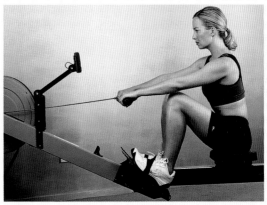
rowing

Cool-down — Total body stretch sequence (*see page 48*)

Workout 2

Workout time 55 mins (5 mins Warmup + 40 mins Exercise sequence + 10 mins Cool-down)

Warmup — 5 mins aerobic exercise, gradually raising heart rate

Exercise sequence	beginner	intermediate	advanced
Incline fly	12rm	10rm	10rm
Chest press	15rm	12rm	10rm
Dips	15	20	to failure
Push-up	to failure	to failure	to failure
Tricep extension	15rm	15rm	15rm
Rest	2 mins	90 secs	60 secs
Repeat the 5 exercises above	**(x2)**	**(x3)**	**(x3–4)**
Back extension	20	20	3 (x10) 5 secs hold
Basic crunch	25	40	50
Bridge	–	30 secs	60 secs
Oblique bridge	–	30 secs each side	60 secs each side
Repeat the 4 exercises above	**(x2)**	**(x4)**	**(x4)**
Shoulder press	15rm	12rm	12rm
Rest	30 secs	30 secs	30 secs
Repeat the exercise above	**(x2)**	**(x3)**	**(x4)**
Lateral raise	15rm	12rm	12rm
Rest	30 secs	30 secs	30 secs
Repeat the exercise above	**(x2)**	**(x3)**	**(x4)**
X-train (focus on arms)	10 mins	15 mins	15 mins

shoulder press

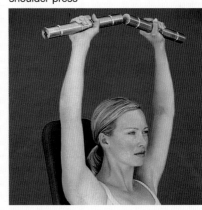

Cool-down — Total body stretch sequence (*see page 48*)

Week 3

In week 3, alternate between workouts 1 and 2 and do each one twice so you work out 4 times a week. Sometimes you will be asked to repeat an exercise or a sequence of exercises within the Exercise sequence.

Workout 1

Workout time 55 mins (5 mins Warmup + 40 mins Exercise sequence + 10 mins Cool-down)

Warmup 5 mins aerobic exercise, gradually raising heart rate

Exercise sequence	beginner	intermediate	advanced
Seated row	20rm	20rm	15rm
Chest press	20rm	20rm	20rm
Lat pull-down (overhand)	15rm	15rm	12rm
Pec fly	15rm	15rm	15rm
Upright row	20rm	20rm	20rm
Push-up	to failure	to failure	to failure
Row (maximum pace)	220yd(200m)@ 80%MHR	330yd(300m)@ 85%MHR	550yd(500m)@ 85%MHR
Rest	2 mins	2 mins	2 mins
Repeat the 7 exercises above	**(x2)**	**(x3)**	**(x4)**
Back extension	20	20	30
Basic crunch	25	40	50
Bridge	–	30 secs	60 secs
Oblique bridge	–	30 secs each side	60 secs each side
Repeat the 4 exercises above	**(x2)**	**(x4)**	**(x4)**

Cool-down Total body stretch sequence (*see page 48*)

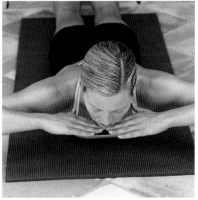

back extension

Workout 2

Workout time 45 mins (5 mins Warmup + 40 mins Exercise sequence + 10 mins Cool-down)

Warmup 5 mins aerobic exercise, gradually raising heart rate

Exercise sequence	beginner	intermediate	advanced
Incline fly	12rm	10rm	10rm
Bicep curl	30rm	50rm	100rm
Lateral raise	20rm	25rm	30rm
Tricep extension	12rm	12rm	12rm
Shoulder press	25rm	25rm	25rm
Straight arm pull-down	12rm	12rm	12rm
Chest press	20rm	25rm	30rm
Single arm row	15rm	12rm	12rm
X-train (focus on arms)	3 mins	3 mins	3 mins
Rest	2 mins	2 mins	2 mins
Repeat the 9 exercises above	**(x2)**	**(x3)**	**(x4)**

Cool-down Total body stretch sequence (*see page 48*)

cross-training

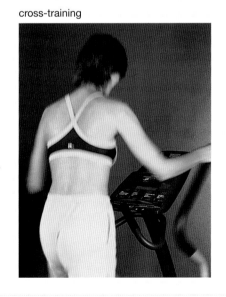

the programs

perfect legs

The aim of a good legs program is to create legs that are toned, firm, and longer-looking. The perfect legs should be shapely, but not too shapely, and certainly not too wide. This program will give you lean legs, but it will also build their strength and endurance. After all, it's no good having great-looking legs if you can't do anything with them.

Benefits

builds strength / tones muscles ✓✓

burns fat / builds aerobic capacity ✓

increases flexibility ✓✓

how the program works

The combination of aerobic and resistance training in this program is crucial – the aerobic work burns fat, while the resistance work creates muscle tone. There are short "blasts" of aerobic activity in the workouts as well as long range of motion, or "dynamic," exercises. These are exercises such as cycling, cross training, walking lunges, and cross country skiing, for example, where the movement is through a number of joints. These exercises will help the legs to look longer because they work the entire length of the muscle rather than just isolating a small part of it, which is what happens with short range of motion exercises.

The muscles in the legs can begin to look bulky if the range of motion in the exercises is too limited. Short range of motion exercises, or isolation exercises, where only small muscle movements are involved, target a small area of the muscle. They tear and then rebuild muscle fibers in this small area, and this is what produces the undesirable "bulky" look. Only using the leg extension machine or doing endless squats would have this effect. Having said this, don't be alarmed if your legs feel bigger 10 days into the program; as you progress, this bulking effect will diminish and you will start to develop leaner legs.

This is a three-week program with three different weekly workouts, each to be performed once a week. Allow a day's rest between workouts. If you want to train more than three times a week, do either 30 minutes of fast walking (*see pages 60–63*) on uneven terrain, or swim for 30 minutes using breaststroke. For diet and cellulite advice, see the perfect buns program, pages 144–45.

Exercise library

Leg press *p111*	Lunge *p106*	Step ups *p109*	Cycle *pp68–9*	X-train *pp70–71*	Run *pp64–7/* fast walk *pp60–63*	Walking lunge *p107*	Leg curl *p111*
Body raise for glutes *p113*	Row *pp70–71*	Squat *p108*	Shuttle runs *pp72–3*	Sideways shuttle runs *pp72–3*	Power lunge *p106*	Fast walk *pp60–63*	

Week 1

Work out 3 times in week 1. Do workouts 1, 2, and 3 once each. Do all 3 circuits in workouts 1 and 2, then stretch to cool down. Have a rest day between each workout day.

Workout 1

Warmup — Workout time 35 mins (5 mins Warmup + 25 mins Exercise sequence + 5 mins Cool-down)
5 mins aerobic exercise, gradually raising heart rate

	circuit 1 beginner	inter/advanced	circuit 2 beginner	inter/advanced	circuit 3 beginner	inter/advanced
Leg press	12rm	10rm	15rm	15rm	20rm	15rm
Lunge	20 each leg	20 each leg	20 each leg	20 each leg	20 each leg	20 each leg
Step ups	20 each leg	30 each leg	15 each leg	25 each leg	10 each leg	20 each leg
Aerobic exercise	Cycle 3mins@75%MHR		X-train 3mins@75%MHR		Run/fast walk 3mins@75%MHR	

Cool-down — Lower body stretch sequence (*see page 49*)

Workout 2

Warmup — Workout time 35 mins (5 mins Warmup + 25 mins Exercise sequence + 5 mins Cool-down)
5 mins aerobic exercise, gradually raising heart rate

	circuit 1 beginner	inter/advanced	circuit 2 beginner	inter/advanced	circuit 3 beginner	inter/advanced
Walking lunge 20lb (10kg) ball	30	40	30	30	30	40
Leg curl	12rm	10rm	12rm	10rm	12rm	10rm
Body raise for glutes	30	30	30	30	30	30
Aerobic exercise	Row 550yd(500m)@75%MHR		X-train 2mins@85%MHR		Row 550yd (500m)@80%MHR	

Cool-down — Lower body stretch sequence (*see page 49*)

Workout 3

Warmup — Workout time 50 mins (5 mins Warmup + 40 mins Exercise sequence + 5 mins Cool-down)
5 mins aerobic exercise, gradually raising heart rate

	beginner	inter/advanced
Fast walk/run	1min@80%MHR, 2mins@65–70%MHR. (x7)	1min@85%MHR, 2mins@65–70%MHR. (x10)
Squat	30	20 (jump)
Shuttle runs 30ft (10m)	30 secs	60 secs
Leg curl	20rm	20rm
Step ups	30 secs each leg	60 secs each leg
Leg curl	20rm	20rm
Sideways shuttle runs 30ft (10m)	30 secs	60 secs
Leg curl	20rm	20rm
Body raise for glutes	15	25
Leg curl	20rm	20rm
Squat	25	40

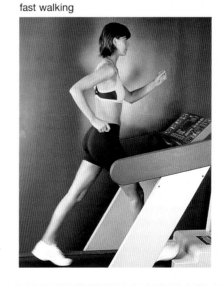

fast walking

Cool-down — Lower body stretch sequence (*see page 49*)

Week 2

Work out 3 times in week 2. Do workouts 1, 2, and 3 once each. For each workout, do all 3 circuits, then stretch to cool down . Rest between each workout day. You should be used to the exercises by now, so concentrate on specific muscles and keep the movements slow and controlled.

Workout 1

Workout time 25 mins (5 mins Warmup + 15 mins circuits + 5 mins Cool-down)

Warmup — 5 mins aerobic exercise, gradually raising heart rate

	circuit 1 beginner	inter/advanced	circuit 2 beginner	inter/advanced	circuit 3 beginner	inter/advance
Leg press	20rm	20rm	20rm	20rm	20rm	20rm
Lunge	20 each leg	25 each leg	20 each leg	25 each leg	20 each leg	25 each leg
Step ups	25 each leg	30 each leg	20 each leg	30 each leg	15 each leg	20 each leg
Aerobic exercise	Cycle 2mins@75%MHR		X-train 2mins@80%MHR		Run/fast walk 2mins@80%MHR	

Cool-down — Lower body stretch sequence (*see page 49*)

Workout 2

Workout time 45 mins (5 mins Warmup + 35 mins circuits + 5 mins Cool-down)

Warmup — 5 mins aerobic exercise, gradually raising heart rate

	circuit 1 beginner	inter/advanced	circuit 2 beginner	inter/advanced	circuit 3 beginner	inter/advanced
Walking lunges	30 with 20lb (10kg) ball	40 with 20lb (10kg) ball	30 with 15lb (6kg) ball	40 with 15lb (6kg) ball	30	40
Leg curl	12rm	10rm	12rm	10rm	12rm	10rm
Body raise for glutes	15	25	15	25	15	25
Steps ups	25 each leg	30 each leg	20 each leg	30 each leg	15 each leg	20 each leg
Aerobic exercise	X-train 2mins@80%MHR Row 550yd(500m)@80%MHR		X-train 2mins@80%MHR Row 550yd(500m)@80%MHR		X-trainer 2mins@80%MHR Row 550yd(500m)@80%MHR	

Cool-down — Lower body stretch sequence (*see page 49*)

Workout 3

Workout time 55 mins (5 mins Warmup + 30 mins aerobic + 15 mins circuits + 5 mins Cool-down)

Warmup — 5 mins aerobic exercise, gradually raising heart rate

	beginner	inter/advanced
Fast walk/run	1min@80%MHR, 2mins@65–70%MHR. (x7)	1min@85%MHR, 2mins@65–70%MHR. (x10)

	circuit 1 beginner	inter/advanced	circuit 2 beginner	inter/advanced	circuit 3 beginner	inter/advanced
Squat	30	40	30	40)	30	40
Sideways shuttle runs 30ft (10m)	30 secs	60 secs	30 secs	60 secs	30 secs	60 secs
Shuttle runs 30ft (10m)	60 secs	75 secs	45 secs	75 secs	45 secs	75 secs
Leg curl	20rm	20rm	20rm	20rm	20rm	20rm

Cool-down — Lower body stretch sequence (*see page 49*)

Week 3

Work out 3 times in week 3. Do workouts 1, 2, and 3 once each. For each workout, do all 3 circuits, then stretch to cool down. Rest between each workout day. The aim in these workouts is to increase the intensity and work for longer and harder.

Workout 1

Warmup
Workout time 30 mins (5 mins Warmup + 20 mins Exercise sequence + 5 mins Cool-down)
5 mins aerobic exercise, gradually raising heart rate

	circuit 1 beginner	inter/advanced	circuit 2 beginner	inter/advanced	circuit 3 beginner	inter/advanced
Leg press	20rm	20rm	20rm	20rm	20rm	20rm
Lunge	20 each leg	25 each leg	20 each leg	25 each leg	20 each leg	25 each leg
Step ups	35 each leg	40 each leg	35 each leg	40 each leg	35 each leg	40 each leg
Aerobic exercise	Cycle 4mins@80%MHR		X-train 4mins@85%MHR		Run/fast walk 2mins@80%MHR	

Cool-down
Lower body stretch sequence (*see page 49*)

Workout 2

Warmup
Workout time 40 mins (5 mins Warmup + 30 mins Exercise sequence + 5 mins Cool-down)
5 mins aerobic exercise, gradually raising heart rate

	circuit 1 beginner	inter/advanced	circuit 2 beginner	inter/advanced	circuit 3 beginner	inter/advanced
Walking lunges	30 with 20lb (10kg) ball	40 with 20lb (10kg) ball	30 with 15lb (6kg) ball	40 with 15lb (6kg) ball	30	40
Leg curl	20rm	20rm	20rm	20rm	12rm	10rm
Body raise for glutes	15	25	15	25	15	25
Step ups	35 each leg	40 each leg	35 each leg	40 each leg	35 each leg	40 each leg
Aerobic exercise	X-train 2mins@70%MHR Row 550yd(500m)@ 70%MHR Walk 2mins@75%MHR		X-train 2mins@70%MHR Row 550yd(500m)@70%MHR Walk 2mins@75%MHR		X-train 2mins@70%MHR Row 550yd(500m)@70%MHR Walk 2mins@75%MHR	

Cool-down
Lower body stretch sequence (*see page 49*)

Workout 3

Warmup
Workout time 55 mins (5 mins Warmup + 30 mins aerobic + 15 mins circuits + 5 mins Cool-down)
5 mins aerobic exercise, gradually raising heart rate

	beginner	inter/advanced
Fast walk/run	1min@80%MHR, 2mins@65–70%MHR. (x7)	1min@85%MHR, 2mins@65–70%MHR. (x10)

	circuit 1 beginner	inter/advanced	circuit 2 beginner	inter/advanced	circuit 3 beginner	inter/advanced
Squat	35	45	35	50	35	45
Sideways shuttle runs 30ft (10m)	30 secs	60 secs	30 secs	60 secs	30 secs	60 secs
Shuttle runs 30ft (10m)	60 secs	90 secs	60 secs	90 secs	60 secs	90 secs
Leg curl	20rm	20rm	20rm	20rm	20rm	20rm

Cool-down
Lower body stretch sequence (*see page 49*)

perfect buns

The aim of this program is to tone the muscles of the butt, shaping the entire area and helping to efffectively "lift" it. An eminent plastic surgeon friend of mine often sends clients to me because surgery can't achieve what the client wants; often exercise can bring about changes in shape that the knife cannot.

the bottom line

The butt is one area of the body that many of my female clients say they would most like to change, but often they find that they have great difficulty in achieving this. Women naturally tend to store fat on the butt, and it can be one of the more stubborn areas to eliminate fat from.

how the program works

The gluteus maximus, the main muscles in the butt, are the biggest single muscles in the body. They are surrounded by a number of other smaller muscles that together define the shape of your butt.

If your main concern is to reduce the size of your butt, you need to focus on burning fat first. The best way to burn fat is by doing aerobic exercise, which raises the heart rate and increases the rate at which you burn fat. Then you can target the butt with exercises that tone and firm the entire buttock area. You won't change the shape of your butt simply by concentrating on the exercises in this program. It's important to burn the fat that sits on top of the muscle first – if you don't, as you start to firm the muscle, you could find that you actually end up making your butt more prominent.

using the program

The exercise sequence is short and simple and targets only the butt, creating tone and shape. For fat burning, do the routine at least three times a week after an aerobic workout where you train for about 20 minutes at 70–80 percent of your maximum heart rate (MHR). Although all aerobic exercise burns body fat, some will actually tone the muscles in the butt as well. Try hill walking, swimming the front crawl, and using the elliptical cross-trainer in the gym. Don't overdo step classes, the Stairmaster, cycling, or rollerblading. These exercises work the muscles of the butt intensively and

can make them appear bulky rather than having a toning effect. Alternatively, to tone the butt, combine this program with the perfect legs program (*see pages 140–43*), which will help to shape the top of the legs as well. Or combine it with another more general program such as the women's or men's general fitness programs (*see pages 156–63*) as these are very effective for fat burning.

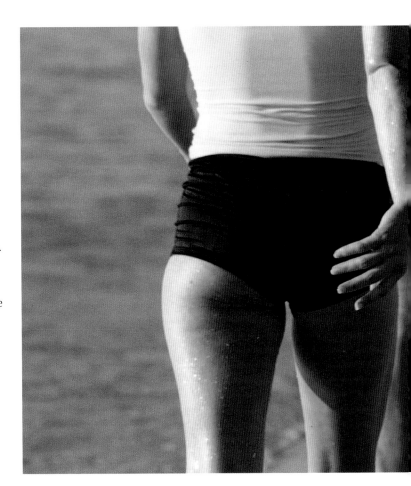

The workout Workout time 10 mins (5 mins Exercise sequence + 5 mins Cool-down)

Exercise sequence   Repetition maximums (rm) or repetitions for each exercise are shown in this order of fitness level:
beginner / intermediate / advanced

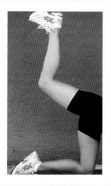 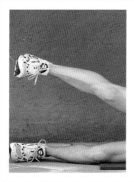 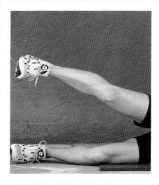 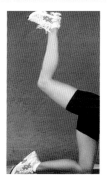

Glute raise *p113*	Abductor raise *p112*	Squats (weights) *p108*	Abductor raise *p112*	Glute raise *p113*
25/30/40 each leg	30/40/40 each leg	25/20/15	30/15/40 each leg	25/30/40 each leg

Cool-down   Lower body stretch sequence (*see page 49*)

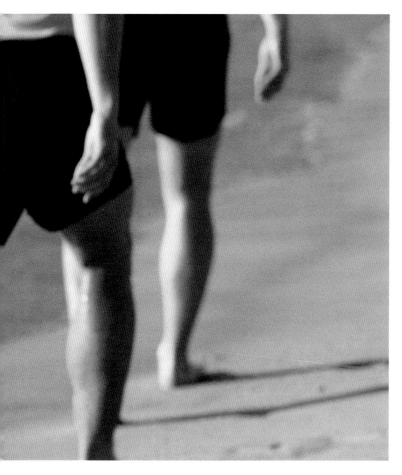

cellulite

This is predominantly a concern for women. Cellulite can develop on the butt and the backs of the thighs and also on the arms. It can give an unpleasant dimpled or "orange peel" effect to skin. It is caused when toxins build up in the fat cells, which causes them to swell and increase in size. They push against the inflexible meshlike interconnective tissue that holds the skin together. The result is cellulite, but there are ways of reducing it:

• Cleanse fat cells of toxins by following the detox diet that accompanies the three-week detox program (*see pages 132–33*) and by drinking plenty of water.

• Improve the elasticity of the interconnective tissue by keeping the skin well hydrated and moisturized.

• Get regular exercise (for example, perfect legs, *pages 140–43*).

• Have a regular massage – this improves circulation, which helps the body to rid itself of toxins, and improves the elasticity of the interconnective tissue.

• Be very wary of miracle creams that claim they can achieve all of this for you.

◄ bottoms up
To burn fat and shape, sculpt and tone the butt, combine regular aerobic workouts with exercises that target the muscles in the butt.

the programs

perfect abdominals

The stomach muscles, or abdominals, must be the area of the body that I get asked about the most. We are all conscious of the flatness or flabiness of our stomach regions. A combination of exercises, aerobic work, and a few alterations to your diet could give you the flat, toned stomach that, up until now, has been elusive.

Benefits

builds strength / tones muscle ✓✓

burns fat / builds aerobic capacity

increases flexibility ✓

how the program works

I am frequently asked the same question: "I do a hundred sit-ups a day, so why is it that I still don't have a flat stomach?". Two questions immediately spring to mind. First, what is the quality of the exercise the person is doing, and second, is this person effectively overloading the stomach muscles by targeting them from several different angles?

The workouts in this program use a variety of exercises to ensure that the abdominals are being continuously challenged and hit from different angles. This way they get an effective workout from each exercise rather than having to perform multiple repetitions of the same exercise with little effect.

Exercise alone won't guarantee you perfect abdominals. People tend to gain and store fat in the stomach area – in fact everyone holds some fat there. And often when you lose weight, the stomach is one of the last places to shed it. This program will certainly help to strengthen and define the stomach muscles, but unless you follow the nutrition tips (*see right*) and lose any excess fat from the area, you'll only ever dream of showing off your perfect abdominals.

using the program

The program consists of two short 15-minute workouts; alternate between them and aim to work out a minimum of three times a week. You can do these workouts at any time, but ideally you should combine them with some aerobic work. Try doing this programme at the end of the women's or men's general fitness programs (*see pages 140–43*).

Be sure to perform the exercises slowly, and maintain control in the stomach rather than using the momentum of the body to make the required number of repetitions. You derive greater benefit from doing fewer high-quality stomach exercises than more low-quality ones.

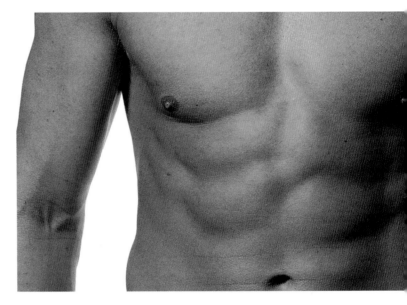

▲ **the six pack**
Endless crunches aren't the answer – it's important to target the abdominal muscles from many different angles.

Nutrition tips

Concentrate on keeping the body well hydrated and eating foods that are easy to digest.

● Ensure that the bulk of your diet is made up of low glycemic/alkaline foods (*see pages 34–5*) since they are easier for the body to digest.

● Avoid high glycemic and heavy starch foods such as potatoes and wheat products.

● Eat early in the evening, preferably at least two hours before you go to bed; if you eat late, eat more alkaline foods. For meal suggestions, see pages 36–7.

● Graze throughout the day rather than eating large meals. Eating lots of smaller meals provides the body with a constant source of energy.

● Cut out alcohol, or reduce intake to a maximum of 8 units for men, 6 for women (*A unit is a glass of wine, a single measure of spirits, or half a pint of beer.*).

● Drink at least 2 quarts (2 liters) of water a day to help flush impurities through your system.

Workout 1

Workout time 15 mins (10 mins Exercise sequence + 5 mins Cool-down)

Exercise sequence   Repetition maximums (rm) or repetitions for each exercise are shown in this order of fitness level:
beginner / intermediate / advanced

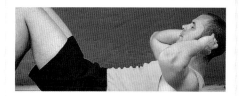 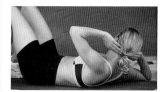 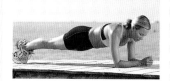

Basic crunch *p102*
15/15/15

Reverse curl *p103*
15/15/15

Oblique crunch *p104*
15/15/15

Bridge *p105*
20/40/25 secs

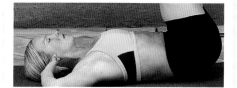 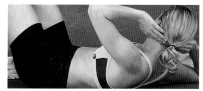 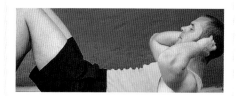

Reverse curl *p103*
10/15/20

Oblique crunch *p104*
10/15/20

Basic crunch *p102*
10/15/20

Cool-down   Total body stretch sequence (*see page 48*)

Workout 2

Workout time 15 mins (10 mins Exercise sequence + 5 mins Cool-down)

Exercise sequence   Repetition maximums (rm) or repetitions for each exercise are shown in this order of fitness level:
beginner / intermediate / advanced

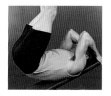 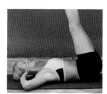 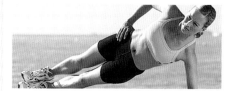 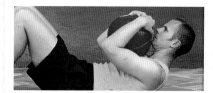

Raised reverse curl
p103 –/15/20

Reverse curl *p103*
15/–/–

Oblique bridge *p105*
20/40/60 secs

Medicine ball crunch *p104*
15/20/25

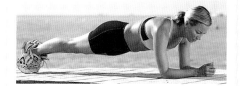 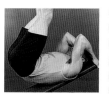 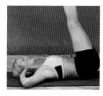 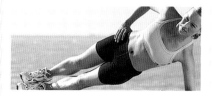

Bridge *p105*
–/40/60 secs

Raised reverse curl
p103 –/15/20

Reverse curl *p103*
10/–/–

Oblique bridge *p105*
20/40/60 secs

Cool-down   Total body stretch sequence (*see page 48*)

the programs

Tim

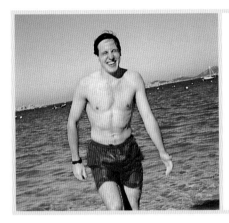

vital statistics

age **26**

profession **journalist**

height **6ft 1in (1.85m)**

weight **178lb (81kg)**

neck measurement **15in (37cm)**

chest measurement **37in (94cm)**

waist measurement **33in (84cm)**

thigh measurement **21in (54cm)**

tim's goal

I was chosen to be the case study for the "Building Mass" program. This was a kind way of saying that, although I had a decent level of aerobic fitness (from regular running, cycling, and soccer), I had the upper-body strength of a 7-year-old girl. My goal was to fill out my arms, chest, and shoulders, without losing the power in my hamstrings and quadriceps.

matt's assessment

Tim is a classic ectomorph. He has always been thin and can eat as much as he likes without putting on weight. He is very active – he regularly cycles and plays competitive soccer. All of this adds up to the worst possible combination for gaining muscle size. Tim had never done any weight-training, so the building mass program would condition his muscles; we then moved on to intense muscle building. This was backed up with a high-energy diet to support muscle growth.

▼ **new to the world of weight training**
Intensive resistance exercises on machines and using weights help to build muscle.

▶ weeks 1–2

The first week was a killer; by far the hardest of the whole program. I had never used weights seriously, and although the sessions themselves are not too tough, the muscular soreness the next day is intense. On the subway, I feel like I've been nailed to my seat and worry that I might miss my stop through a sheer inability to stand up and walk to the exit. Rarely used muscles like the triceps groan as I perform simple tasks like pushing a door open. By week two, the technique on the machines is starting to feel a lot more natural, and the pain in my muscles after each session is

thankfully much reduced. I am training three times a week, for one hour a time. Although I have continued to cycle, I have decided to take a break from running.

▶ weeks 3–5

At my initial assessment, Matt scrutinized my diet. It was just about satisfactory (naturally, I gave a heavily edited version), but to aid with muscle building and recovery, he suggested some changes. White pasta, baked potatoes, red meat, bananas, and honey were out. In come wild rice, wholemeal pasta, hummus, and

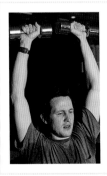
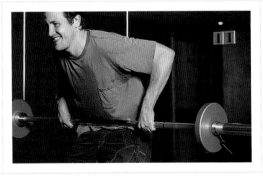
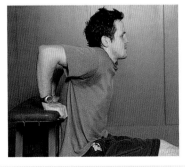
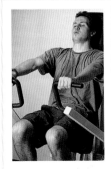

▶ bigger and stronger
Hard work to begin with, but the building mass program paid off.

apples. The goal is to eat food that will give me a slow and consistent release of energy to avoid highs, lows, and mid-afternoon lulls. By week five, the post-session stiffness has basically gone.

▶ weeks 6–8

I'm starting to notice changes! The aim of the training was to start with the core areas (like stomach, chest, and shoulders) before blitzing the smaller muscle groups (like the biceps and triceps). My chest is the first area to show improvements: definitely bigger, firmer, and stronger. Carrying groceries and luggage is much easier than it used to be, and taking my bike up and down stairs no longer gets me out of breath. Due to the heavy lifting, my body needs a lot more calories than before; I eat five or six small meals a day. I do, however, feel much better for it. The dip in energy that I would experience between 2–4pm has gone.

▶ weeks 9–12

At the start of the program I was lifting small weights and reaching muscular failure quickly. Now, as well as lifting bigger weights, I can feel my body responding to the extra demands I'm placing on it. My arms have started to follow the progress made by chest and shoulders. Apart from moments where I've felt like heading out on a head-clearing run through the park, there have been no low points to speak of.

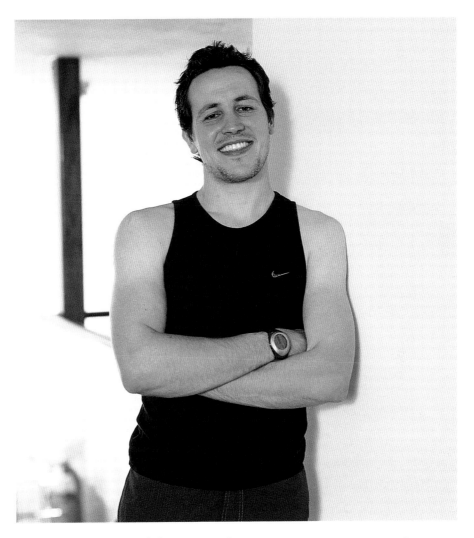

"My girlfriend wants to write a personal letter of thanks to Matt Roberts."

beyond the program

• For a man of slight build, Tim has achieved great results. However, he has only just turned the corner in terms of what he could achieve.
• Tim should continue with the program for at least another 12 weeks. By then he could bulk up considerably.

vital statistics

weight **187lb (85kg)**
an increase of 8½lb (4kg)

neck measurement **16in (40cm)**
chest measurement **39in (98.5cm)**
waist measurement **32in (82cm)**
thigh measurement **22in (56.5cm)**

the programs

building mass

The aim of this program is to create muscle. Many people think that working with weights will guarantee this. In fact, building mass is one of the more difficult goals to achieve, partly because your degree of success is dependent on your body type. Assess your body type (*see pages 76–7*) before embarking on this program; that way you can set yourself realistic goals.

Benefits

builds strength / tones muscles ✓✓✓

burns fat / builds aerobic capacity

increases flexibility ✓

using the program

The program is broken down into routines for the shoulders, arms, chest, back, and legs. Aim to work out four times a week, and to work each of these body parts at least twice a week. For each workout, aim to target two or three body parts, and choose a routine from the relevant program. Mix and match programs so you work your entire body. Try to avoid repeating exercises in a workout, and don't target one area of the body at the expense of the rest of the body.

Keep the movements slow and controlled as you perform these exercises. This way the muscles work hard during the whole movement, and you will see better results from your workouts. Keep increasing your weights so you continuously challenge your muscles and maximize the effectiveness of your workouts.

warming up

Before each workout, do an intense five- to six-minute aerobic session that raises the heart rate quickly and warms up the muscles you are going to work. There is no point in doing 10 minutes of running and then starting a chest routine.

protein

Protein is essential for muscle growth and helps the body to rebuild and repair itself. High-intensity workouts actually damage the muscles to encourage the body to rebuild them bigger and stronger, so you need to supply the body with adequate protein to help it with its repair work. However, the liver and kidneys can't cope with very high levels of protein, and it should not come from red meat, dairy products, or eggs as they contain high levels of saturated fat (*see below*).

Program ideas
Below is a suggested 4-week program based on 4 workouts a week. It combines routines from the different body part workouts to give a good total body workout.

Workout 1	Chest 1, Arms 2
Workout 2	Back 1, Legs 2, Shoulders 1
Workout 3	Chest 2, Back 3
Workout 4	Legs 1, Shoulders 2, Arms 3
Workout 5	Chest 4, Arms 1
Workout 6	Back 2, Legs 4, Shoulders 2
Workout 7	Chest 5, Back 4
Workout 8	Legs 3, Shoulders 3, Arms 4
Workout 9	Chest 5, Arms 1
Workout 10	Back 1, Legs 2, Shoulders 1
Workout 11	Chest 6, Back 3
Workout 12	Legs 1, Shoulders 2, Arms 3
Workout 13	Chest 4, Arms 2
Workout 14	Back 2, Legs 4, Shoulders 2
Workout 15	Chest 5, Back 1
Workout 16	Legs 2, Shoulders 3, Arms 4

Nutrition tips

The intensive workouts in these programs require plenty of energy to fuel them. If you do not supply the body with sufficient nutrients, your workouts will be ineffective and you will struggle to build mass.

● Mesomorphs and endomorphs should follow my basic nutrition guidelines, and aim to eat a varied diet consisting mainly of low-glycemic, alkaline foods (*see pages 34–5*).

● Men should consume about 3000 calories a day, and women about 2000, but add 500 calories to your daily requirement when following this program. Get these calories from low-glycemic carbohydrates or good quality, low-fat proteins.

● Ectomorphs in particular should eat lots of smaller snack-size meals; this spreads calories through the day and provides the body with a constant source of energy.

● Protein should make up 10–20 percent of the diet, and as much as possible, this should come from grains, beans, and nuts, but you can also include some chicken and fish.

● Eat a good source of protein, such as nuts or fish after a workout; there are also some good high-protein postworkout bars available.

● Drink at least 2 quarts (2 liters) of water a day.

shoulder program

To create good shapely shoulders, you need to concentrate work on the deltoids. These form a cuplike shape at the top of the shoulder and are made up of three different sections of muscle. A common mistake when building muscle in the shoulders is to concentrate work on the front section and to forget about adding dimension to the middle and back of the shoulder. The exercises that follow target all sections of the deltoid and will help to create an even rounded shape. You also need to work on the trapezius muscles, which run from the top of the neck across the the top of the back and shoulders. This muscle can build quickly in some people – particularly mesomorphs and endomorphs – and can give a bulky appearance to the neck, which may not be desirable. None of the exercises in the routines that follow will overemphasize the trapezius muscles. If your trapezius muscles are not pronounced, building them up can develop good defined shape at the top of the shoulders. If this is your goal, put more emphasis on routines 1 and 4.

Shoulder routines   Each of these routines takes between 8 and 12 mins

Routine 1

Lateral raise	12rm, 45 secs rest
Shoulder press	14rm, 45 secs rest
Upright row	16rm, 90 secs rest
Lateral raise	10rm, 45 secs rest
Shoulder press	12rm, 45 secs rest
Upright row	14rm, 90 secs rest
Lateral raise	8rm, 45 secs rest
Shoulder press	10rm, 45 secs rest
Upright row	12rm

Routine 2

Lateral raise	12rm (drop set), 60 secs rest
Lateral raise	10rm (drop set), 60 secs rest
Lateral raise	8rm (drop set), 60 secs rest
Shoulder press	16rm, 45 secs rest
Shoulder press	18rm, 45 secs rest
Shoulder press	20rm

Routine 3

Cable lateral raise	14rm, 45 secs rest, 12rm, 45 secs rest
Reverse fly	10rm (drop set), 45 secs rest
Reverse fly	8rm (drop set), 45 secs rest
Lateral raise	10rm, 8rm, 60 secs rest between sets

Routine 4

Shoulder press	16rm, 12rm, 10rm, 8rm, 16rm, 45 secs rest between sets
Inward thumb lateral raise	14rm, 45 secs rest
Upright row	10rm, 45 secs rest
Inward thumb lateral raise	12rm, 45 secs rest
Upright row	8rm

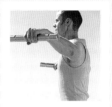

Lateral raise *p86*

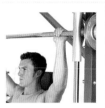

Shoulder press *p88*

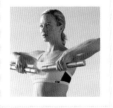

Upright row *p89*

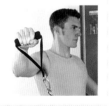

Cable lateral raise *p87*

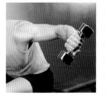

Reverse fly *p90*

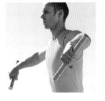

Inward thumb lateral raise *p87*

the programs

arm program

Toned, defined arms are in fashion, and people always ask me what exercises they can do to achieve them. A combination of the right exercises and the right training techniques gives the best results. I have used drop sets (*see page 80*) and matrix 7s here, a training technique where you divide exercises into half and full movements. Here, you do 7 full barbell curls, then 7

half barbell curls where you stop when your arm is bent at 90 degrees. You then perform 7 curls starting at the halfway point and ending in the finish position at the top of the shoulder. You finish by doing 7 full curls, or as many as you can complete before your muscle reaches fatigue. Combine these routines with routines for other parts of the body for a great all over workout.

Arm routines   Each of these routines takes between 15 and 20 mins

Routine 1

Dips	max
Bicep curl with barbell	12rm
Dips	max
Bicep curl with barbell	12rm
Dips	20
Hammer curl	12
Dips	20
Hammer curl	12
Tricep overhead	10
Close pull-up	max
Tricep overhead	10
Close pull-up	max

Routine 2

Tricep pushdown thumbs in	10rm, 8rm
French press	10rm, 8rm
Dips	10 reps or max
Tricep extension	10 reps (drop set)
Bicep curl with barbell	12rm
Bench supported hammer curl	10rm
Bicep curl with barbell	10rm
Bench supported hammer curl	8rm
Bicep curl with dumbbell	25rm

Routine 3

Dips	max
Close hand push-up	max
Tricep pushdown thumbs up	14rm, 10rm, 8rm, 6rm, 14rm
Seated row	16rm, 14rm
Dips	max
Close hand push-up	max
Bicep curl with barbell	7s matrix (see above)
Bicep curl with ball	12rm
Barbell matrix	7s
Bicep curl with ball	12rm
Close pull-up	max

Dips
p98

Bicep curl with barbell *p96*

Tricep pushdown thumbs in *p99*

Hammer curl *p97*

Tricep overhead *p98*

Close pull-up *p92*

Tricep pushdown thumbs up *p99*

French press *p100*

Tricep extension *p101*

Bench supported hammer curl *p97*

Dumbbell curl *p96*

Close hand push-up *p100*

Bicep curl with ball *p96*

Seated row *p94*

chest program

Nothing enhances a man's torso better than well defined pectoral muscles. In women, strong pectorals can give breasts a firm, toned appearance. With any chest routine, it's important to use a variety of exercises and training techniques that target different parts of the chest, as this creates a symmetrical shape.

Some routines use drop sets (*see page 80*), where you do one set of reps, then do a set with the same number of reps, but at 75 percent of the initial weight. This overloads the muscle and is one of the most effective techniqes for gaining muscle and strength. Some of the exercises isolate the pectorals, while others work the pectorals assisted by other muscle groups. This enables greater overload of the pectorals as you can work them for longer and so achieve better results.

These routines are suitable for those with intermediate to advanced fitness levels who have been following a general gym program for at least six to eight weeks.

Chest routines Each of these routines takes between 12 and 16 mins

Routine 1 — **Intermediate**
Pec fly	10rm (x2)
Chest press with barbell	10rm, 8rm
Dips	to failure or 10rm (x2)

Routine 2 — **Intermediate**
Chest press with barbell	12rm, 10rm, 8rm, 60 secs rest between sets
Incline fly	10rm, 8rm, 60 secs rest between sets
Machine fly	14rm, 12rm, 60 secs rest between sets

Routine 3 — **Advanced**
Machine chest press	14rm
Pec fly	12rm, 10rm, 8rm, 60 secs rest between sets
Chest press	10rm (drop set) (x2)
Push-up	to failure

Routine 4 — **Advanced**
Chest press	14rm, 10rm, 8rm, 6rm, 16rm, 60 secs rest between sets
Incline fly	12rm (x2)
Decline fly	to failure (x2), 30 secs rest between sets
Dips	to failure or 10

Routine 5 — **Advanced**
Pec flys	12rm (drop set), 10rm (drop set), 8rm (drop set), 60 secs rest between sets
Push-ups	to failure
Chest press machine	20rm (x2), 90 secs rest between sets

Routine 6 — **Advanced**
Chest press with barbell	16rm (drop set)
Incline fly	8rm (x2)
Decline fly	max
Dips	max (x2)

Pec fly
p82

Chest press with barbell *p96*

Dips
p98

Incline fly
p84

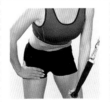
Machine fly
p82

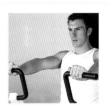
Machine chest press
p83

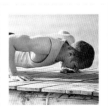
Push-up
p85

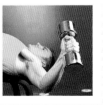
Decline fly
p84

back program

The back is made up of many different muscles, but the routines that follow target the latissimus dorsi, the rhomboids, and the trapezius muscles. If you build up these muscles and improve their tone and definition, you create a well proportioned back with a broad, muscular shape. Generally, people aim for one of two effects when building a muscular back: a wide back with an open V-shape or a thick-set back with greater girth. For a wide back, concentrate on pull-ups and lat pull-downs that emphasize the latissimus dorsi muscles (the lats). For thickness, you need to concentrate on the lats and the rhomboids: reverse flys, seated rows, and bent-over rows will all emphasize these muscles.

Back routines Each of these routines takes between 12 and 16 mins

Routine 1	Intermediate
Lat pull-down	10rm (x2)
Single arm row	8rm, 10rm
Reverse fly	12m (x2)
Close pull-up	12+ (if able to lift body weight for more than 12)

Routine 2	Intermediate
Single arm row	10rm
Straight arm pull-down	12rm
Single arm row	8rm
Straight arm pull-down	10rm
Wide pull-up	10 or to failure

Routine 3	Advanced
Reverse fly	12rm
Seated row	10rm (drop set)
Reverse fly	10rm
Seated row	8rm (drop set)
Upright row	16rm

Routine 4	Advanced
Reverse fly	16rm
Bent-over barbell row	16rm, 12rm, 10rm, 8rm, 16rm
Lat pull-down	10rm (x2)
Back extension	15 (x2)

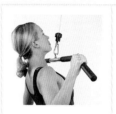

Lat pull-down
p90

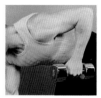

Single arm row
p91

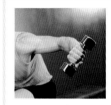

Reverse flye
p90

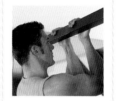

Close pull-up
p92

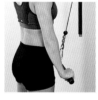

Straight arm pull-down *p94*

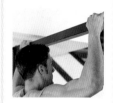

Wide pull-up
p92

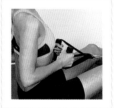

Seated row
p94

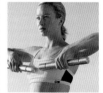

Upright row
p89

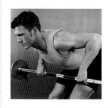

Bent-over barbell row *p91*

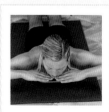

Back extension
p95

leg program

The routines that follow will improve and define the shape of the entire lower body, but they target the legs in particular. For many people, training with the goal of building bulk on the legs can be very frustrating. This is particularly true for ectomorphs, who may work hard and yet see no initial gain at all. It's generally the case that if you were born with thin legs,

you will always have thin legs. It's particularly difficult to bulk up the calves, but small calves can still be strong and powerful. You can, however, improve tone and muscle definition, which will enhance their shape. It can take longer to achieve results with the legs than with other parts of the body. Persevere; you need well-shaped legs to balance a strong upper body.

Leg routines   Each of these routines takes between 15 and 20 mins

Routine 1

Squat	14rm, 12rm, 10rm, 60 secs rest between sets
Leg curl	14rm, 12rm, 10rm, 45 secs rest between sets
Lunge	12rm each leg (x2), 60 secs rest between sets
Single leg calf raise	16rm, 14rm, 45 secs rest between sets

Routine 2

Leg extension	14rm
Power lunge	12rm each leg
Static squat	60 secs, 60 secs rest
Leg extension	10rm
Step-ups	20 each leg
Static squat	60 secs, 60 secs rest
Leg extension	8rm
Power lunge	14rm each leg
Static squat	60 secs

Routine 3

Leg curl	12rm
Lunge	10rm each leg
Ball squat	14rm, 60 secs rest
Leg curl	10rm
Lunge	10rm each leg
Ball squat	12rm

Routine 4

Lunge	14rm each leg
Squat	10rm
Single leg calf raise	14rm each leg, 60 secs rest
Lunge	12rm each leg
Squat	10rm
Single leg calf raise	12rm, 60 secs rest
Lunge	8rm each leg
Squat	8rm
Single leg calf raise	12rm each leg

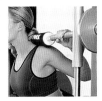

Squat
p108

Leg curl
p111

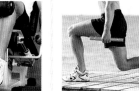

Lunge
p106

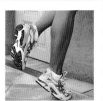

Single leg calf raise
p112

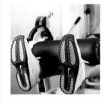

Leg extension
p110

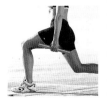

Power lunge
p106

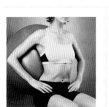

Ball squat
p108

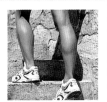

Step-ups
p109

the programs

men's general fitness

Sometimes you have a specific health and fitness goal to aim for, and other times you just want to be generally healthy and maintain good overall fitness. Use the periods when you don't have the pressure of a specific goal to take stock of where you are and work on your general fitness before the next challenge begins.

> **Benefits**
>
> builds strength / tones muscles ✓✓
>
> burns fat / builds aerobic capacity ✓✓
>
> increases flexibility ✓✓

setting goals

With a maintenance program, the most difficult task can be setting clear goals. Your goal, in effect, is to stay the same: to maintain your level of fitness, keep your muscles toned and strong, and prevent weight gain.

Start by taking circumference measurements of your chest, waist, hips, arms, and legs so you have starting points against which to compare later measurements. The danger on any maintenance program is that, even though you are working out, your body can become accustomed to the program and, as it is challenged less and less, you actually become less fit. Be careful not to get stuck in an exercise rut. Keep increasing your weights as you find them easier to work with, and keep pushing yourself that little bit further.

how the program works

The program consists of three workouts, each one to be performed once a week, so you work out a total of three times a week. If you want to train four times a week, repeat one of the workouts, but repeat a different one each time so you continue to introduce variety.

The resistance exercises in this program build muscle mass and tone the upper body, while also sculpting the waist and defining the abdominals to create a "six pack." In workout 2, I have introduced a different training technique where you perfrom exercises for a specified number of seconds, rather than using repetition maximums (rm). Do as many repetitions as you can, being sure to maintain good form and posture. Where a weight is required for an exercise, choose one that allows you to do the specified number of repetitions, but the

last few repetitions should be difficult. It's worth taking time to experiment and find the appropriate weight. Once you've found your starting weight, increase your weights and your number of repetitions as your strength improves. Using a time target encourages you to extend yourself beyond your comfortable limits. Focus on technique, and keep pushing until the time is up.

This program can also help to keep your weight stable if you follow it alongside a healthy balanced diet (*see pages 24–37*).

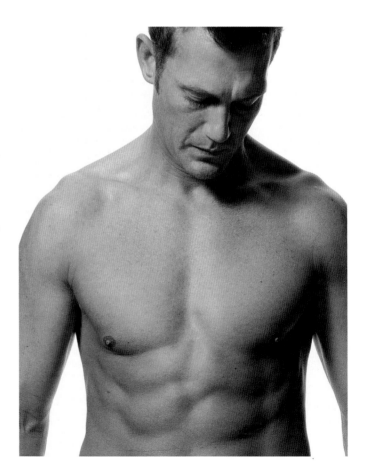

▶ **sculpt your body**
The program provides comprehensive overall workouts that will keep you trim and maintain good muscle tone. Keep challenging the body to get the most out of the program.

Exercise library

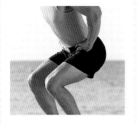

Squat
p108

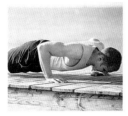

Push-up
p85

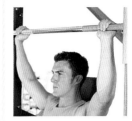

Leg curl
p111

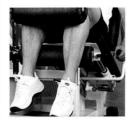

Shoulder press
p88

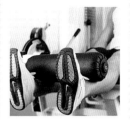

Leg extension
p110

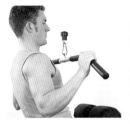

Lat pull-down
p90

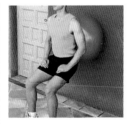

Ball squat
p108

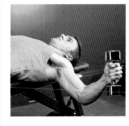

Pec fly
p82

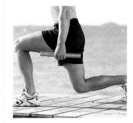

Power lunge
p106

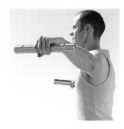

Lateral raise
p86

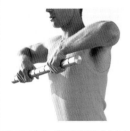

Upright row
p89

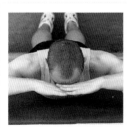

Back extension
p95

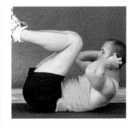

Full crunch
p102

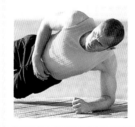

Oblique bridge
p105

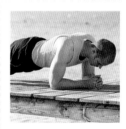

Bridge
p105

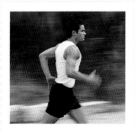

Walk *pp60–63*/run
pp64–7

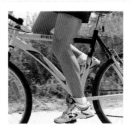

Cycle
pp68–9

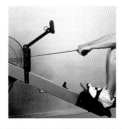

Row
pp70–71

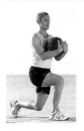

Walking lunge
with ball *p107*

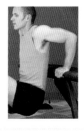

Dips
p98

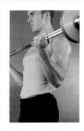

Bicep curl
barbell *p96*

Workout 1   Workout time 55 mins   (5 mins Warmup + 35 mins Aerobic exercise + 5 mins Cool-down + 10 mins Stretch)

Warmup   5 mins aerobic exercise, gradually raising heart rate

Aerobic exercise	beginner	intermediate	advanced
X-train	1min@70%MHR, 1min@85%MHR. (x5)	1min@70%MHR, 1min@90%MHR. (x6)	1min@70%MHR, 1min@90%MHR. (x7)
Walk with gradient	10mins@75%MHR	8mins@85–90%MHR	5mins@80%MHR
Row	550yd(500m)@75%MHR	1100yd(1000m)@80%MHR	1600yd(1500m)@80%MHR
Run	440yd(400m)@80%MHR	880yd(800m)@85%MHR	1100yd(1000m) as fast as possible

Cool-down   5 mins slow walking, gradually lowering heart rate

Stretch   Total body stretch sequence (*see page 48*)

Workout 2   Workout time 45 mins   (5 mins Warmup + 35 mins Exercise sequence + 5 mins Cool-down)

Warmup   5 mins aerobic exercise, gradually raising heart rate

For the following exercises, select a weight that works the muscles to near fatigue in the time period specified; rest for 30 seconds after each exercise.

Exercise sequence	beginner	intermediate	advanced
Squat	30 secs	45 secs	60 secs
Push-up	30 secs	45 secs	60 secs
Walking lunge	30 secs	45 secs	60 secs
Shoulder press	30 secs	45 secs	60 secs
Leg extension	30 secs	45 secs	60 secs
Lat pull-down	30 secs	45 secs	60 secs
Step-ups	30 secs each leg	45 secs each leg	60 secs each leg
Pec fly	30 secs	45 secs	60 secs
Leg curl	30 secs	45 secs	60 secs
Rest 2 mins			
Repeat the 9 exercises above	(x3)	(x5)	(x5–6)
Lateral raise	15rm	12rm	12rm
Upright row	15rm	12rm	12rm
Back extension	20	20	30
Full crunch	25	40	50
Oblique bridge	–	30 secs	60 secs
Repeat the 5 resistance exercises above	(x2)	(x4)	(x4)

Cool-down   Total body stretch sequence (*see page 48*)

lateral raise

Workout 3   Workout time 45 mins (5 mins Warmup + 35 mins Exercise sequence + 5 mins Cool-down)

Warmup   5 mins aerobic exercise, gradually raising heart rate

	beginner	**intermediate**	**advanced**
Walk/run	6mins@75%MHR	8mins@75%MHR	10mins@75%MHR
Pec fly	15rm	15rm	15rm
Leg extension	15rm	15rm	15rm
Lat pull-down	15rm	15rm	15rm
Leg curl	15rm	15rm	15rm
Cycle	6mins@75%MHR	8mins@75%MHR	10mins@80%MHR
Pec fly	15rm	15rm	15rm
Leg extension	15rm	15rm	15rm
Lat pull-down	15rm	15rm	15rm
Leg curl	15rm	15rm	15rm
Row	1100yd(1000m)@ 75%MHR	1600yd(1500m)@ 75%MHR	2700yd(2500m)@ 80%MHR
Shoulder press	15rm	15rm	15rm
Lunge with ball	15 each leg	20 each leg	25 each leg
Dips	15	20	25
Bicep curl barbell	15rm	15rm	15rm
Repeat the 4 resistance exercises above			

Cool-down   Total body stretch sequence (*see page 48*)

cycling

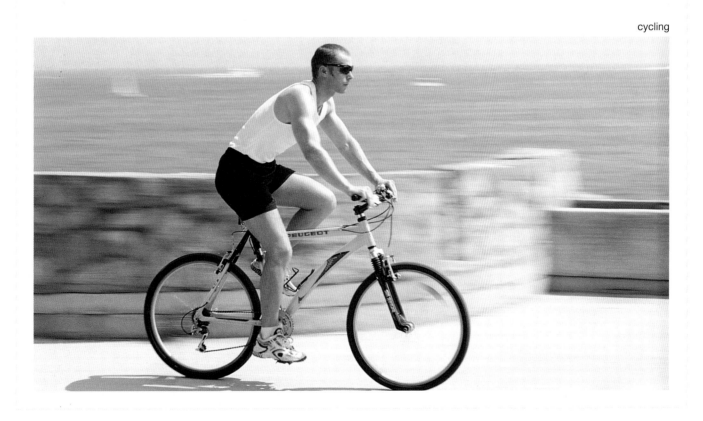

women's general fitness

You may not have a specific fitness goal in mind, or perhaps you have just completed another program; just because you aren't working toward a particular goal doesn't mean that you don't want to stay in shape and healthy. This program will help you in your "maintenance" time, however long that may be.

Benefits

builds strength / tones muscles ✓✓

burns fat / builds aerobic capacity ✓✓

increases flexibility ✓✓

how the program works

The wonderful thing about fitness is that once you have reached a certain level, maintaining it is relatively easy. This program works all the major muscle groups and tests your heart and lungs regularly and to a significant enough level to keep body fat low while also maintaining muscle tone. The exercises target and tone typical problem areas for women, namely the stomach, hips, butt, thighs, and the tops of the arms. This is a good program to move on to after compling the postnatal program (*see pages 186–7*), or if you have just achieved a fitness goal such as running a marathon, for example.

The program consists of three workouts. Aim to work out three to four times a week. Do workouts 1, 2, and 3 once each week, and repeat one of the workouts for your fourth training session. Always repeat a different workout each week, so you introduce variety into your exercise routine and continue to challenge the body.

Follow my nutritional guidelines (*see page 24–37*) alongside this program to help control your weight and keep you feeling fit and healthy.

setting goals

Although you don't have a clear goal to work toward in this program, you still need to monitor your progress. Rather than weighing yourself, take circumference measurements of your chest, waist, hips, arms, and legs. Remeasure yourself regularly to ensure that you maintain your shape and that your body is continuing to be challenged by the program. The danger with a maintenance program is that you settle into the routine and stop pushing yourself to work harder.

▶ **keep working at it**
You may not have a clear goal in mind, but it's still important to challenge the body, and enjoy yourself while doing it.

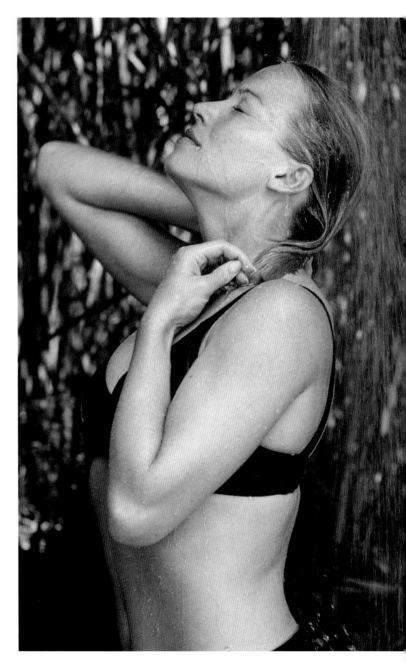

Exercise library

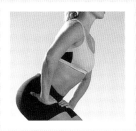

Squat
p108

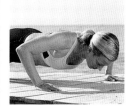

Push-up
p85

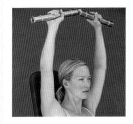

Walking lunge with
ball *p107*

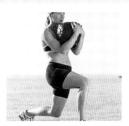

Shoulder press
p88

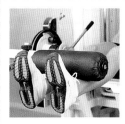

Leg extension
p110

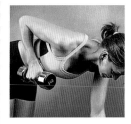

Single arm row
p91

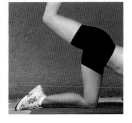

Glute raise
p113

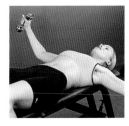

Pec fly
p82

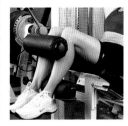

Leg curl
p111

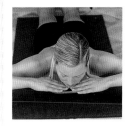

Back extension
p95

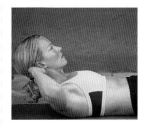

Basic crunch
p102

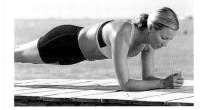

Bridge
p105

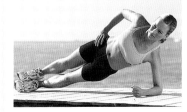

Oblique bridge
p105

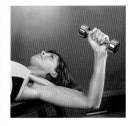

Chest press
p83

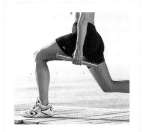

Lunge
p106

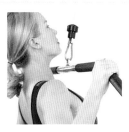

Lat pull-down
p90

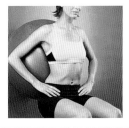

Ball squat
p108

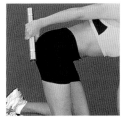

Tricep extension
p101

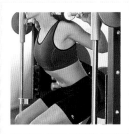

Leg press
p111

the programs

Workout 1

Workout time 55 mins (5mins Warmup + 35mins Exercise sequence + 5mins Cool-down + 10mins stretch)

Warmup	5 mins aerobic exercise, gradually raising heart rate		

Aerobic exercise	beginner	intermediate	advanced
Cycle	5mins@80%MHR	8mins@85%MHR	12mins@85%MHR
Run/walk	8mins@80%MHR,	10mins@85%MHR,	12mins@85%MHR,
X-train	1min@80%MHR.	1min@85%MHR.	1min@90%MHR.
	1 min rest	1 min rest	1 min rest
	(x5	(x6)	(x6)
Walk with gradient	10mins@75%MHR	8mins@80%MHR	5mins@85–90%MHR
Row	550yd(500m)	800yd(750m)	1100yd(1000m)
Run	660yd(600m)@80%MHR	800yd(750m)@85%MHR	1100yd(1000m) as fast as possible

Cool-down	5 mins slow walking to gradually lower heart rate
Stretch	Total body stretch sequence (*see page 48*)

Workout 2

Workout time 50 mins (5 mins Warmup + 35 mins Exercise sequence + 10 mins Cool-down)

Warmup	5 mins aerobic exercise, gradually raising heart rate

For the following exercises, select a weight that works the muscles to near fatigue in the time period specified; rest for 30 seconds after each exercise.

Exercise sequence	beginner	intermediate	advanced
Squat	30 secs	45 secs	60 secs
Push-up	30 secs	45 secs	60 secs
Walking lunge with ball	30 secs	45 secs	60 secs
Shoulder press	30 secs	45 secs	60 secs
Leg extension	30 secs	45 secs	60 secs
Single arm row	30 secs	45 secs	60 secs
Glute raise	30 secs each leg	45 secs each leg	60 secs each leg
Pec fly	30 secs	45 secs	60 secs
Leg curl	30 secs	45 secs	60 secs
Repeat the 9 exercises above	(x3)	(x5)	(x5–6)
Back extension	20	20	30
Basic crunch	25	40	50
Bridge	–	30	60
Oblique bridge	–	30 secs	60 secs
Repeat the 4 exercises above	(x2)	(x4)	(x4)

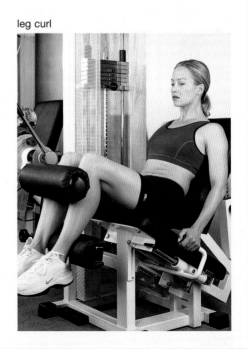

leg curl

Cool-down	5 mins slow walking to gradually lower heart rate
Stretch	Total body stretch sequence (*see page 48*)

Workout 3

Workout time 50 mins (5 mins Warmup + 35 mins Exercise sequence + 10 mins Cool-down)

Warmup   5 mins aerobic exercise, gradually raising heart rate

Exercise sequence	beginner	intermediate	advanced
Walk/run	6mins@75%MHR	8mins@75%MHR	10mins@75%MHR
Chest press	15rm	15rm	15rm
Lunge	15rm each leg	15rm each leg	15rm each leg
Lat pull-down	15rm	15rm	15rm
Ball squat	15rm	15rm	15rm
Cycle	6mins@75%MHR	6mins@75%MHR	10mins@80%MHR
Chest press	15rm	15rm	15rm
Lunge	15rm each leg	15rm each leg	15rm each leg
Lat pull-down	15rm	15rm	15rm
Ball squat	15rm	15rm	15rm
Row	1100yd(1000m)@75%MHR	1600yd(1500m)@75%MHR	2200yd(2000m)@80%MHR
Shoulder press	15rm	15rm	15 rm
Glute raise	15 each leg	20 each leg	25 each leg
Tricep extension	10rm	15rm	20
Leg press	15rm	15rm	15rm
Repeat the 4 resistance exercises above			

Cool-down   Total body stretch sequence (*see page 48*)

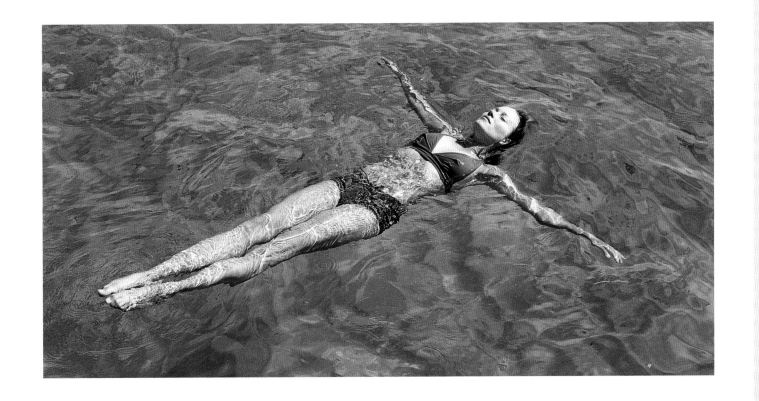

tennis fitness

I am often asked if playing tennis is enough to stay in shape, but it really depends on the level of tennis a person plays, how often they play, and whether they play singles or doubles. I usually answer that tennis is a great sport to play, but you should be fit to play it, you shouldn't play it to get fit. This program will improve your fitness and strength – and your game.

Benefits
builds strength / tones muscles ✓✓
burns fat / builds aerobic capacity ✓✓
increases flexibility ✓

Exercise library

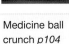
Cycle *pp68–9*/ run *64–7*/ X-train *70–71*

Row *pp70–71*

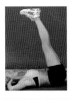
Chest press *p83*

Seated row *p94*

Pec fly *p82*

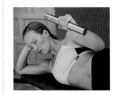
Straight arm pull-down *p94*

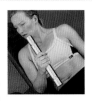
Lateral raise *p86*

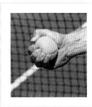
Dips *p98*

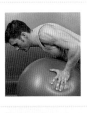
Ball push-up *p85*

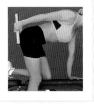
Bicep curl *p96*

Tricep extension *p101*

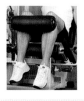
Leg extension *p110*

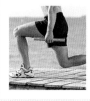
Leg curl *p111*

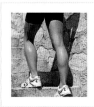
Power lunge *p106*

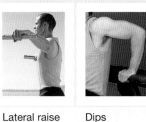
Step-ups *p109*

Leg press *p111*

Lunge *p106*

Forearm front *(see opp.)*

Forearm back *(see opp.)*

Oblique bridge *p105*

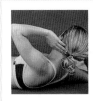
Oblique crunch *p104*

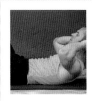
Basic crunch *p102*

Medicine ball crunch *p104*

Reverse curl *p103*

Raised reverse curl *p103*

Bridge *p105*

Outward rotator cuff *p93*

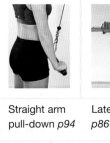
Inward rotator cuff *p93*

Ball squeeze *(see right)*

forearm front *strengthens wrist and forearm stroke*

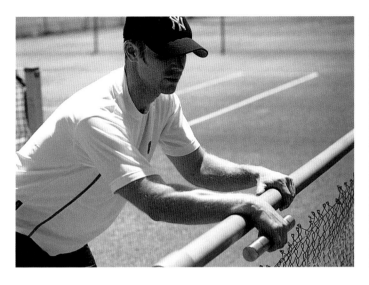

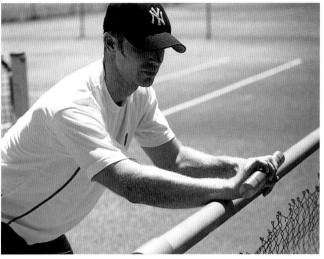

1 ▲ Hold a weight in your hand. Place your arm on a rail or bench so the underside of your wrist is supported and your forearm is parallel to the ground. Relax your wrist so your hand drops down.

2 ▲ Using the muscles in your forearm to control the movement, raise the weight as high as possible. Hold for 2 seconds, then return to the start position. Repeat on other side.

forearm back *strengthens forearm*

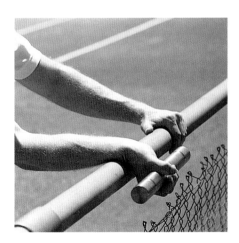

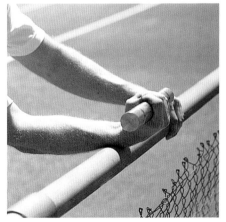

ball squeeze
strengthens grip

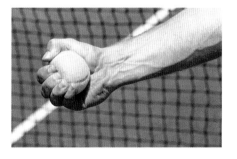

1 ▲ Hold a weight in your hand. Place your arm on a rail or bench so the top of your wrist is supported and your forearm is parallel to the ground. Relax your wrist so your wrist joint opens up.

2 ▲ Using only the muscles in your forearm, raise the weight to the highest point possible. Hold for 2 seconds, then return to the start position. Repeat on the other side.

▲ Hold a tennis ball firmly in your hand. Squeeze it, hold for 2 seconds, then release for 2 seconds. Repeat.

the aim

This program is suitable for anyone who plays tennis, regardless of the level of your game. The aim is to bring your fitness up to a level that will help improve your game, give more strength and power to your strokes, and prevent any tennis injuries.

aerobic fitness

A good game of tennis can go on for as long as four hours. The nature of the game means that it stops and starts and involves short bursts of energy and short periods of rest. You need to be flexible, able to move around the court quickly, and able to change direction quickly as well. A good tennis training program should prepare you for this long energy requirement and build stamina as well as endurance.

muscular strength

You also need a good level of strength in your core postural muscles – the erector spinae and the abdominals – as both the forehand and backhand strokes require balance, which comes from the trunk of the body. The forehand stroke requires strength from the shoulders, chest, and arms; while the backhand stroke requires strength through the rear shoulder, back, forearms, upper arms, and thighs. A good serve requires strength in nearly all of the muscles of the upper body.

The most common tennis-related injuries affect the elbows, lower back, knees and shoulders. An effective tennis training program needs to build strength in all of these muscles and take all of the physical demands that a game makes on a player into consideration.

using the program

The program is divided into three workouts, each one to be performed once a week, so you work out three times a week. The workouts provide you with a good aerobic workout to build your cardiovascular strength, while also building strength in the relevant muscles, which helps to reduce your risk of injury. Over the weeks, work on improving the speed at which you perform the exercises, and increase your weights as you progress.

Workout 1   Workout time 60 mins (5 mins Warmup + 45 mins Exercise sequence + 10 mins Cool-down)

Warmup	5 mins aerobic exercise, gradually raising heart rate		
Exercise sequence	**beginner**	**intermediate**	**advanced**
Cycle/run/X-train	1min@80%MHR, 2mins@65%MHR. (x5)	1min@80%MHR, 1min@65%MHR. (x7)	1min@80%MHR, 1min@70%MHR. (x10)
Row	550yd (500m)	550yd (500m)	550yd (500m)
Cycle/run/X-train	1min@80%MHR, 2mins@65%MHR. (x5)	1min@80%MHR, 1min@65%MHR. (x5)	1min@80%MHR, 1min@70%MHR. (x7)
Row	550yd (500m)	800yd (750m)	1100yd (1000m)
Chest press	16rm	16rm	16rm
Seated row	16rm	16rm	16rm
Pec fly	–	16rm	16rm
Straight arm pull-down	–	16rm	16rm
Lateral raise	15rm	15rm	15rm
Dips	15	20	20
Ball push-ups	–	10	15
Bicep curl (dumbbell)	16rm	16rm	16rm
Tricep extension	16rm	16rm	16rm
Cool-down	Total body stretch sequence (*see page 48*)		

Workout 2   Workout time 55 mins (5 mins Warmup + 40 mins Exercise sequence + 10 mins Cool-down)

Warmup   5 mins aerobic exercise, gradually raising heart rate

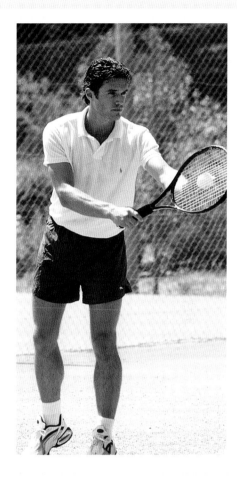

Exercise sequence	beginner	intermediate	advanced
Cycle	5mins@75%MHR	5mins@80%MHR	5mins@80%MHR
Leg extension	20rm	20rm	20rm
Chest press	16rm	16rm	16rm
Leg curl	16rm	16rm	16rm
Run/walk	6mins@75%MHR	6mins@80%MHR	6mins@80%MHR
Power lunge	15 each leg	20 each leg	20 each leg
Seated row	16rm	16rm	16rm
Step-ups	15 each leg	20 each leg	20 each leg
Row	550yd (500m)	800yd (750m)	1100yd (1000m)
Leg press	15rm	15rm	15rm
Dips	15	20	25
Lunge	15rm each leg	15rm each leg	15rm each leg
Run/walk	10mins@70%MHR	10mins@75%MHR	10mins@75–80%MHR
Forearm front	20rm	20rm	20rm
Forearm back	20rm	20rm	20rm
Oblique bridge	–	30 secs	45 secs
Oblique crunch	15	15	20
Basic crunch	15	20	20
Medicine ball crunch	–	–	15
Reverse curl	10	15	20
Raised reverse curl	–	–	15
Bridge	30 secs	45 secs	60 secs

Cool-down   Total body stretch sequence (*see page 48*)

Workout 3   Workout time 65 mins (5 mins Warmup + 40–50 mins Exercise sequence + 10 mins Cool-down)

Warmup   5 mins aerobic exercise, gradually raising heart rate

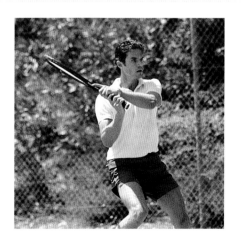

Exercise sequence	beginner	intermediate	advanced
Cycle/run/X-train/walk	30mins@ 75%MHR	35mins@ 75%MHR	45mins@ 75–80%MHR
Outward rotator cuff	20rm	20rm	20rm
Inward rotator cuff	20rm	20rm	20rm
Forearm front	20rm	20rm	20rm
Forearm back	20rm	20rm	20rm
Ball squeeze	20 (x2)	30 (x2)	40 (x2)

Cool-down   Total body stretch sequence (*see page 48*)

the programs

golf fitness

Most golfers want to be able to hit the ball farther and with more control. Good upper body strength will improve your swing and reduce the likelihood of back injury. Use this program in conjuction with a general fitness program (*see pages 156–63*).

Benefits
builds strength/tones muscles ✓✓
burns fat/builds aerobic capacity
increases flexibility ✓✓

Golf exercises Workout time 20 mins (5 mins Warmup + 10 mins Exercise sequence + 5 mins Cool-down)

Warmup   5 mins aerobic exercise, gradually raising heart rate

Exercise sequence   Repetition maximums (rm) and repetitions for each exercise are shown in this order of fitness level: beginner / intermediate / advanced

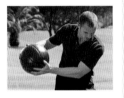
Medicine ball swing
(*see right*)
15/20/30

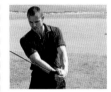
X-tube pull-down
(*see right*)
15/20/30

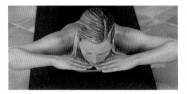
Back extension *p95*
15/20/25

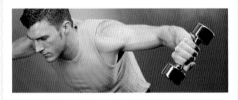
Reverse fly *p90*
15/15/15 rm

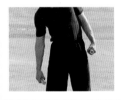
Side bend (*see right*)
15/15/15 rm

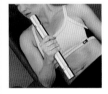
Inward rotator cuff
p93 15/15/15 rm

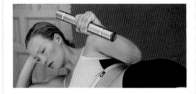
Outward rotator cuff *p93*
15/15/15 rm

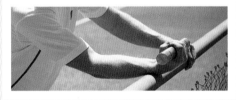
Forearm strength *p165*
15/15/15 rm

Cool-down   Golf stretch (*see below*)

Golf stretch Perform this 5-minute stretch sequence to loosen the muscles prior to a game of golf or as a cool-down after the exercise sequence above. Hold times are suggested minimums.

Back *p44*
20 secs hold

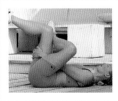
Glutes *p46*
20 secs hold

Spine rotation
p45 10 secs hold

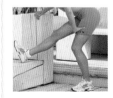
Hamstring stretch
p46 20 secs hold

Quads *p46*
15 secs hold

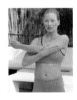
Shoulders *p42*
15 secs hold

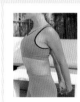
Chest *p43*
15 secs hold

medicine ball swing
for swing control

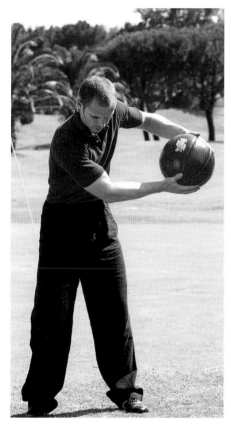

◄ ▼ Stand with feet shoulder-width apart, knees slightly bent. Hold the medicine ball with both hands in front of you and lean forward slightly. Swing the ball to the left until your rear arm is at shoulder height. Hold for 1 second, then swing slowly to the right and hold for 1 second. Repeat.

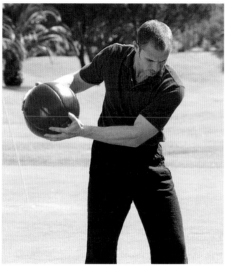

side bend
for postural strength

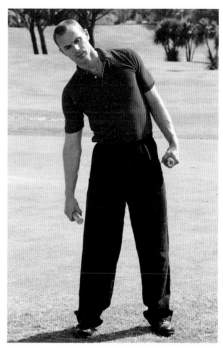

▲ Stand with arms by sides, a weight in each hand. Lower the weight down toward the knee. Use the obliques to pull the body back up. Repeat on other side.

X-tube pull-down *for swing strength*

▶ Tie an X-tube to a tree or pole slightly higher than shoulder height. Stand with feet hip-width apart, knees slightly bent, as if about to perform a golf swing.

▶▶ Hold the handle with both hands and, keeping your back straight, pull the tube across the front of the body. Slowly return to the start position. Repeat on the other side. Alternatively, use the cable machine at the gym to perfrom this exercise.

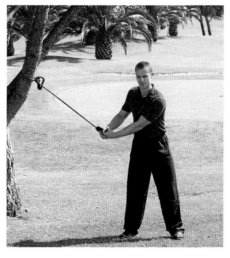

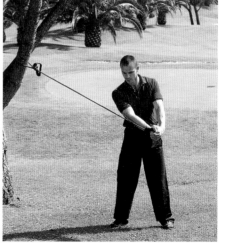

skiing fitness

For many of us skiing is a sport that we take part in once a year for a week or two, at most. Often it isn't until we hit the slopes, and are reminded of how physically demanding skiing is, that we suddenly wonder why we haven't done some special training in preparation. This program will make you a stronger skiier and, as a result, reduce your risk of injury on the slopes.

Benefits

builds strength / tones muscles ✓✓

burns fat / builds aerobic capacity ✓✓

increases flexibility ✓

how the program works

Ideally, you should start this program at least four weeks before going skiiing; but the earlier you start, the stronger and more physically prepared you will be. The program consists of two workouts to be done at the gym three times a week. Each week, do workout 1 twice and workout 2 once. If you want to train four times a week, add another workout 2 to your schedule. The program will help to strengthen the major muscles used for skiing, in particular the muscles that support the knee. It will also build stamina so you'll be able to work at a high intensity for short bursts – like when you meet a difficult section of a slope – and still recover quickly.

Workout 1   Workout time 55 mins (5 mins Warmup + 45 mins Exercise sequence + 5 mins Cool-down)

Warmup	5 mins aerobic exercise, gradually raising heart rate
Exercise sequence	Repetition maximums (rm) or repetitions for each exercise are shown in this order of fitness level: beginner / intermediate / advanced

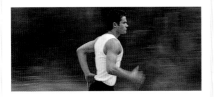 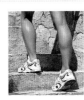 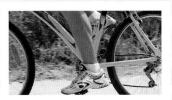

Walk *pp60–3*/run *pp64–7*
1min@80%MHR, 2mins@70%MHR (x5)/
2mins@80%MHR, 2mins@70%MHR (x5)/
2mins@80%MHR, 1min@rest (x7)

Ball squat *p108*
20/20/20 rm

Leg curl *p111*
15/15/15 rm

Step-ups *p109*
15/15/20 each leg

Cycle *pgs68–9*/X-train *pgs70–71*
1min@80%MHR, 2mins@70% (x4)/
2mins@80%MHR, 2mins@70% (x4)/
2mins@85%MHR, 1min@rest (x7)

     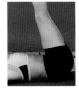

Leg extension *p110*
15/15/15 rm

Knee raise *p110*
10/15/20 each leg

Static squat *p108*
20/40/60 secs hold

Power lunge *p106*
10 (x2)/15 (x2)/
20 (x3) each leg

Basic crunch
p102
10/15/20

Reverse curl
p103
10/15/20

Oblique crunch
p104
10/15/20

Cool-down	Lower body stretch sequence (*see page 49*)

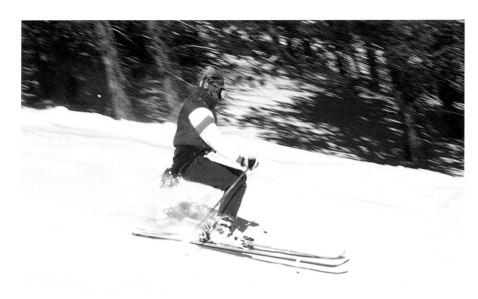

Nutrition tips

As much as possible, eat low glycemic alkaline foods (*see pages 34–5*).

Breakfast

Have a good breakfast of low/medium glycemic foods to give you energy through your morning skiing and take you up to lunchtime. Try hot cereal, wheat-free muesli (*see page 36*), or wholemeal toast.

Drink lots

Try to keep yourself well hydrated on the slopes. Water is not always the most appealing drink on a cold day skiing, however it is still important to keep fluid levels high.

◀ **fit for the slopes**
Work out before you go skiing and last longer on the slopes.

Workout 2

Workout time 55 mins (5 mins Warmup + 40 mins Exercise sequence + 10 mins Cool-down)

Warmup	5 mins aerobic exercise, gradually raising heart rate
Exercise sequence	Repetition maximums (rm) or repetitions for each exercise are shown in this order of fitness level: beginner / intermediate / advanced

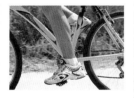

Aerobic exercise *pp50–73*
20mins@70%MHR/
25mins@75%MHR/
30mins@75%MHR

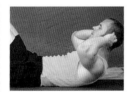

Basic crunch *p102*
10/15/20

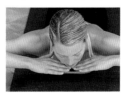

Back extension *p95*
10/15/20

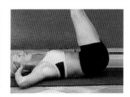

Reverse curl *p103*
10/15/20

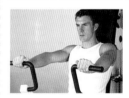

Chest press *p83*
15(x2)/15(x3)/15(x3) rm

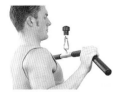

Lat pull-down *p90*
15 (x2)/15 (x3)/15 (x3) rm

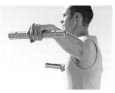

Lateral raise *p86*
15 (x2)/15 (x3)/15 (x3) rm

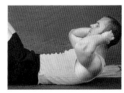

Basic crunch *p102*
10/15/20

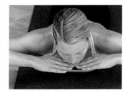

Back extension *p95*
10/15/20

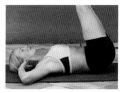

Reverse curl *p103*
10/15/20

Cool-down	Total body stretch sequence (*see page 48*)

sports agility and power

Whether you play a sport for fun or at a serious level, there are two factors that affect your performance and risk of sustaining an injury. Agility, your ability to move around quickly and nimbly, and power, the force or strength you can put behind a movement. Any skilled athlete will take time to hone these skills, since they can be the difference between winning and losing.

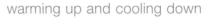

Benefits

builds strength / tones muscles ✓✓

burns fat / builds aerobic capacity ✓

increases flexibility ✓

power and agility in sport

Most sports require power in some degree, but many athletes don't concentrate on this aspect of sport as a skill that can be worked on and improved. The need for power is obvious in some sports – a sprinter, for example, relies on power to get her to the finish line. But even sports such as golf and tennis require power. Tiger Woods has a powerful swing; as a result he can hit the ball farther than anyone else. By putting power behind their serves, tennis players can often hit the ball at speeds of over 140 miles (225km) per hour.

Good agility is probably one of the main reasons why some people succeed as sportspeople while others fail. Agility on the sports field is crucial to success. You may not be the fastest or the most skillful, but if you are agile, you give yourself a strong advantage. Good agility is obvious in gymnasts, but it's also impressive in sports such as basketball

and tennis. Agility helped Michael Jordan to dominate the basketball court for a decade. In tennis, Andre Aggasi's agility means he can return a serve where others might not be able to, and reach a ball quickly, wherever it lands on the court.

Power and agility go hand in hand and can certainly produce astonishing improvements in performance if you take the trouble to work on them.

how the program works

The first five exercises work on your speed and power and will help you to produce dynamic movement. The last two drills will help your mobility and agility. You can perform all of the exercises in a circuit, or choose particular exercises that improve skills needed for a specific sport. The aim of these exercises is to make you the powerhouse of your team or to make you individually awesome when playing your sport.`

warming up and cooling down

Before performing any of these exercises or drills, warm up by doing 8 to12 minutes of aerobic exercise (*see pages 50–73*). It's important to warm up thoroughly as these are intensive exercises where the muscles have to work very hard. Follow the warmup with the standing stretch sequence (*see page 49*).

At the end of your workout, cool down gradually for 6 to 10 minutes by jogging slowly or walking. Then repeat the standing stretch sequence as your cool-down stretch. Hold each stretch for 20 to 30 seconds.

a word of caution

These are high-impact exercises. They should be performed on a shock absorbent surface such as a football field or grass in order to protect the joints. Wear shoes with high shock absorbency and good support.

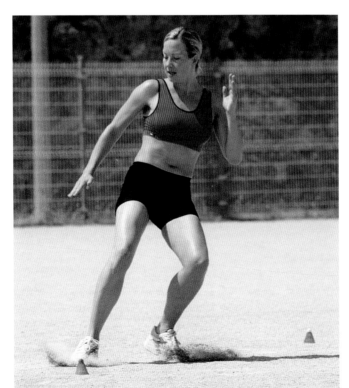

distance bounding
for all team sports, sprinting, gymnastics

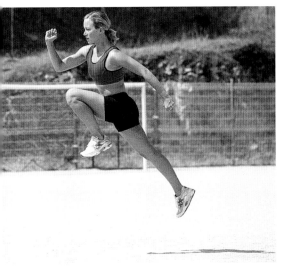

◀ **A power-building exercise** for sprinters, it can help to improve stride power when sprinting at full speed. The action is a little like overstriding when running. Place markers at the start and finish points, and distance bound the specified distances. From a standing start, leap forward, exaggerating the length of your stride and making it as long as possible. The best sprinters can achieve bounding stride lengths of up to nearly 13ft (4m) compared to their maximum sprint stride length of more like 8–10ft (2.5–3m). Try to "hang" in the air to achieve length as you stride.

	intermediate	advanced
Distance	100–130ft (30–40m)	165–200ft (50–60m)
No of lengths	8–10	15–20
Rest between lengths	30 secs	30 secs

depth jumps
for tennis, track and field, basketball, volleyball

▼ **Good for creating explosive power,** this exercise helps you to move away from a point quickly and improves acceleration. Stand on a step, or a box or bench about 20–24in (50–60cm) high. Jump down from the step or bench, making sure to land evenly, on both feet. Bend your knees to help shock absorption, but no lower than about 90 degrees. When you land, spring back up as high as you can and land in the same way. Get back onto the step or bench and repeat the exercise. Minimize the amount of time your feet spend on the ground.

	intermediate	advanced
No of reps	15	25
Rest	90 secs	60 secs
No of sets	5	8–10

vertical bounding
for basketball, track and field, soccer

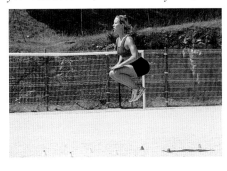

◀ **This exercise develops the power** in your jump, but it will also help to improve acceleration. Line up markers with approximately 3ft (1m) distance between them. Start with markers, then progress to low hurdles (collapsible ones are safest) as you improve. Bound over each marker, keeping your feet together and your back straight. Use your abdominals to lift your knees to your chest as you jump. Aim to get as much height as possible. If you have to stop or pause, start again.

	intermediate	advanced
No of hurdles	6–8	8–10
No of reps	5	6–8
Rest between sets	2 mins	3 mins
No of sets	3	4

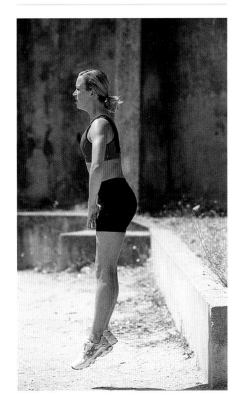

overhead throw
for tennis, golf, soccer, field events

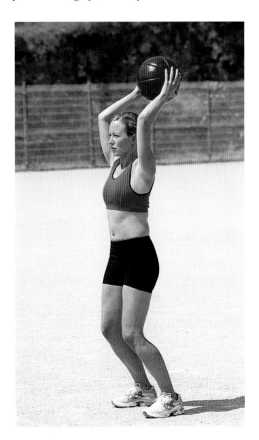

▲ **A great power builder** for the upper body, the overhead throw is great training for most sports. You need a partner who can throw the ball back to you; stand 5ft (1.5m) apart, but progress to 7–10ft (2–3m) apart as you get stronger. Stand with feet hip-width apart and parallel, or position one foot slightly forward for stability. Hold the ball up and slightly behind your head with elbows slightly bent. Use an overhead throw similar to a soccer "throw-in" to pass the ball to your partner. Straighten your arms as you bring the ball up above your head, and put as much power behind your throw as possible (this will concentrate work on the triceps). Release the ball when it is just forward of your head.

	intermediate		advanced	
	Men	Women	Men	Women
Weight of ball	9lb (4kg)	6lb (3kg)	13lb (6kg)	9lb (4kg)
No of throws	20	20	20	20
Rest between sets	60 secs	60 secs	30 secs	30 secs
No of sets	4	4	6	6

rotational throw
for tennis, golf, rugby

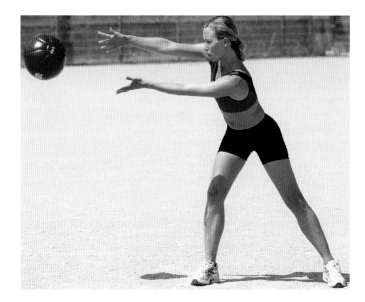

▲ **This exercise builds strength** for upper body rotational movements. You need a partner who can throw the ball back to you. Your partner should stand alongside you, about 7–10ft (2–3m) away. Stand with feet just wider than shoulder-width apart for stability, and hold the ball in front of you with both hands. Keeping your arms straight, bring the ball up to one side until it is level with your shoulder (as if you were performing the first phase of a golf swing). Then bring the ball down and across your body, and throw the ball sideways to your partner. Use the rotational movement to put as much power behind the throw as possible.

	intermediate		advanced	
	Men	Women	Men	Women
Weight of ball	11lb (5kg)	9lb (4kg)	16lb (7.5kg)	11lb (5kg)
No of throws	20	20	20	20
Rest between sets	1 min	30 secs	30 secs	30 secs
No of sets	4	4	6	6

around the clock

for all team sports and racket sports

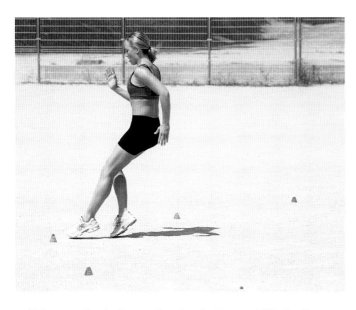

▲ **This exercise helps to develop better mobility** in all directions and will vastly improve your reaction time. Use markers to indicate the numbers of an imaginary clock face on the ground with a radius of 13–20ft (4–6 meters). Mark the central point of the clock. You need a partner who can shout out instructions to you. Start in the middle of the clock, facing the upper half of the clock face (make sure you face this way at all times). Your partner shouts out numbers between 1 and 12 representing the numbers of the clock, and you must run to the number and then back to the start position as quickly as possible. Run straight forward to numbers 10, 11, 12, 1, and 2; stride sideways to numbers 3, 4, 8, and 9; and run backward to number 5, 6, and 7. Your partner can penalize you with 10 push-ups if you fail to use the correct procedure. You can alter the radius of the circle to suit your sport. For example, a badminton player's radius of movement is less than a tennis player's or a soccer player's.

	beginner	intermediate	advanced
Time	45 secs	60 secs	60 secs
Rest between sets	2 mins	60 secs	60 secs
Reps	4	8	10–12

shuttle runs

for all team sports and racket sports

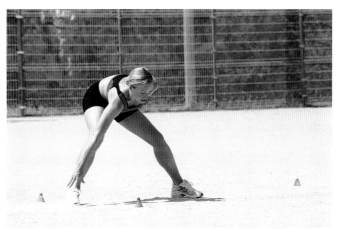

▲ **Use shuttle runs to improve agility and speed.** Measure out a 60ft (20 meter) lane and place 5 markers at 12ft (4 meter) intervals along it. You can do this exercise in 3 ways, i) facing forward at all times, ii) facing forward to run one direction and backward to return, iii) sideways, using side strides. Or combine the three styles, depending on the sport you are training for. Run to the first marker, then run back to the start. Then run to the second marker, and run back to the start. Repeat this for all the markers. As you become more advanced, try using medicine balls as markers and as resistance for this drill. You will need 5 medicine balls of different weights: 4lb (2kg), 9lb (4kg), 13lb (6kg), 18lb (8kg) and 22lb (10kg). You can also use medicine balls of the same weight. Place the heaviest ball closest to you and the lightest farthest away. Run to the first ball, pick it up, and bring it back to the start line. Do the same for the remaining balls until all are at the start line. Run as fast as possible between the markers or balls, and use speed on your turns to improve your agility.

	beginner	intermediate	advanced
No of sets	4	6	8
Rest between sets	2 mins	90 secs	60 secs

jo

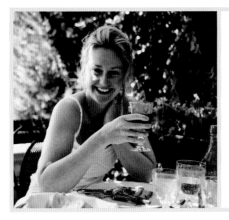

vital statistics

age **31**

profession **magazine comissioning editor**

height **5ft 7in (1.72m)**

weight **140lb (63kg)**

body fat **29%**

dress size **10**

jo's goal

The decision to run the Berlin Marathon was easy, especially as I made it following several glasses of wine. At the time the vigorous exercise that running 26 miles entailed didn't look a problem. In the cold light of day I had to admit that the last "vigorous" exercise I did was at school, and that was over 15 years ago.

matt's assessment

Jo set the ultimate goal of running a marathon. For someone who had never run before, this was going to be a big undertaking.

The initial aim of the program was to strengthen her legs to prepare her for the intense training ahead, and also to reduce her risk of injury. We then worked on gradually building up her running time to prepare her for the actual event. I also suggested some alterations to Jo's diet to help cleanse her body and increase her energy levels.

the cool-down
Gentle stretching helps to ease any muscle tension after a run.

▶ week 1

The first time I meet Matt Roberts he explains what lies ahead in the four months of training. To start with he tests my blood, saliva, and urine, which makes me feel guilty. Will he be able to detect the litany of abuse I have put my body through? He's very polite and points out that I'd benefit from a detox diet. Caffeine-, alcohol-, and wheat-free, lots of fish and fruit and vegetables.

I go straight on to the running machine. We begin aerobic work in the gym and weight-training for my muscles and joints interspersed with running sessions outside.

Matt asks me how I'm feeling – I want to lie to him. I admit to some pains. I've had a terrible headache from detoxing, and it's mortifying to feel my flabby body flying around me.

▶ week 2

I suddenly have hard muscles. Scared I'm going to start looking like a Russian shot putter. I haven't lost any weight, but Matt reassures me it will drop off later.

▶ weeks 3–4

Each time we meet he increases the intensity of the session, and it's *never* easy.

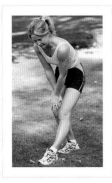
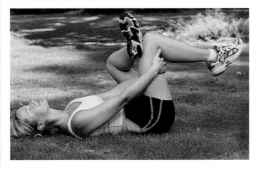
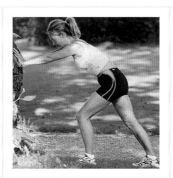
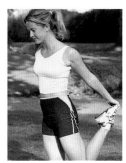

But I've started looking forward to the sessions the night before. It's knowing that I can do the running, and that I'll feel good afterward. I have newfound energy, I'm much more awake, and I still haven't run farther than four miles. But I have to admit to having food fantasies about melted mozzarella and chocolate.

▶ weeks 4–7

Go for the first run on my own. Something I have *never* done before. I discover there's a world of runners out there I've never noticed before and suddenly I'm one of them. By week 7 I've lost seven pounds, my clothes are too big, and people compliment me on how I look. I can run for one and a half hours now, just three times that is the

marathon. My heart rate stays steady and low. Running is taking over my life – I've even got the right shoess.

▶ weeks 10–16

I can now run without thinking about it. Start running for two, then three hours –

even on my own. The longer distances are tough, my knees hurt and my lungs feel like they're about to burst. But I'm so far into the training now that I want it to be hard in order to know what I'm up against. I've put so much into it, I want to know if my no-longer badly abused body is up to it.

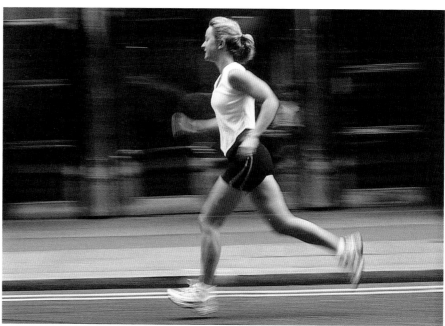

▼ ▶ start with shorter runs
Work up to the big event by gradually increasing the length of your runs.

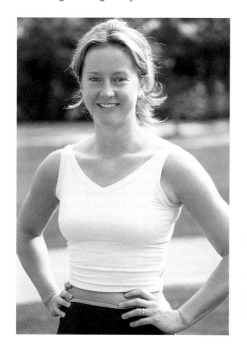

"I have newfound energy and I'm much more awake. Running is taking over my life."

marathon report

• Jo ran the Berlin marathon in 4 hours, 44 minutes, an excellent time for a first marathon.
• Having successfully completed a marathon, it's important to maintain a fitness routine afterward. Jo could follow the women's general or lunchtime programs.

vital statistics

weight **125lb (57kg)**
a loss of 13lb (6kg)

dress size **8**
a drop of one dress size

body fat **24%**
a loss of 5%

the programs

your first marathon

To complete a full marathon – 26 miles (42km) – or even a half marathon – 13 miles (21km) – is a great personal achievement. It is also very difficult, so it's important to approach the event with a comprehensive training program that allows your body enough time to prepare for the challenge. Allow at least four months to properly prepare for your first marathon.

Benefits

builds strength ✓

aerobic ✓✓✓

flexibility ✓

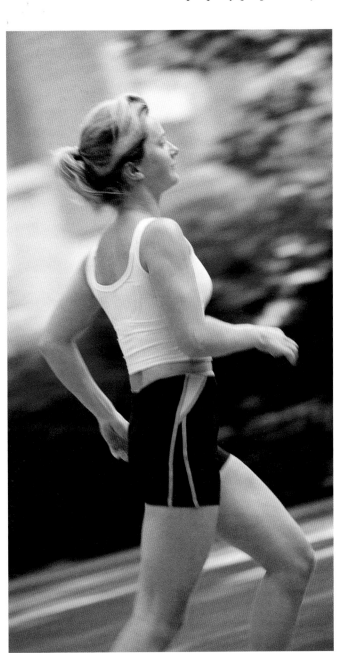

preparing for a marathon

You can never fully convey the mixture of joy, pride, relief, fatigue, and pain that comes with completing a marathon. After a first marathon, most people find that they're looking forward to the next one.

You should finish your first marathon feeling as strong and as well as possible. The aim is to run through the finishing line, not walk across it or fail to finish at all. To achieve this, you need a well planned and well structured training program that will adequately prepare your body for the challenge ahead. The most common mistake that people make when training for their first marathon is leaving their longest run to the day of the marathon itself. Very often, people do a lot of running in preparation, but over short distances. Even if you leave your long runs until a week or two before the marathon, you don't allow your body enough time to build up to the level of endurance required to run 26 miles (42km).

how the program works

This program builds muscle strength as well as aerobic endurance and speed. You start with short runs and work up to longer ones; I have also built in essential recovery time, which should never be overlooked. Training for a marathon is hard work, and there is always the risk of injury.

The program guides you day-by-day toward the main event and stretches over four months, the minimum amount of time you can allow yourself to prepare adequately for a marathon. Unless you are already in great shape, training for any less than this will make the marathon less than enjoyable.

◀ **run a marathon**
The program builds strength in the legs, then develops aerobic fitness. Start with shorter runs and build up to running longer distances.

pre-marathon tips

The program eases in pace as you approach the day of the marathon itself, but make sure you get plenty of rest in the week before the race.

It has long been the standard procedure to carbohydrate load by eating pasta – usually the white durum wheat variety – the night before a run, but this is not the best food to eat.

• There is some sense in eating carbohydrates as they are slow energy releasers, but try healthier options such as brown rice, wild rice, wholemeal pasta, or wheat-free pasta with a light noncreamy sauce.

• Drink plenty of water the night before – that way you won't need to drink as much in the morning. Finding toilets at marathon start lines can be very difficult.

the big day

If you have followed the program, your body should be in peak form and ready to meet the challenge ahead. The following tips will help you on the day of the marathon:

• Leave at least an hour and a half between breakfast and the start of the race. Have a bowl of hot cereal or wheat-free muesli made with oats. Add low glycemic fruits such as apples, pears, kiwis, and apricots, if desired.

• Drink a little water before you set off so your body is adequately hydrated, and drink lots of water during the marathon. Aim to drink water every couple of miles.

• Don't be taken along by the crowd at the starting line as you might start too fast and exhaust yourself early on, then struggle to finish the race; find your own pace.

after the marathon

You will need to replace lost energy and minimize muscle ache in the aftermath of the marathon. When you finish:

• Have an energy drink and a high glycemic snack such as bananas, pretzels, or hard candy to lift your energy levels.

• Stretch thoroughly at the end of the race. This will help prevent any unwanted muscle aches in the days that follow.

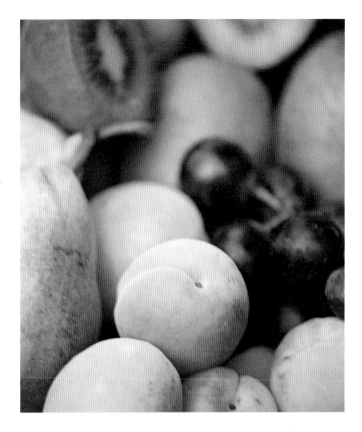

Nutrition tips

During your training period keep to the general nutrition guidelines (*see pages 24–37*). This program is very physically demanding, so you need to increase your calorie intake, but get them from healthy foods. Eat low glycemic foods such as fresh fruit and vegetables, grains, and beans (*see pages 34–5*).

Keep the body hydrated – aim to drink 2 quarts (2 liters) of water a day. Reduce or cut out the following drinks – most will only dehydrate the body:

● Tea
● Coffee
● Sugary drinks (be wary of drinks that pass themselves off as sports drinks)
● Alcohol (especially in the month before the marathon).

Increase your intake of fruit and vegetables high in vitamins A,C, and E as they contain anti-oxidants, which help to reduce toxin buildup in the body. Eat lots of the following:

● Noncitrus fruits such as strawberries, cherries, and pears.
● Brightly colored vegetables such as peppers, carrots, and eggplant.
● Green vegetables, especially broccoli, zucchini, and spinach.

Eat the following foods as they are high in essential fatty acids, which help protect joints:

● Oily fish, especially tuna, salmon, mackerel, and sea bass.
● Sunflower and pumpkin seeds, almonds and walnuts.

Replace energy lost while training in the 30 minutes after your workout. Eat low glycemic fruit such as apples and pears.

Your first marathon

Start each workout by doing 5 mins aerobic exercise (*see pages 50–73*) to raise the heart rate. Unless otherwise specified, finish with the lower body stretch sequence (*see page 49*) or the total body stretch sequence (*see page 48*).

Day	Exercise
Week one	
1	Workout 1, Week 3 from perfect legs program (*see page 143*) + aerobic exercise 30mins@65–70%MHR
2	Off
3	Aerobic exercise 30mins@70%MHR
4	Off
5	Workout 1, Week 3 from the perfect legs program (*see page 143*) + cycle or X-train 3mins@75%MHR, 2mins@65%MHR. (x5)
6	Off
7	Run or walk 30mins@70–75%MHR
Week two	
8	Off
9	Workout 1 from skiing fitness (*see page 170*) + total body stretch (*see page 48*)
10	Off
11	Cycle 30mins@75–80%MHR
12	Off
13	Workout 1 from skiing fitness (*see page 170*) + total body stretch (*see page 48*)
14	Off
Week three	
15	Run/fast walk 45mins@70%MHR
16	Off
17	Workout 1 from skiing fitness (*see page 170*) + total body stretch (*see page 48*)
18	Off
19	Aerobic exercise (not running) 35mins@75%MHR
20	Off
21	Workout 1 from skiing fitness (*see page 170*) + total body stretch (*see page 48*)
Week four	
22	Off
23	Run/fast walk 45mins@70%MHR
24	Off
25	Workout 1 from skiing fitness (*see page 170*) + total body stretch (*see page 48*)
26	Off
27	Off
28	Run 60mins@70%MHR

Day	Exercise
Week five	
29	Off
30	Workout 1, Week 3 from perfect legs program (*see 143*)
31	Run/fast walk 35mins@75–80%MHR
32	Off
33	Workout 1 from skiing fitness (*see page 170*) + total body stretch (*see page 48*)
34	Off
35	Run 60mins@70%MHR
Week six	
36	Off
37	Off
38	Aerobic exercise (not running or walking) 50mins@70%MHR
39	Off
40	Workout 1 from skiing fitness (*see page 170*) + total body stretch (*see page 48*)
41	Off
42	Run/fast walk 60mins@70%MHR
Week seven	
43	Off
44	Off
45	Workout 1 from skiing fitness (*see page 170*) + total body stretch (*see page 48*)
46	Off
47	Run 45mins@75%MHR
48	Off
49	Off
Week eight	
50	Run 60mins@70%MHR
51	Off
52	Aerobic exercise (not running) 45mins@75%MHR
53	Off
54	Workout 1 from skiing fitness (*see page 170*) + total body stretch (*see page 48*)
55	Off
56	Run 30mins@75%MHR
Week nine	
57	Off
58	Run/fast walk 2hours@70–75%MHR

Your first marathon
After every long run, take time to perform the total body stretch sequence (*see page 48*).

Day	Exercise
59	Off
60	Workout 1 from skiing fitness (*see page 170*) + total body stretch (*see page 48*)
61	Off
62	Aerobic exercise (not running) 45mins@75%MHR
63	Off

Week ten
Day	Exercise
64	Off
65	Run/fast walk 2hours@75%MHR
66	Off
67	Workout 1, Week 3 from perfect legs program (*see page 143*) + run 30mins@75–80%MHR
68	Off
69	Aerobic exercise (not running) 45mins@75%MHR
70	Off

Week eleven
Day	Exercise
71	Off
72	Run 60mins@70–75%MHR
73	Off
74	Aerobic exercise (not runnning) 60mins@70%MHR
75	Off
76	Aerobic exercise 5mins@85%MHR, 3mins@70%MHR. (x3)
77	Off

Week twelve
Day	Exercise
78	Run 5mins, walk 2mins for 16miles (25km)
79	Off
80	Off
81	Workout 1 from skiing fitness (*see page 170*) + total body stretch (*see page 48*)
82	Off
83	Run 60mins@70%MHR
84	Off

Week thirteen
Day	Exercise
85	Aerobic exercise (not running) 30mins@75–80%MHR
86	Off
87	Off
88	Run 2hours@70%MHR
89	Off
90	Off

Day	Exercise
91	Run 60mins@75%MHR
92	Off

Week fourteen
Day	Exercise
93	Off
94	Aerobic exercise (not running) 60mins@70–75%MHR
95	Off
96	Workout 1 from skiing fitness (*see page 170*) + total body stretch (*see page 48*)
97	Off
98	Off

Week fifteen
Day	Exercise
99	Off
100	Run 18miles (29km)@70–75%MHR
101	Off
102	Off
103	Off
104	Aerobic exercise (not running) 45mins@75%MHR
105	Off

Week sixteen to main event
Day	Exercise
106	Run 30mins@75–80%MHR
107	Off
108	Workout 1, Week 3 from perfect legs program (*see page 143*)
109	Off
110	Run 50mins@75%MHR
111	Off
112	Off
113	Run 30mins@75–80%MHR
114	Off
115	Off
116	Workout 1, Week 3 from perfect legs program (*see page 143*)
117	Off
118	Off
119	Run 30mins@70–75%MHR
120	Off
121	Off
122	Main Event

the programs

back care workout

Back problems are one of the top three reasons for days lost at work in the US and Europe. We spend more time sitting at desks and in front of computers, both of which hunch our bodies into unnatural positions. Often the back is the first place to feel the strain. The exercises in this program will help to strengthen your back muscles and prevent back problems.

Benefits

builds strength /tones muscles ✓✓
burns fat /builds aerobic capacity
increases flexibility ✓

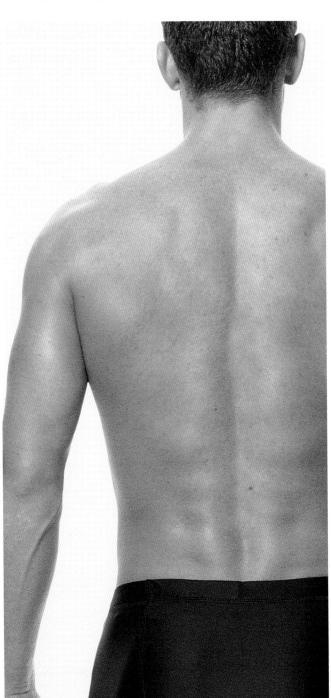

what causes back problems?

Back problems that gradually build up cause more problems than those that result from one poorly executed lift. Failing to bend your knees when lifting a heavy object can put your back out, but these days it's more likely to be sedentary workers who complain of back pain. Sitting at a desk for hours on end can put the body out of balance and cause long-term back problems. In the sitting position, muscles in the back are lengthened and the shoulders roll forward, while the hamstrings shorten and the abdominals become weak. These muscular imbalances can eventually cause the spine to curve, which creates points of weakness along the spine and resulting back pain.

Incorrect technique when performing exercises can also put unneccessary strain on the back and cause pain. Always try to keep the position of your back in mind whenever you exercise, and try to maintain good posture at all times.

If you are currently suffering from back pain, consult your doctor or a physiotherapist before starting this program.

how the program works

This simple 20-minute series of exercises targets the different muscles in the back. It can be performed three times a week as a quick workout on its own, or used once a week in conjunction with other programs to help improve posture and strengthen the lower back.

Note: When you are doing the seated row, reverse fly and lat pull-down for the second times, use a lighter weight since the muscles will be overloaded from performing the exercises the first time around.

◀ back to basics
Make a conscious effort to maintain good posture at all times, as this helps to prevent unnecessary strain on the back.

The workout

Workout time 20 mins (5 mins Warmup + 10 mins Exercise sequence + 5 mins Cool-down)

Warmup 5 mins aerobic exercise, gradually raising heart rate

Exercise sequence Repetition maximums (rm) or repetitions for each exercise are shown in this order of fitness level: beginner / intermediate / advanced

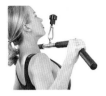

Lat pull-down *p90*
15/15/15 rm

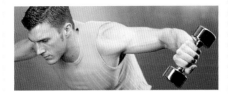

Reverse fly *p90*
15/15/15 rm

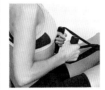

Seated row *p94*
15/15/15 rm

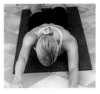

Dorsal raise *p95*
15/20/25 rm

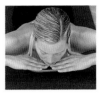

Back extension *p95*
10/15/20 rm

Reverse curl *p103*
10/15/20

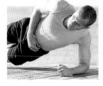

Oblique bridge *p105*
– /30/60 secs

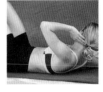

Oblique crunch *p104*
14 each side / – / –

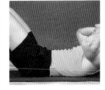

Basic crunch *p102*
10/15/20 all slow

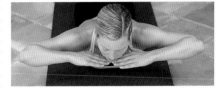

Back extension *p95*
10/15/20

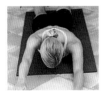

Dorsal raise *p95*
15/20/25

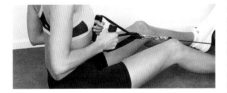

Seated row *p94*
15/15/15 rm

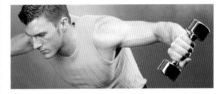

Reverse fly *p90*
15/15/15 rm

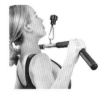

Lat pull-down *p90*
15/15/15 rm

Cool-down Total body stretch sequence (*see page 48*)

back extension

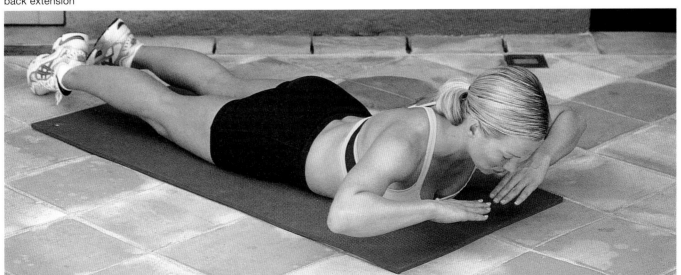

prenatal program

At one of the most physically trying times in a woman's life, fitness and health couldn't be more important. For many years the standard advice given to pregnant women was to do nothing for nine months. Now we know that women who exercise in pregnancy often feel more physically prepared for the birth – and tend to recover more quickly after it.

Benefits
builds strength / tones muscles ✓
burns fat / builds aerobic capacity ✓✓
increases flexibility ✓

how the program works

This program will help you to keep your energy levels up during your pregnancy and help to prevent excessive weight gain. It will also help you to maintain a good, strong posture as well as minimizing swelling and circulatory problems.

The program consists of one workout for each trimester. Aim to work out two to three times a week, but five times a week maximum. In the second and third trimesters, exercises should be performed sitting down where possible (with the exception of the glute raise, which should be performed standing), as this helps control blood pressure. Don't overheat; don't work at more than 70 percent of your maximum heart rate.

The key to exercising when pregnant is to listen to your body. If you experience any discomfort while working out, stop immediately. I advise against using the leg curl and leg extension machines during pregnancy as they can raise blood pressure, which may reduce blood flow to the fetus. Seek advice from your doctor before embarking on this program.

1st trimester Workout time 50 mins (5 mins Warmup + 40 mins Exercise sequence + 5 mins Cool-down)

Warmup	5 mins aerobic exercise, gradually raising heart rate

Aerobic exercise	all levels
Cycle	5mins@70%MHR
Walk	2mins@75%MHR, 2mins@65%MHR (x3)
X-train	10mins@70%MHR
Row	280yd (250m)@70%MHR

Exercise sequence	intermediate	advanced
Chest press p83	15rm	15rm
Tricep extension p101	15rm	15rm
Box push-up p85	80% of maximum effort and number	
Squat (no weights) p108	20	20
Walking lunge (no ball) p107	20	20
Standing glute raise p113	25 each leg	25 each leg
Abductor raise p112	25 each leg	25 each leg
Repeat the 7 exercises above		
Basic crunch (feet on bench) p112	30	30
Oblique crunch p104	20 each side	20 each side
Back extension p95	15	15
Repeat the 3 exercises above	(x2)	(x3)

Cool-down	Short standing stretch sequence (see page 49)

squat

tricep extension

2nd trimester Workout time 60 mins (10 mins Warmup + 45 mins Exercise sequence + 5 mins Cool-down)

Warmup	10 mins aerobic exercise @ 70%MHR

Aerobic exercise	both levels
Cycle	5mins@65%MHR
Walk	2mins@70%MHR, 2mins@60%MHR (x4–5)
X-train	2mins@70%MHR, 1min@60%MHR (x4)

Exercise sequence	intermediate	advanced
Squats (no weights) p108	20	20
Chest press p83	20	20
Lat pull-down (underhand) p90	15	15
Cat stretch p45	15	15
Standing glute raise p113	20 each leg	20 each leg
Rest 30 seconds		
Repeat the 5 exercises above	**(x3)**	**(x4)**
Bicep curl p96	20rm	20rm
Tricep extension p101	20rm	20rm
Lateral raise p86	15rm	15rm
Shoulder press p88	15rm	15rm
Repeat the 4 exercises above	**(x2)**	**(x3)**

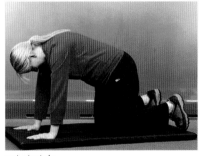
cat stretch

Cool-down	Short standing stretch sequence (*see page 49*)

3rd trimester Workout time 60 mins (10 mins Warmup + 40 mins Exercise sequence + 10 mins Cool-down)

Warmup	10 mins aerobic exercise @ 70%MHR

Aerobic exercise	both levels
Walk	15–20mins@65%MHR
X-train	10–12mins@65%MHR

Exercise sequence	intermediate/advanced
Chest press p83	15rm
Lat pull-down p90	15rm
Repeat the 2 exercises above	**(x3)**
Bicep curl p96	15rm
Tricep extension p101	15rm
Repeat the 2 exercises above	**(x3)**
Squat (no weights) p108	20 rest for 30 secs
Cat stretch p45	20 (hold each position for 5 secs)
Repeat the 2 exercises above	**(x3)**
Lateral raise p86	20rm
Standing glute raise p113	20 each leg
Repeat the 2 exercises above	**(x3)**

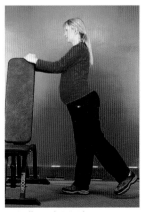
standing glute raise

Cool-down	Short standing stretch sequence (*see page 49*)

the programs

postnatal program

Chances are that you're feeling exhausted, so don't feel you have to rush into an exercise routine. If you exercised regularly before you became pregnant, you're probably impatient to get back to it and to get to work on your body. Seek advice from your doctor, but don't do anything more strenuous than your daily routine demands for the first four weeks following the birth.

> **Benefits**
>
> builds strength / tones muscles ✓
>
> burns fat / builds aerobic capacity ✓✓
>
> increases flexibility ✓

If you had a straightforward noncesarean delivery, it's usually safe to embark on a moderate exercise program in the fifth week following the birth, but seek advice from your doctor. In weeks five to eight, your joints will still be soft from the effects of relaxin in the system (*see page 40*) so extreme stretching is not advisable. By week nine, you can begin to step up the pace a little, but stay within comfortable limits.

The program is divided into two phases: five to eight weeks after the birth and nine to 12 weeks after it. There are two workouts in each phase, and each workout is to be performed twice a week, so you should aim to work out four times a week. Whether you've been left with 10 pounds to lose or 40 pounds, your goal in the first phase of the program is the same: get your body moving and work on gradually getting your aerobic fitness back. By the end of week 12, you won't have your old body back yet, but you will have regained enough of your fitness to move on to another program. Assess your goals and choose accordingly.

Don't diet during this program; concentrate on good general nutrition, not calorie reduction. Your body needs plenty of nutrients for milk production if you're breastfeeding, but also to repair itself and keep energy levels up.

Weeks 5–8

Workout 1 time 45 mins (5 mins Warmup + 30 mins Exercise sequence + 10 mins Cool-down)
Workout 2 time 60 mins (5 mins Warmup + 45 mins Exercise sequence + 10 mins Cool-down)

Workout 1

Warmup — 5 mins aerobic exercise, gradually raising heart rate

	all levels		
Fast walk	20–30mins@75%MHR		
Exercise sequence	**beginner**	**intermediate**	**advanced**
Squat p108	20	25	30
Push-up or box push-up p85	12–15	15–20	20–30
Lunge p106	15 each leg	20 each leg	25 each leg
Upright row p89	15rm	15rm	15rm
Leg extension p110	12rm	12rm	12rm
Shoulder press p88	20rm	20rm	20rm
Walking lunge (no weights) p107	20	30	30
Rest 1min			
Repeat the 7 resistance exercises above	(x2)	(x3)	(x4)

Cool-down — Total body stretch sequence (*see page 48*)

Workout 2

Warmup — 5 mins aerobic exercise, gradually raising heart rate

	all levels		
X-train	1min@80%MHR, 1min@70%MHR. (x10)		
Walk	1min@80%MHR, 1min@70%MHR. (x10)		
Row	1000metres@75–80%MHR		
Exercise sequence	**beginner**	**intermediate**	**advanced**
Basic crunch p112	25	40	50
Reverse curl p103	15	20	25
Back extension p95	12	15	20
Repeat the 3 resistance exercises above	(x3)	(x4)	(x5)

Cool-down — Total body stretch sequence (*see page 48*)

Weeks 9–12

Workout 1 time 70 mins (5 mins Warmup + 55 mins Exercise sequence + 10 mins Cool-down)
Workout 2 time 70 mins (5 mins Warmup + 55 mins Exercise sequence + 10 mins Cool-down)

Workout 1

Warmup 5 mins aerobic exercise, gradually raising heart rate

	all levels		
Jog or fast walk	45mins@75–80%MHR		

Exercise sequence	beginner	intermediate	advanced
Basic crunch *p112*	30	50	60
Bridge *p105*	20 secs	45 secs	60 secs
Back extension *p95*	20	25	30
Rest 30 secs			
Repeat the 3 resistance exercises above	(x3)	(x4)	(x5)

Cool-down Total body stretch sequence (*see page 48*)

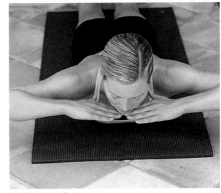
back extension

Workout 2

Warmup 5 mins aerobic exercise, gradually raising heart rate

	all levels		
Jog or fast walk	30mins@75–80%MHR		

Exercise sequence	beginner	intermediate	advanced
Squat *p108*	20	25	30
Walking lunge *p107*	20 each leg	30 each leg	30 each leg
Leg curl *p111*	15rm	15rm	15rm
Step-ups *p109*	30 secs	45 secs	60 secs
Push-up *p85*	12–15	15–20	20+
Lat pull-down *p90*	15	12	12
Lateral raise *p86*	12	12	12
Shoulder press *p88*	20rm	20rm	20rm
Row	280yd (250m)	280yd (250m)	280yd (250m)
Rest	2 mins	90 secs	60 secs
Repeat the 9 exercises above	(x2)	(x4)	(x4)
Cycle	6mins@75%MHR	10mins@75%MHR	12–15mins@75%MHR
Basic crunch *p112*	30	50	60
Bridge *p105*	20 secs	45 secs	60 secs
Back extension *p95*	20	25	30
Rest 30 secs			

Cool-down Total body stretch sequence (*see page 48*)

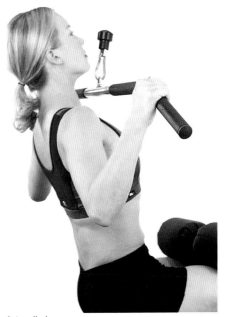
lat pull-down

the programs

park program

On a nice day, what's better than getting outside in the fresh air and making a local park into your gym. This program provides a good, aerobic workout that conditions the heart while also working and toning the muscles. You alternate between short bursts of aerobic exercise and toning sequences so the heart rate is maintained at a healthy elevated level.

Benefits

builds strength / tones muscles ✓✓

burns fat / builds aerobic capacity ✓

increases flexibility ✓

how the program works

The resistance training sequences in this program use the principle of peripheral heart action (PHA) training (*see page 56*). This is where you use resistance training to tone the muscles, but you move the exercises up and down the body, which helps to condition the heart. So, for example, when you do a leg exercise, the heart has to work to control blood supply to the legs. If you then do a chest exercise, it has to immediately supply blood to that part of the body. This change in direction of blood flow works and strengthens the heart while simultaneously toning the muscles. In effect you are doing two workouts in the same amount of time as it would normally take to do one.

using the program

This is a great outdoor workout, but, of course, you could also perform it indoors in the gym. When doing the workout, try to move as quickly as possible from one exercise to the next, to ensure that your heart rate is elevated for the duration of the workout. If you are using a heart rate monitor, aim to keep your heart rate between 65 and 85 percent of your maximum heart rate (MHR). There are aerobic bursts of running and fast walking in the program. Beginners should always work at 75 percent of MHR, and intermediate and advanced levels should work at 80 percent MHR.

This program offers a good, high-intensity, overall workout. Performed three times a week, it will build stamina and burn fat. More advanced exercisers might want to extend the length of their workout. If this is the case, treat the workout as a circuit and repeat it.

If you do this workout outside, choose grass or another surface that absorbs shock and so minimizes high-intensity impact on the joints.

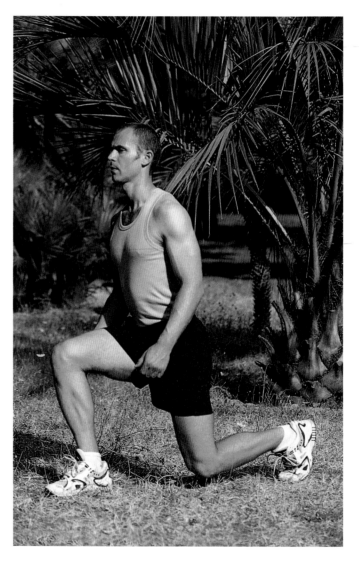

▲ **escape the confines of the gym**
Take your exercise routine outdoors when the weather is good.

Workout 1

Workout time 45–60 mins (5 mins Warmup + 35–50 mins Exercise sequence + 5 mins Cool-down)

Warmup   5 mins aerobic exercise, gradually raising heart rate

Exercise sequence   Repetition maximums (rm) or repetitions for each exercise are shown in this order of fitness level: beginner / intermediate / advanced

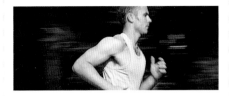

Run *pp54–7*/Walk *pp60–3* 5mins@75%MHR
7mins@80%MHR / 10mins@80%MHR

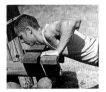

Push-up *p85*
10/20/30

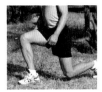

Lunge *p106*
10/15/20 each leg

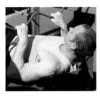

Pull-up *p92*
10/15/20

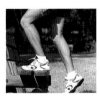

Step-ups *p109*
10/15/20 each leg

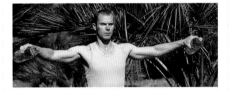

Lateral raise *p86*
15/20/25 rm

Run *p54* /walk *p60*
5/7/10 mins

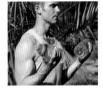

Bicep curl *p96*
15/20/25 rm

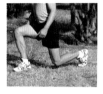

Power lunge *p106*
10/15/20 each leg

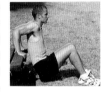

Dips *p98*
10/20/25

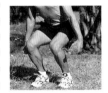

Squat *p108*
15/20/25

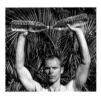

Shoulder press *p88*
15/20/25

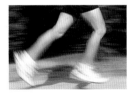

Run *p54*/walk *p60*
5/7/10 mins

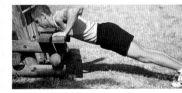

Push-up *p85*
10/20/30

Lunge *p106*
10/15/20 each leg

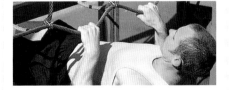

Pull-up *p92*
10/15/20

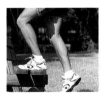

Step-ups *p109*
10/15/20 each leg

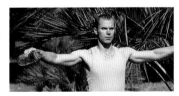

Lateral raise *p86*
15/20/25

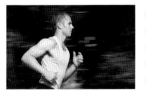

Run/walk *p54*/*p60*
5mins@75%MHR/
7mins@80%MHR/
10mins@80%MHR

Cool-down   3 mins aerobic exercise, gradually lowering the heart rate
Stretch   Total body stretch sequence (*see page 48*)

the programs

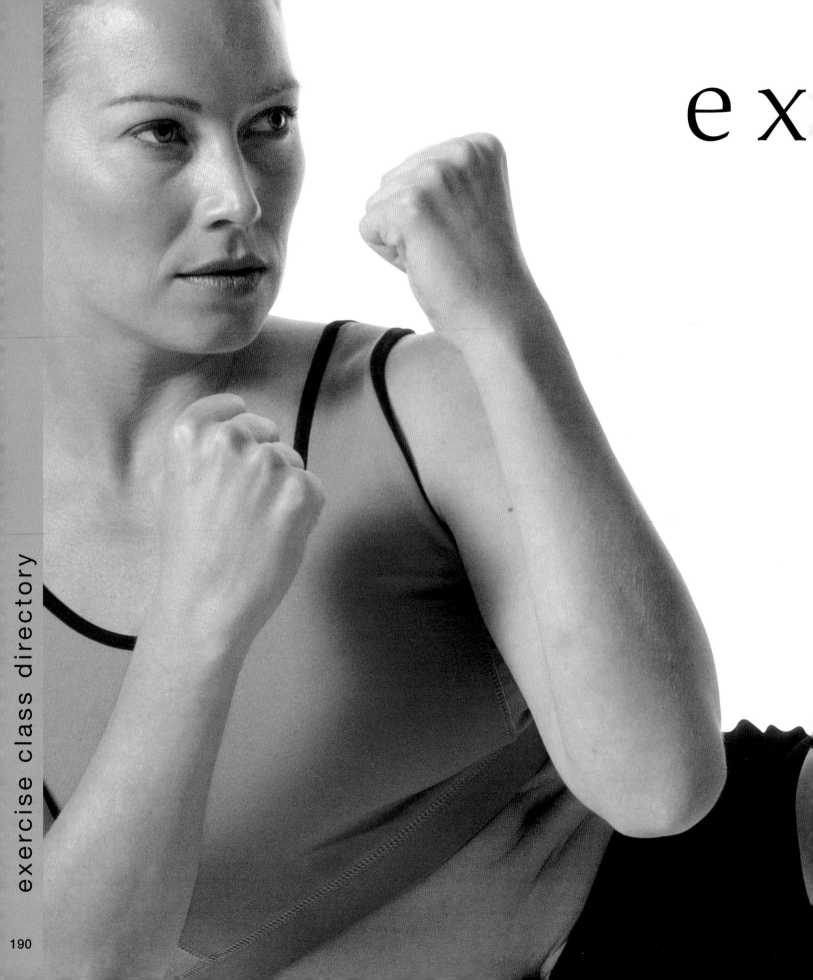

ercise class
directory

Exercise classes are a great – and indeed more sociable – way to get and stay in shape. Some people prefer to exercise as part of a class because they find that it increases their motivation levels. This directory tells you what to expect from a class and assesses each one for its ability to: burn fat, build aerobic strength, build muscle, increase flexibility, and tone muscle. It also indicates the degree of coordination needed. The classes are rated as follows: fair ✓ good ✓✓ excellent ✓✓✓.

aerobic

It could be said that the whole fitness boom of the past few decades started with the simple aerobics class. Now there is a range of class styles to suit all tastes, including classes that use music to keep you motivated and make your workout more interesting.

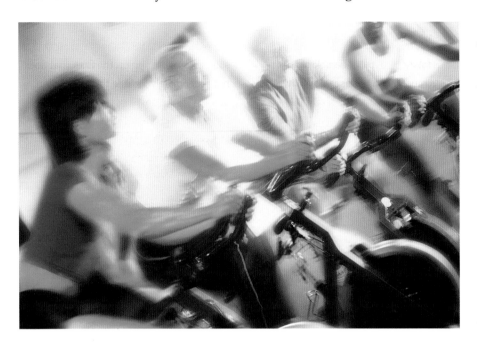

High impact aerobics

burns fat ✓✓   **builds aerobic strength** ✓✓
builds muscle   **increases flexibility** ✓
tones muscle ✓   **needs coordination** ✓✓

One of the most popular classes, high impact aerobics can be used to raise the intensity of your workouts.

Class structure After a warmup, the exercises build to an intensive aerobic peak that lasts for 20–40 minutes, depending upon the level of the class. The movements are high impact – both feet leaving the ground – and low impact. The last 5–10 minutes is a gradual cool-down. Abdominal work is often included at the end and should always be followed by stretching.

The benefits This class improves your cardiovascular fitness, burns fat, and develops muscular endurance and some explosive power in the lower body. Hand-eye coordination is vastly improved.

What to wear Wear something that will keep you cool – cotton or cotton/lycra shorts and a cotton t-shirt, crop-top, or vest. Shoes should have shock-absorbent soles and be supportive around the ankle.

Signs of a good instructor A good teacher will check the class for any injuries and take these conditions into account, giving individual as well as group instructions. Overdoing these classes can lead to joint and muscle injuries, so a good instructor should check to make sure you have no problem in these areas.

Not suitable for Anyone with soft tissue (cartilage or ligament) knee injuries, or a history of achilles tendon or back problems. Osteoporosis sufferers should check with their doctor before attending this class.

Jazzercise

burns fat ✓   **builds aerobic strength** ✓
builds muscle   **increases flexibility** ✓
tones muscle ✓   **needs coordination** ✓✓

As its name suggests this exercise is a combination of choreographed jazz dancing and workout.

Class structure The class warms up with some simple jazz moves, performed to music. After the warmup and stretch, the class moves on to the main body of the session. This is broken down into single dance moves that are gradually added together to form a longer sequence. After this sequence, the class cools down with some slow flowing movements and ends with a dance-style stretch.

The benefits Although the workout feels light at first, when the class is learning the moves, Jazzercise has a good cardio-vascular benefit. The concentration needed to put the moves together may interest those who find regular exercise classes unstimulating. Jazzercise has no real toning benefit to the upper body, but it will have a minor effect on the lower body. This type of class is best considered as part of an overall fitness routine.

Who goes Jazzercise is aimed at those who enjoy dance and have good coordination.

What to wear Anything from professional dancewear to baggy t-shirts and sneakers.

Signs of a good instructor A good instructor will be able to keep the class together as a unit, yet be able to cope with different levels of ability within the class.

Low impact aerobics

burns fat ✓✓   builds aerobic strength ✓✓

builds muscle   increases flexibility ✓

tones muscle   needs coordination ✓

Like high impact aerobics, this class is a mainstay of modern health clubs.

Class structure After a warmup, the exercises build to an aerobic peak that lasts for 20–40 minutes, depending upon the level of the class. The main aim of the workout is to raise the heart rate and work the body without resorting to high impact movements. The last 5–10 minutes is a gradual cool-down. Abdominal work is often included at the end and should always be followed by stretching.
The benefits The benefits are similar to high impact aerobics except that the workout programs are designed to reduce the strain on the joints.
What to wear As for high impact aerobics.
Signs of a good instructor As for high impact aerobics.
Not suitable for Anyone with soft tissue (cartilage or ligament) knee injuries.

Salsarobics

burns fat ✓   builds aerobic strength ✓

builds muscle   increases flexibility ✓

tones muscle   needs coordination ✓✓

This is another form of dance that has been modified into an exercise class.

Class structure Salsarobics is very dance based and requires good coordination.

The class warmup includes some aerobics and salsa steps and is followed by a quick stretch. The main part of the session involves slowly combining new salsa moves into a longer sequence. This part can last 20–30 minutes and will vary in difficulty depending on the ability of the class. The class finishes with a quick standing stretch.
The benefits For avid dance fans, it is a great way of working the cardiovascular system. The intensity of the sessions is low but effective if done regularly.
Who goes Classes are usually mainly female and cover a wide range of ages.

Spinning

burns fat ✓✓   builds aerobic strength ✓✓✓

builds muscle ✓   increases flexibility

tones muscle ✓   needs coordination ✓

Spinning is an intensive workout done on stationary bicycles in a studio.

Class structure After setting up the bikes, the class starts with a gentle warmup. Next the instructor talks you through hill climbs, sprint races, time trials, and group races. Some classes include upper body and abdominal work. Classes last 45–60 minutes and vary in size from five to 50.
The benefits A good spinning class gives the heart and lungs a hard workout while also building strength in the legs. It is one of the best classes for fat-burning.
Who goes Spinning is for those who already have a very good level of fitness, but want to be pushed a bit further. You need to feel confident on a bike. Classes are usually an even male/female split.
What to wear Choose something that lets your skin breathe, or wear layers that you can take off easily. Consider wearing padded cycling shorts and make sure you take plenty of water with you.
Signs of a good instructor Good instructors should screen the class at the start for medical problems and make sure that the exercise bikes are set up properly.
Not suitable for People who are generally unfit or have a low level of fitness.

Step aerobics

burns fat ✓✓   builds aerobic strength ✓✓

builds muscle ✓   increases flexibility ✓

tones muscle ✓   needs coordination ✓✓

This is a choreographed workout with many variations such as "pump and step," "jazz step," or "step and tone."

Class structure The class should always start with a warmup on the floor that does not immediately include the hard action of stepping up and down on the step. After the warmup there is a prework stretch.
The benefits This class improves your cardiovascular fitness, burns fat, and develops muscular endurance and some explosive power in the lower body. Hand-eye coordination is vastly improved.
Who goes The class is fairly tough and is not recommended for beginners. Classes usually attract a female following.
What to wear Wear something that will keep you cool – cotton or cotton/lycra shorts and a cotton t-shirt, crop-top, or vest. Shoes should have shock-absorbent soles and be supportive around the ankle.
Signs of a good instructor A good teacher will check the class for any injuries and take these conditions into account, giving individual as well as group instructions.

Stomp

burns fat ✓✓   builds aerobic strength ✓✓✓

builds muscle   increases flexibility ✓

tones muscle ✓   needs coordination

Like spinning, this exercise uses only one piece of gym equipment, the step machine or Stairmaster.

Class structure Once the class is set up correctly on the machines, the warmup begins. This involves low intensity stepping followed by a quick stretch. The class aims to use visualization, competition, and class involvement to keep the exercises interesting and the work rate high.

The benefits Motivation is by far the biggest advantage of this class. Although the workout does involve some arm movements, these are little more than token gestures and do not have much effect on toning the upper body.

Who goes The class is fairly tough and is not recommended for beginners. There is usually an even male/female split.

What to wear Normal gym clothes in layers that you can take off easily.

Signs of a good instructor Personality and a creative mind are both required.

Tae bo

burns fat ✓✓   **builds aerobic strength** ✓✓
builds muscle ✓   **increases flexibility** ✓
tones muscle ✓✓   **needs coordination** ✓✓

Tae bo is the invention of Billy Blanks and combines a series of martial arts moves with aerobics steps.

Class structure The class is like a normal exercise class and is performed to music.

You warm up with some funky dance steps and low level kicks and punches. The main section of the workout consists of different types of kicks and punches and Tae kwon do based moves that are put together into sequences. The workout then alternates between these quick-moving martial arts moves and modern dance steps at a high intensity. After the cool-down there are some effective, if pedestrian, stomach toning exercises.

The benefits The class is a good aerobic workout at a high intensity. Tae Bo is good for motivation and fat burning, but less effective at toning muscles.

Who goes Although mixed, there are usually more women than men in the classes. Some of the aerobics steps require reasonable coordination.

What to wear Normal studio workout gear and supportive shoes because there are plenty of moves that require stability through the ankles.

toning

These classes aim to tone, build, or define various parts of your body. They should all be used as part of an overall program that also challenges your cardiovascular system, although done on their own they provide quick solutions for problem areas.

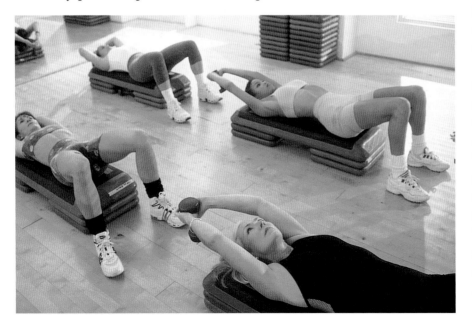

Abs class

burns fat   **builds aerobic strength**
builds muscle ✓   **increases flexibility** ✓
tones muscle ✓✓   **needs coordination**

This is essentially a quick blitz class for the abdominals, and very good for someone who wants to target that part of the body alongside their existing workout routine.

Class structure Abs classes are usually about 30–40 minutes long. The structure varies but will often include some form of warmup that is aerobic in nature. This prepares the body for the muscle conditioning part of the routine. The main section of the routine starts with some relatively low intensity abdominal exercise. This will become more intensive and include variations of isolation abdominal exercises (those that concentrate only the abdominals) with compound exercises (those that use a number of muscle groups as well as the abdominal muscles). This variation gives the abdominal area the chance to work through intensive and moderate cycles. Classes also target muscle groups near the abdominals such as the obliques (sides) and lower back muscles to create a tighter torso. Exercises for other body areas allow the abdominals a chance to rest, recover and then perform again at high intensity. The session finishes with a stretch for the back, abdominals, and any other areas that may have been worked during the session.

The benefits Strengthening the abdominal muscles is a crucial part of any well-rounded workout program. This type of class is not really effective on its own. If you want to tone your abs and lose weight in the abdominal area you really need to incorporate abdominal training into an aerobic training program. Another benefit of the class is that the strength of your torso has a direct bearing on your performance in other activities and sports. The torso is the main axis of the body, supplying both stability and balance.

What to wear Any comfortable exercise clothing such as shorts or leggings with a t-shirt. Take off or put on layers to keep your body at a comfortable temperature.

Signs of a good instructor There are two things to look out for. First, the instructor should gradually build the session to a series of intensive peaks that you work through and then recover from to repeat again during the class. Second, the session should become progressively easier during the last 8–10 minutes so that although you are tired, you are able to squeeze the last efforts out of the muscle fibers.

Not suitable for Pregnant women in the second and third trimesters, and anyone with chronic back complaints or neck and shoulder problems.

Bums and tums

burns fat   builds aerobic strength
builds muscle ✓   increases flexibility ✓
tones muscle ✓✓✓ needs coordination

The bums and tums class, or one of its numerous variations, is a key class in any studio timetable. As the name suggests, its aim is to work the butt and torso areas of the body. A great many people seem concerned about these two parts, so Bums and tums classes are always pretty full.

Class structure This class usually starts with a warmup in an aerobics style followed by a quick stretch for the target areas before the main work begins.

The main section of the class can vary greatly in structure according to the style of the instructor. However, most classes will start with the big dynamic exercises that are performed standing up, that is lunges and squats. These use the whole weight of the body, and advanced classes may add hand weights or bars to make the exercises even harder. After the standing exercises come the abdominal exercises and the prone glute exercises on the floor. These exercises are normally performed in quick succession to each other and will tire the muscles quite quickly.

Once all of these specific exercises are done, the session is completed with a long stretch for the worked muscles.

The benefits Taught in the correct fashion, this class is a great way of maintaining the muscle structure and making these areas of the body look more toned and shapely.

It is important to realize that a bums and tums-style class cannot offer every answer to shaping those specific areas of the body. As well as toning muscle, you also need aerobic exercise to burn body fat.

The desired effect is achieved only with a combination of fat burning and toning. If this class is part of a program with plenty of aerobic training, it is an effective way to improve the shape of these parts of the body. However, overdoing this style of class can exaggerate any problem you feel you have with these areas.

What to wear Typical gym wear or any comfortable exercise clothing such as shorts or leggings with a t-shirt.

Signs of a good instructor The instructor should move the exercises on quickly, alternating from muscle group to muscle group so that no single group becomes over-fatigued too quickly.

Who goes This class is usually dominated by women in a wide range of ages and fitness levels.

Callanetics

burns fat   builds aerobic strength
builds muscle   increases flexibility ✓
tones muscle ✓   needs coordination

Callanetics is a still-popular exercise system developed by an American, Callan Pinckney, as a result of her own back and knee problems. Her aim was to devise a no-impact form of exercise that would tone muscles and give greater strength to the body.

Class structure The class starts with some large fluid movements intended to warmup the muscles and prepare them for the work ahead. This part of the session is not particularly stressful but it is still effective in achieving the desired aim.

After the warmup, the class moves on to small repetitive movements, performed to target specific muscle groups.

The special feature of Callanetics is that the exercises all work in a very small range

exercise class directory

of motion and are performed up to 100 times in any one position. The small movements build up a high level of lactic acid in the muscles which soon causes a burning effect. The session gradually works its way around the different areas of the body building high levels of lactic acid and creating the "burn" in the muscles.

At the end of the class there is a stretching session to ease and relax all the muscles used in the workout.

The benefits Callanetics will have a toning effect on muscles that have not been exercised for some time. However, because of the small range of movement used in each exercise, it does not achieve effective muscle conditioning. The burning sensation coupled with the feeling of fatigue that follows lactic acid buildup gives the impression that the muscles have been through a really serious workout. However, this is primarily a psychological effect that lasts longer than any actual physical effect.

Who goes This class is usually attended by novice exercisers or those who are returning to a regular exercise routine after a long break.

What to wear Any comfortable gym wear such as leggings and a t-shirt.

Lower body toning

burns fat	builds aerobic strength	
builds muscle ✓	increases flexibility ✓	
tones muscle ✓✓	needs coordination	

This is another popular class on any gym's studio program, aimed at building tone and strength in the muscles of the legs and butt area.

Class structure The overall format is fairly standard, although there are, of course, many minor variations depending on the instructor and their particular preferences.

The class starts with a vigorous 5–10 minute warm up using walking and choreographed aerobics moves to work the large muscles of the lower body. This warmup is designed to increase the flow of blood to the muscles to prepare them for the more specifically targeted work ahead. After the warmup the class performs quick standing stretches.

The main section of the workout consists of standing exercises and floor exercises. The standing exercises come first and include squats and lunges, with variations such as bench step-ups and lateral squats. They are performed in quick combinations that train the muscles in different positions, and make them work harder by alternating between rest and work. These sequences can be intense, and you will almost certainly feel the muscles "burn" during this phase of the workout because you are constantly lifting your entire body weight. With so many muscles used in each movement, these are some of the most comprehensive workout exercises you can perform.

The next stage involves floor exercises that are designed to concentrate the workload on the inner and outer thighs and the butt. There are also some small exercises that aim to target small and very specific areas of the lower body. This section is also very intense and, if taught correctly, should move quickly from muscle to muscle so that hard work is followed by rest period and the sequence repeated.

The main body of this class can last between 15 and 40 minutes depending on the teacher and the level of the class.

Once the hard work is over the class normally goes through a long and necessary period of stretching to ease all the tension accumulated during the preceding long work phase.

The benefits This class is designed to tone every muscle of the lower body, and with the right teacher it can be very effective.

The only problem that can arise is that if someone is particularly self-conscious about part of their lower body, they can be tempted to attend too many of these classes. This can sometimes lead to over-development of these muscles without the necessary fat loss to match the body's shape change. If this happens, the problem area can actually become bigger – usually the opposite of the desired effect.

Who goes The class has elements that would suit anyone; however, it is nearly always attended by women.

What to wear Regular workout gear, whether it be a loose t-shirt and leggings or top-of-the-line lycra exercise gear.

Signs of a good instructor A good teacher will motivate the class and keep it moving quickly from exercise to exercise so that boredom does not set in. Lower body toning classes can be monotonous if the teacher does not use all of their creative abilities to keep the class interested.

Pump

burns fat ✓	builds aerobic strength	
builds muscle ✓✓	increases flexibility ✓	
tones muscle ✓✓✓	needs coordination	

Pump is a style of class that originated in New Zealand and was devised by fitness legend Les Mills. Its aim is to combine the benefits of aerobic exercise performed in the dance studio with gym-based resistance activity.

Class structure The purpose of the class is to tone the muscles as effectively as a workout in the gym. To achieve this, it uses body weight and an adjustable barbell to increase the intensity of the exercises.

After a warmup, the class stretches before starting the main part of the session. The class quickly moves from one controlled weight training exercise to another, constantly moving around the body from one muscle group to another. This allows a muscle group to be hit hard but then rested while another area of the body is targeted. The exercises used are varied but include squats, shoulder press, bicep curls, lunges, and bench presses. Although you are able to increase the weights, the class is still a toning class rather than a muscle bulking class. with repetitions of each exercise remaining high. Once the whole body has been really well worked, the class cools down and stretches.

The benefits In the hands of a good instructor, the class format offers great motivation compared to training on your own in a gym. Using the hand weights and barbells builds fantastic tone into the upper body muscles and gives a great shape to the upper arms and shoulders. This workout also strengthens the heart and increases the pulse rate because of all the extra blood that has to be moved to the muscles, although it is not as effective as a specific aerobic routine.

Who goes One of the positive aspects of this class is that it doesn't discriminate between men and women: it works equally well for both. It also does not require any coordination, so everyone can enjoy it.

What to wear Usual gym gear and a good pair of cross-trainers.

Signs of a good instructor This can be a difficult style of class to teach, because there is not much moving around and the exercises are quite static. A degree of self-motivation is still required, and it therefore takes a really good teacher to keep the interest and motivation high.

Not suitable for This class can be adapted to suit anyone. However, if you have joint problems or are pregnant, make sure that you are given alternative moves as and when appropriate. Additionally, if you have high blood pressure, get advice from your doctor before signing up, and inform the instructor of your condition.

aerobic and toning

Probably the current most popular form of class that combines aerobic with resistance training for a whole-body workout. Aerobic and toning classes are favored particularly by people in a hurry, and those who just want to attack all areas of their bodies at once.

Aquarobics

burns fat ✓   builds aerobic strength ✓
builds muscle ✓ increases flexibility ✓
tones muscle ✓✓ needs coordination ✓

The resistance of the water is what makes this workout so effective.

Class structure Although the class takes place in water, it is like a basic aerobics class. After a warmup, the aerobic section involves running, jumping, and making dynamic movements against the water's resistance to raise the heart rate. Floats, webbed mittens or paddles can be used to increase the resistance.

Next comes the toning section of the class which is incredibly effective because the water adds resistance in every direction: many exercises work two muscle groups in one movement. The class finishes with a quick stretch. Stretching is not so effective in water as the body quickly gets cold.

The benefits While toning the muscles, this class doesn't make you hot and sweaty because of the cooling effect of the water. It might feel that you are not working hard enough, but the body is usually exercising at the correct rate. Another benefit is that the body is lighter in water and so there is far less stress on the joints, which makes it an excellent class for anyone with joint

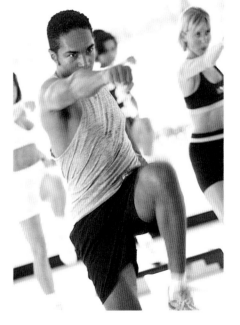

problems. With its combination of reduced stress to joints and the cooling effect of water, this is a good class for pregnant women, even in the third trimester.

What to wear Your usual comfortable swimsuit; skimpy bikinis are not really appropriate for this class.

Signs of a good instructor The class must be taught from the side of the pool because if the teacher is in the water, the class can't see what he or she is doing. This makes motivation slightly harder and the ability to keep to the speed of the class vital.

Boot camp/military fitness

burns fat✓✓   builds aerobic strength✓✓
builds muscle ✓✓ increases flexibility ✓
tones muscle ✓✓✓ needs coordination ✓

This workout derives from the tough physical training of the army.

Class structure This is a back to basics session involving exercises such as squat thrusts, squat thrusts, sprinting, and sit-ups. The class starts with a warmup and standing stretch. The rest of the training is a circuit format that requires you to perform a set exercise for either a certain amount of repetitions or a set period of time. The class can last from 45 minutes to 2 hours with as many as four trainers at a time. Just when you feel like dropping, it is time to stretch and the session is over.

The benefits This class works the heart, lungs, and muscles, and it works them hard. In terms of cardiovascular benefit, muscle toning, and motivation it is a great class, if you like being shouted at. If not, it may be a bit extreme. An important point to bear in mind is that you feel comfortable with the exercises you are asked to do. Sometimes, in the interests of pushing you to the limit, the instructor may require moves that are potentially harmful to the muscles.

Who goes Participants are generally quite fit and are there to be pushed hard. The classes are fairly evenly split between men and women with an age range of 25–40 for men and 20–35 for women.

What to wear Workout gear that you don't mind getting dirty.

Signs of a good instructor The best are trained in military fitness. A good teacher will instruct the class rather than just shout and push people to their limits.

Not suitable for Pregnant women and those with high blood pressure or a low level of general fitness.

Cardio-pump

burns fat ✓✓   builds aerobic strength ✓✓
builds muscle ✓ increases flexibility ✓
tones muscle ✓✓ needs coordination ✓

Also called (among other names) Aero-pump and Tonerobics, this is basically a combination of a traditional aerobics class and resistance exercises.

Class structure The format is very versatile, but the basics remain the same. It starts with a choreographed warm up that lasts for 5 to 10 minutes.

The main part of the workout combines resistance and aerobic exercises in one of two ways. The most common is to keep alternating between raising the pulse and targeting the muscles. The other way is to have separate sessions of aerobics and toning. Both styles use body weight, hand weights, and rubber exercise bands during the toning section.

The class finishes with a thorough stretch to lengthen the worked muscles.

The benefits Taught well, this is a fantastic class to attend – it has a cross-training effect of hitting cardiovascular fitness, strength, toning, and flexibility all in one workout. It is also a great motivational class, especially if taught in the interval style where the teacher moves from aerobic to resistance throughout the class. The whole of the body is targeted rather than one particular area. This is important if you wish to avoid building up one part of your body out of proportion to the rest.

Who goes Anyone can go, but be sure to get advice as to which level to start at.

What to wear Wear cool clothes: you can get pretty hot in this class. Be sure to wear cross-trainers with good cushioning across the whole of the foot, not just front or back.

Signs of a good instructor This can be a tough class to teach, but a good one will be able to control the actions of the whole class at all times. He or she should spend time going around encouraging and assisting class members individually rather than just staying at the front of the class.

Not suitable for This style of class is not recommended for pregnant women since the body tends to get very hot; nor is it suitable for anyone who has a history of ankle or joint problems. Always consult the teacher or your doctor if you have any concerns about trying Cardio-pump.

Circuit training

burns fat ✓   builds aerobic strength ✓✓
builds muscle ✓ increases flexibility ✓
tones muscle ✓✓ needs coordination

This class provides a motivational form of exercise that is suitable for anyone.

Class structure The class begins with an aerobic warmup. It then consists of a series of exercises in a circuit that test different parts of the body. The exercises are performed for a certain length of time, usually monitored by the instructor. Upper body exercises should be alternated with lower body exercises to allow one part of the body to recover while another is being worked. Some circuit classes may be upper or lower body circuits only, or they may be strength circuits or agility circuits.

exercise class directory

The benefits Circuit training is one of the most generalized ways of working on your fitness and can be adapted to give a wide variety of benefits, whether toning, cardiovascular, flexibility, or strength.

What to wear Wear something that will keep you cool, and wear shoes that are supportive in all areas.

Signs of a good instructor A good teacher is able to motivate the class to work through the longer or more difficult areas of the circuit. He or she should be able to devise a circuit that matches your personal goals and objectives.

Not suitable for There should be a style of class to suit almost all people, but if you are in doubt or unsure, always consult your instructor or doctor.

Step and pump

burns fat ✓✓   **builds aerobic strength** ✓✓
builds muscle ✓   **increases flexibility** ✓
tones muscle ✓✓ **needs coordination** ✓

Step and pump combines step classes with a good all-over toning element.

Class structure This class is similar to Cardio-pump. It starts off with a warmup, off the step, and builds up to a stretch.

The class can be performed either as alternating high intensity stepping routines and strength moves or as a step session followed by a toning session. It finishes with a long stretching session.

The benefits Taught the right way, this is a great class style with all the elements of cross training. The class is best if the toning section uses exercise bands or weights when strengthening the muscles. Using step as the aerobic element means that you do not need good coordination.

Who goes Regular exercisers attend this class, so it can be a high intensity number.

What to wear Wear shoes that have good support for the foot and ankle, and cool clothes or easily removable layers.

Signs of a good instructor An instructor needs to keep the class together, no matter what level of fitness, and teach the class up close rather than just standing at the front.

Not suitable for This is suitable for anyone, except perhaps women in the early stages of pregnancy (at that time it is important to keep the body's core temperature low).

martial arts and combat

These classes are a great way to get the combined benefits of aerobic workout, muscle toning, and stress-busting, and as such they have seen an enormous growth in popularity. They are high energy, and have a contemporary feel despite their classical roots.

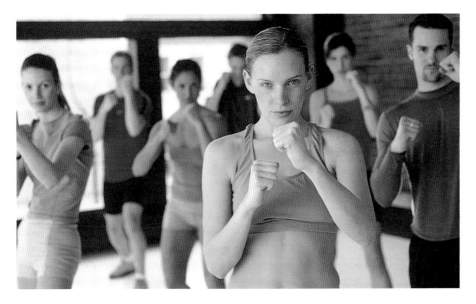

Boxercise

burns fat ✓   **builds aerobic strength** ✓✓
builds muscle ✓   **increases flexibility** ✓
tones muscle ✓✓ **needs coordination** ✓✓

Boxercise mixes boxing movements with aerobic and toning exercises.

Class structure The class is similar in format to an aerobics class starting with a warmup followed by an "aerobic peak" and finishing with a cool-down and stretch. Boxercise is an enjoyable way of using the benefits of boxing without the contact. It can be high intensity and includes an array of exercises to condition the abdominals and upper and lower body.

The benefits Boxercise provides a good full body workout that is a nice variation to the usual routine. Although noncontact, the

classes can still provide a great stress release. Your cardiovascular system will get an intense workout and your upper body strength in particular will be tested.
What to wear Shorts or leggings, t-shirt, and supportive training shoes.

Boxing

burns fat ✓✓   **builds aerobic strength** ✓✓
builds muscle ✓✓ **increases flexibility** ✓
tones muscle ✓✓ **needs coordination** ✓✓

Growing in popularity, boxing can be contact or noncontact depending upon your personal requirements.

Class structure Sessions usually include skipping in various forms, some target pad work, some work on a heavy punching bag, and a lot of body conditioning. You will probably be trained as part of a group, but there will be some one-to-one time mixed with work that you are expected to do on your own. The session has a number of high and low intensity periods as different skills or body areas are worked on.
The benefits Your cardiovascular system and upper body are worked hard during this class. Special attention is paid to the torso and shoulders, where the prime muscles in your punching action are. Hand-eye coordination is tested to improve accurate movement of body, legs, and fists.
What to wear Shorts, t-shirt, and training shoes that support your ankles.
Signs of a good instructor The teacher should be affiliated with a body such as the Amateur Boxing Association and must carry appropriate insurance. He or she must be able to work you at the level that is right for you rather than just providing one workout for everyone.
Not suitable for Anyone who has back or shoulder problems, or is pregnant.

Capoeira

burns fat ✓   **builds aerobic strength** ✓✓
builds muscle ✓   **increases flexibility** ✓✓
tones muscle ✓   **needs coordination** ✓✓✓

This spectacular dancelike Brazilian martial art is performed to music.

Class structure Capoeira takes place within a marked out circle in which fighters perform gymnastic moves and cartwheels to get away from each other. This requires great strength and balance. Beginners start by practising the moves and balancing on their hands and feet before getting to a combat stage.
The benefits This martial art burns a lot of calories but does take patience to master. As a result, beginners might worry about making slow progress. However, the skills soon develop after the first few sessions and the training greatly improves fitness.
What to wear The sessions are stop–start, so wear easily removable layers.
Signs of a good instructor See the "links" at planetcapoeira.com for a group near you.
Not suitable for This is not recommended for anyone lacking patience or coordination.

Jet kun do

burns fat ✓   **builds aerobic strength** ✓✓
builds muscle ✓   **increases flexibility** ✓✓
tones muscle ✓   **needs coordination** ✓✓

Bruce Lee, the most famous martial artist of all time, devised Jet kun do by combining various Eastern martial arts with modern fighting techniques.

Class structure The class structure mixes the discipline and structure of Karate with the fighting practice of Tae kwon do.

After a quick warmup, you practice combat moves such as kicks, punches, and defensive blocks. These are performed at high pace and repeated. This high intensity work soon tires the muscles. Next you get a chance to put the moves into practice against an opponent of equal skill.
The benefits The hybrid nature of this class, with touches of Karate, Boxing, Tae kwon do, and other forms of martial art, makes this an interesting format. Jet kun do will increase the body's stamina, improve flexibility, and build strength, although not necessarily muscle tone.
What to wear When starting simply wear loose clothes. You will need dedicated gear if you decide to continue.
Who goes This class generally attracts people who want to learn how to fight like Bruce Lee rather than simply get in shape in an interesting way. The classes attract men and women, although men predominate.
Sign of a good instructor There is a Jet kun do association; however, it is not usually recognised by other martial arts.

Jiu jitsu

burns fat ✓✓   **builds aerobic strength** ✓✓
builds muscle ✓ **increases flexibility** ✓
tones muscle ✓ **needs coordination** ✓

Jiu jitsu combines the grappling style of Judo with the kicks and punches of Tae kwon do and weapons of Kendo.

Class structure The art of Jiu jitsu is to use joint locks, pressure points, and killer blows to defeat an opponent. The moves and disabling holds are practiced with a partner or instructor until mastered. Next, they are used against an opponent before going on to learn the moves using weapons.
The benefits The combat situations are very explosive and would certainly improve stamina. However, as a beginner you do not do that much combat work, so it would

make sense to get in shape before starting Jiu jitsu rather than using it as a fitness class. If you are looking to learn a martial art and are confused by the vast choice of styles, Jiu jitsu is worth looking at because it uses such a wide range of techniques.
Who goes Although classes are popular with men between late teens and mid-thirties, this art is suitable for anyone.
What to wear Choose loose comfortable clothes until you get to a point that you want to buy the correct fighting outfit.

Judo

burns fat ✓✓ **builds aerobic strength** ✓✓
builds muscle ✓ **increases flexibility** ✓✓
tones muscle ✓ **needs coordination**

Judo is a contact martial art that uses holds and throws against an opponent.

Class structure The Judo session always starts with exercises to warmup the major muscles and elevate the heart rate.

The main session involves spending a few minutes at a time learning each hold or throw and about five minutes practicing them. These periods of high intensity work followed by periods of rest develop great stamina. The holds and throws also require a great amount of upper body strength.
The benefits Judo builds dynamic strength in the upper body and is a great form of aerobic training because of the constant high intensity bursts. Judo suits those who lack patience and want to quickly put their developing skills to use because there is grappling and wrestling from the outset.
What to wear As with most martial arts there is a set outfit to wear. However, when starting wear comfortable workout clothes.
Signs of a good instructor A good Judo teacher should be affiliated to their appropriate martial arts association.

Karate

burns fat ✓ **builds aerobic strength** ✓✓
builds muscle ✓ **increases flexibility** ✓
tones muscle ✓ **needs coordination** ✓✓

Karate promotes the use of the entire body to the unarmed person to protect themselves.

Class structure Karate is based on the control and constant practice of different moves on your own, or with a partner, until the correct level of control is achieved. Less aggressive than other martial arts, Karate has a major rule that you must not injure a training partner. Karate also aims to teach students how to draw energy from inside the body to give greater power to any movement. Experts demonstrate this by breaking wooden blocks and so on.
The benefits This graceful martial art is more about control than actual fighting. Like the other martial arts it builds a good level of stamina and a reasonable level of upper body strength.
Who goes Karate does not require as much actual fighting as other martial arts, which makes it suitable for all who want to try it.
What to wear Start with loose clothes; if you decide to continue, then buy the outfit.

Kendo

burns fat ✓✓ **builds aerobic strength** ✓✓
builds muscle ✓ **increases flexibility** ✓
tones muscle ✓✓ **needs coordination** ✓

Kendo is a very complex martial art. It aims to provide not only a style of fighting but also a code for living life based on ancient Japanese teachings.

Class structure This is a sword fighting art now performed with bamboo swords and heavy protective body armor. Kendo moves

are vigorous, unlike the delicate and subtle moves of fencing.

The class itself is divided into practice time and fight time. All of the moves are broken down into short routines and these are practiced and repeated until mastered. With the weight of the suit, these moves rapidly tire you out. Once you are proficient in some of the moves, you then move on to combat. This is performed in the center of the room with two opponents facing each other. The intensity of combat further raises the heart rate and expends more energy.
The benefits This type of martial art is fantastic for stamina. It is probably the most explosive of all the martial arts and the weight of the armor means that the body has to work at a high energy level, improving upper body and torso strength. Kendo requires complete physical control and mental discipline.
Who goes These classes tend to attract those who are serious about learning a martial art. They are usually disciplined, and as focused on the spiritual element of Kendo as the physical art. Age and sex are not a barrier to enjoying this martial art.
What to wear Choose loose clothes: the protective outfit will be provided at the session. Serious devotees buy their own armor, but it is very expensive.

Kickboxing

burns fat ✓✓ **builds aerobic strength** ✓✓
builds muscle ✓ **increases flexibility** ✓✓
tones muscle ✓✓ **needs coordination** ✓

Kickboxing can be anything from a class based workout to a full contact session.

Class structure Many of the warmup exercises are rehearsals for the main program which involves kicking and punching moves that increase in speed and difficulty. This is an exercise class that needs great coordination to keep up with the fast changing drills and routines. As the routine picks up speed, the heart rate rises and the workout becomes aerobic. The class also involves stretching the legs and back to increase mobility.

The benefits Kickboxing provides an aerobic workout. In addition it increases coordination and lower body power.

What to wear Shorts, t-shirt, and training shoes that support your ankles.

Signs of a good instructor Look for a teacher who is affiliated to the appropriate organization and carries insurance.

Not suitable for Anyone who is pregnant or has joint trouble.

Tae kwon do

burns fat ✓   builds aerobic strength ✓✓
builds muscle ✓   increases flexibility ✓
tones muscle ✓✓ needs coordination ✓✓

Tae kwon do is, in martial arts terms, a relatively modern, dynamic form.

Class structure Tae kwon do combines karate moves with grappling and sparring like Judo or Thai boxing.

A Tae kwon do session starts with a general warmup and then moves on to sessions of learning and fighting, like Judo. The main differences are that the work phases of Tae kwon do last longer than Judo, and the jumping and kicking is far more dynamic. A session can last from 60 to 90 minutes at a basic to intermediate level and is very hard work.

The benefits Tae kwon do is mainly a stamina-based exercise with interval training of intensity work and rest periods.

What to wear Shorts, t-shirt, and training shoes that support your ankles.

Sign of a good instructor He or she should be affiliated to a Tae kwon do association.

Not suitable for Anyone who is pregnant or has joint trouble.

mind and body

Classes in this category are good for reducing stress, improving posture and increasing flexibility, so they're particularly suitable for people who sit at a desk all day. Yoga has a huge celebrity following which has helped bring it into the exercise mainstream.

Alexander technique

burns fat   builds aerobic strength
builds muscle   increases flexibility ✓
tones muscle ✓   needs coordination

Alexander technique has many loyal followers who attend the classes seeking postural correction and relief from back problems and tension.

Class structure Classes perform a series of postural exercises aimed at correcting poor posture and developing more control of the body's movements. The exercises are done in isolation and will repetitively work on a specific area to increase local strength in a balanced way. The core strength of the body is developed creating a balance between opposing sets of muscles.

The benefits These classes are not really for toning muscles or increasing fitness, but they will improve your posture.

What to wear Shorts or tracksuit bottoms, t-shirt and training shoes.

Signs of a good instructor A good teacher should produce a thorough screening of your body to analyze areas of imbalance. He or she should work with individual class members to ensure that the postures are done correctly.

Not suitable for Suitable for all unless a doctor specifically advises otherwise.

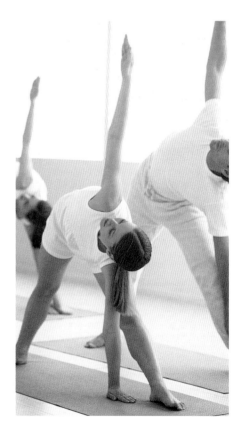

Ashtanga yoga

burns fat ✓   builds aerobic strength
builds muscle ✓   increases flexibility ✓✓✓
tones muscle ✓✓   needs coordination ✓✓

This flowing form of yoga is also known as Power or Dynamic yoga.

Class structure Classes generally begin with gentle yoga movements to warmup. Depending upon your level of expertise, the class increases the variety of postures and the speed at which they are performed providing a higher intensity workout than other yoga forms. There can be some fairly extreme postures that really test your flexibility. As with all yoga forms, controlled breathing is a key element of Ashtanga yoga. Each session generally finishes with some meditation exercises and stretches.
The benefits Ashtanga yoga increases your core body strength and flexibility and also gives a low level aerobic workout.
What to wear Tracksuit bottoms or leggings (preferably cotton) and a t-shirt.
Signs of a good instructor The instructor should give individual attention, positioning your body correctly for difficult postures. He or she should screen you before the start and take account of existing illness or injury.
Not suitable for Individuals with back, hip, or knee injuries or anyone with excessively low blood pressure.

Hatha yoga

burns fat   builds aerobic strength
builds muscle   increases flexibility ✓✓✓
tones muscle ✓   needs coordination ✓✓

Hatha yoga is the most popular of the yoga classes and aims to increase mobility and blood flow around the body through holding postures and controlled breathing techniques.

Class structure Hatha yoga movements form the basis of all physical yoga styles. The sessions involve a gradual buildup of sets of postures performed either standing or sitting. These sets become slowly more challenging but involve less rapid changes between standing and sitting postures than Ashtanga yoga, which gives this type of yoga wider appeal. At the end of each session some meditative work may be done as a relaxing finale.
The benefits Reduced blood pressure and stress, and improved mobility.
What to wear Tracksuit bottoms, leggings or shorts (preferably cotton), and a t-shirt.
Signs of a good instructor The teacher will display good hands-on techniques to increase your mobility and correctly position your body. He or she will screen you before starting and tell you how to modify the postures to take account of existing illness or injury.
Not suitable for Individuals with chronic back, hip, or knee injuries.

Iyengar yoga

burns fat   builds aerobic strength
builds muscle ✓   increases flexibility ✓✓✓
tones muscle ✓   needs coordination ✓✓

Iyengar yoga is a precise form of yoga that concentrates on perfecting each of the postures.

Class structure Because of the emphasis on precision, Iyengar yoga postures are taught in a very strict fashion and are held for a long period of time so that each one is fully utilized and improved. This style of yoga uses a variety of props such as a belt, folded blanket, wooden block, or chair to help you achieve the postures particularly if you lack flexibility. The attention to detail means that Iyengar yoga is taught at a far more leisurely pace than Ashtanga yoga and the aim of the class is a lower intensity workout that is noncompetitive. Holding the postures for a long time gives the muscles enough time to stretch and really develop in length and elastic strength.
The benefits Iyengar yoga is fantastic at developing flexibility in all areas of the body and creating greater body awareness. Of all the styles of yoga, Iyengar is the one that focuses most attention on perfecting the postures.
Who goes Classes include a wide range of ages, both men and women. Anyone can do this form of yoga.
What to wear Loose, warm clothes in layers that you can take off.

Meditation

burns fat   builds aerobic strength
builds muscle   increases flexibility
tones muscle   needs coordination

The basic principle of meditation is to harness the power of your mind and be able to "close out" the world. Many people believe that if we could control our minds, we could prevent some illnesses and actually perform better.

Class structure Meditation has many different forms and can be taught in anything from a yoga chanting style to a more relaxing visualization style. It is therefore important to experiment and find the style that will suit you best.

In a yoga-style meditation class you start by concentrating on your breathing and learning how to control it. This teaches greater physical awareness and is a start to achieving control of your mind. Once you have got to a state of controlled breathing, you then turn your thoughts to a set chant. These chants are taken from yoga writings and repeating these words over and over concentrates your thoughts to the one area of the chant. This combined controlled breathing and chanting has an amazing effect that completely removes you from the outside world and allows you to relax.

The visualization style of meditating normally starts off by using controlled breathing techniques to slow down the body and focus the mind. From there the teacher will talk the class through a visualization in which each member of the class immerses themselves. This can last any length of time and include other sensory aids such as sounds or music.

The benefits True relaxation and the ability to clear the mind of everyday thoughts is a very undervalued skill. A good meditation routine is a wonderful way of achieving this much needed escape and is something that would benefit everybody. Some people feel embarrassed when attending this type of class, but if you allow yourself to relax into it the results can be surprising.

Who goes Absolutely anyone can go to these classes regardless of sex, age, and physical fitness.

What to wear Wear comfortable clothes that will keep you warm.

Pilates

burns fat	builds aerobic strength
builds muscle ✓	increases flexibility ✓✓
tones muscle ✓✓	needs coordination ✓

Pilates (Pi-lah-tees) was originally devised by Joseph Pilates to enable professional dancers with back injuries to recover quickly and get back to work. Pilates has become a popular form of exercise with benefits for everyone, not just for dancers. This exercise class concentrates primarily on developing strong stomach and back muscles.

Class structure There are several different versions of Pilates, but the authentic form will be taught in a specially designed area and will use various pieces of equipment to provide resistance and make the muscles work hard. To start, you will be introduced to the principles of Pilates such as postural stance and correct breathing. Once you have an understanding of this, you then move from one piece of equipment to another repeating a set move against resistance so that you are making large movements that require the core muscles of the stomach and lower back to exert control. These are all carried out in a controlled fashion and are repeated many times to work the relevant muscles.

The Pilates principles have also been devised for use in a studio environment, where the exercises are done on a mat, usually without equipment although some are performed with the aid of a padded metal ring to provide resistance. All the movements aim to develop and maintain core body strength.

The strict Pilates follower may not approve of some of the studio adaptations that are on offer. However, for many people these classes are easier to find and more accessible than the authentic form.

The benefits Pilates is incredibly good for building strength in the postural muscles, and has an impressive success rate in toning and shaping the body provided you work with an experience instructor and can stick to the strict regime. Pilates may also improve your flexibility over time, but it is not effective as a fat burning exercise and has little aerobic benefit.

Who goes The authentic form of Pilates is still popular with dancers and is particularly favored by people seeking relief from back problems. Modern interpretations attract a wide spectrum of men and women.

What to wear Loose, comfortable clothes that also keep you warm. The class is not fast moving and therefore you do not build up a great deal of body heat.

Qi gong

burns fat	builds aerobic strength
builds muscle	increases flexibility ✓
tones muscle ✓	needs coordination ✓

Qi gong is an ancient practice that has its roots in Chinese medicine. Its moves seem similar to those of Tai chi, but its cultural background is not the same, and it is performed to give a slightly different result.

Class structure Because its roots are in medicine, Qi gong puts great emphasis on stimulating the body's tissues, muscles, and organs. This is achieved largely through breathing and meditation.

The class starts with breathing techniques for the lower, middle, and upper stomach area, which are very relaxing. The aim is to feel at one with your body and give yourself the ability to control your breathing and the flow of energy, or *qi*, around your body. Next come larger movements that further enhance the flow of energy. These movements are also intended to stimulate the organs and energy centers which, according to Qi gong, are located in different areas of the body. In general the moves are far simpler and have a more meditative quality than those performed in Tai chi.

At the end of the class you feel relaxed and energized with a wonderful, almost warm feeling throughout your body.

The benefits This class teaches you to channel your thoughts away from everyday anxieties, an interlude that can prove very refreshing and help to restore energy.

Because it is easier to perform than Tai chi, you don't need the same level of patience to enjoy the class and to feel that you are doing the movements correctly. If you feel the need to have an active way of relaxing yourself but find Yoga too difficult or Tai chi too time consuming, Qi gong is the perfect class for you.

What to wear A tracksuit or warm workout clothes to avoid getting cold; the moves are not fast, so you will not build up a great deal of body heat. As for your feet, the best way to enjoy the class is barefoot.

Signs of a good instructor Any good teacher will be affiliated to one of several Qi gong associations in China.

Stretch and relaxation

burns fat	builds aerobic strength
builds muscle	increases flexibility ✓✓✓
tones muscle	needs coordination

This is a class that more people should try to attend as part of a fitness program. There are two aims: first to stretch and lengthen all the main muscles of the body, and second to use controlled breathing to calm the body and reduce or resolve stress.

Class structure This class will always start with a warmup to provide blood to the muscles so that they can be stretched more easily and effectively. The warmup will normally last 5–8 minutes and can take a variety of forms from walking around while moving the arms and upper body to performing an aerobic exercise to music.

Typically, the main section of the class starts with all the stretches you can do while standing. This will include the arms, chest, back, and legs. These stretches should all be performed slowly, and each one should be held ideally for a minimum of 10

seconds. Once all the standing stretches are completed the class then moves down onto exercise mats and gets ready to perform all of the prone stretches.

This is where the strongest stretches for the legs and back will be done, and the most important stretches for the protection of the lower back and postural muscles. These stretches will be held for up to 40 seconds each, so that the maximum effect can be achieved.

After this long period of stretching it is quite usual for the class to remain lying down and concentrate on deep breathing or even perform a relaxation process either by visualization or by muscle tightening followed by relaxing.

The benefits This class offers wonderful relaxation opportunities and at the same time helps you develop greater flexibility and longer muscles, something from which we would all benefit.

Who goes Men and women of all ages and levels of fitness.

What to wear Comfortable, stretchy or baggy clothes that let you move freely. The class is slow and relaxed, so you will not overheat. It is a good plan to take an extra top in case you feel cold.

Signs of a good instructor An effective class should be taught in a strong fashion with all stretches performed slowly and in a controlled manner. Look for a teacher who gains your confidence and knows what you want to achieve.

Tai chi

burns fat	builds aerobic strength
builds muscle	increases flexibility ✓
tones muscle	needs coordination ✓

This is an ancient Chinese exercise characterized by slow, graceful movements and practiced by millions

every morning in China. In Chinese philosophy, *chi* is the energy force that gives the body vitality. Tai chi is believed to help maintain clear *chi* channels through the body, promoting good health and wellbeing. It is not strenuous exercise, so do not expect to work up a sweat. Tai chi is meditative and the emphasis is on inner health.

Class structure The class begins with an initial warmup to stimulate pressure points and the internal systems of the body. The teacher then takes the class through a number of different "forms" or sequences of movements and poses, many of which require great strength and concentration to hold. It is therefore a more demanding exercise form than Qi gong.

The benefits Each movement is intended to work harmoniously with a different internal body system, such as the nervous and cardiovascular systems, stimulating the body's flow of energy. The concentration on performing each movement slowly and deliberately excludes the outside world and has a very calming effect on the mind. Tai chi also helps with body alignment, balance, and understanding the body's rhythm and movement. Regardless of your level of ability, you should feel noticeably calmer after a session of Tai chi.

Who goes Men and women of all ages and levels of fitness. Tai chi was once considered more of a "spiritual" class, but its popularity is now widespread.

What to wear Loose clothes that keep you warm. No shoes, or very soft shoes.

Signs of a good instructor Your teacher should help you to understand your body through movement, and explain the philosophy behind the different poses.

Not suitable for People who lack concentration and patience.

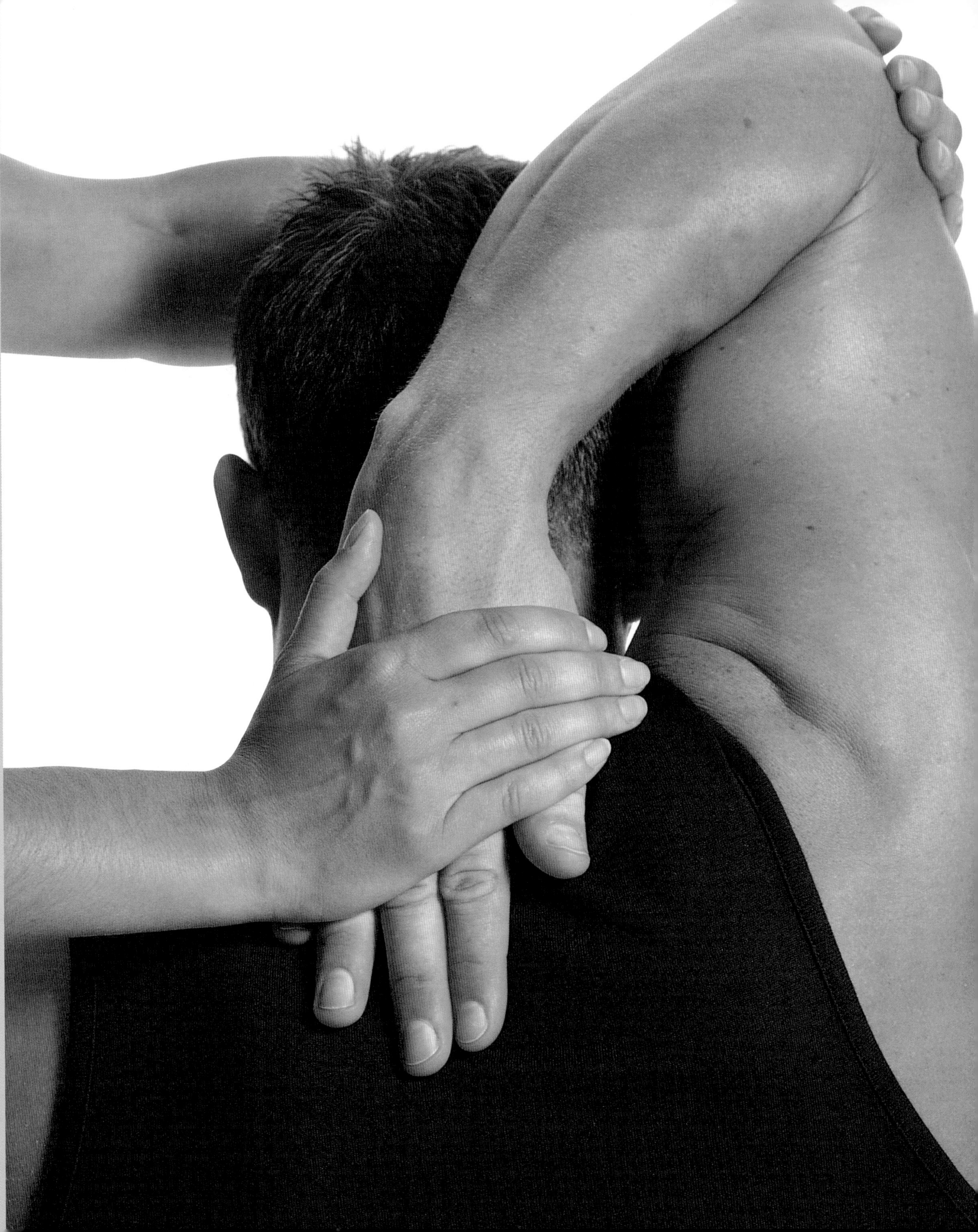

making the right choices

I hope that reading this book will inspire you to embrace a healthier lifestyle, and encourage you to become more fit by making exercise part of your daily routine. You may well decide to join a gym or hire a personal trainer, or even buy some fitness equipment to use regularly at home. The aim of this section is to point you in the right direction so that you know what to look out for and what to ask yourself when making decisions in all of those areas. Then you will know that you have made wise choices that positively benefit your health, fitness, and well-being.

choosing a gym

Today, there are so many gyms around that the choice can seem overwhelming. Finding one that fullfils your requirements and feels comfortable to you is an essential step to achieving your fitness objectives, because it is all too easy to come up with reasons for not going to the gym. By thinking ahead and carefully assessing your needs, you should be able to find a suitable gym that will make exercising and working out an enjoyable and rewarding experience.

analyze your requirements

If you are unsure about your choice of gym, ask if they will let you try out the facilities before you join. Aim to visit at the time you would usually go to the gym. Try several gyms this way. A little effort at the beginning can ensure that you do not end up wasting a large quantity of time and money.

size

The size of the club, the range of its facilities, and the ratio of gym staff to members should be taken into account. Here are some points to consider.

• Social aspect: Is going to the gym for you as much about socializing as it is about exercising? Will others inspire you to go regularly? A large club is likely to bring you into contact with a wider group of people who have more varied interests.

• Privacy: If you are worried about exercising alongside a host of other people, choose a small club or find out if the gym has a quiet time that suits you.

• Attention: It is crucial that the gym staff are able to give you enough attention for your personal needs. If you have a high level of self-motivation, a large club may be satisfactory. If you need to be guided and pushed through a routine, a smaller, more service-oriented club might be better to help you achieve your goals.

• How busy does it get?: Always ask about the size of the club's membership and the average number of people that attend at the times you intend to visit. Even the best facilities have a maximum capacity and you don't want to be prevented from using what you are paying for because of overcrowding.

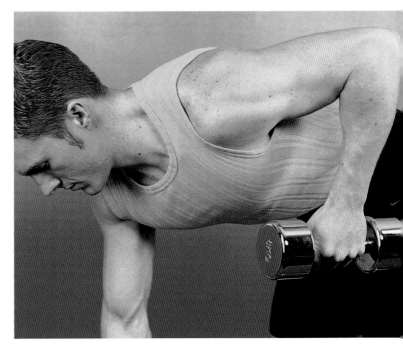

▲ **free weight facilities**
For training and toning specific muscle groups, it is important that a gym has a large variety of free weights and fixed weight machines.

facilities

Choosing a gym that matches your training goals and lifestyle will get you well on the way to achieving your aims.

• Your personal goals: If your goal is to increase muscle size, then you will need a gym that provides an extensive array of fixed weight machines and free weights. If your goal is to lose weight, a club with a large selection of aerobic equipment such as treadmills, cycles, and rowing machines is better suited to your purpose. If your goal is to complete a triathlon you will need a swimming pool; if you enjoy exercise classes, the gym should have one studio and possibly more for variety.

• Your short- and long-term goals: These will change naturally along with your interests, commitments, and lifestyle, and the gym should be able to provide you with a broad sweep of alternatives, particularly if you are tied in through advance payments or joining fees which you lose through moving clubs.

• Ease of use: This is a very important consideration. Does the club have opening hours that suit you, including evenings and weekends? Can you park your car – and do you have to pay extra? Is the club close to local transportation? Are amenities such as showers, towels, and toiletries provided so that you have less stuff to haul around with you? Are trainers and therapists available when you want them?

value

Unless money is no object, it is important to consider all the financial implications carefully and read the small print so you know what you are signing up for.

• Budget requirements: Work out your budget and stick to it because you can be tied in to a contract for a period of time. Don't forget to take into account the joining fee.

• Joining fees and monthly payments: To make life easier, find out if the club you are considering has a monthly payment plan. You may be able to negotiate the joining fee because the full amount often applies only if the club is confident of being booked to capacity all of the time.

• Hard sell: Don't be fooled by sales incentives and tactics, and make sure you have had your orientation before you sign.

staff

Helpful and knowledgeable staff can make all the difference, so do talk to them and check out their qualifications.

• Reception: Are the reception staff able to answer all of your questions? These people are your main route to all areas of the club, and a poor receptionist may prevent you from being able to make the most of everything that is on offer.

• Gym staff: Are the gym staff qualified through an accredited organization? Always choose a club with properly qualified personnel. If you feel that your level of fitness or desired goals demand intensive attention and personal training, find out if the club offers this service.

It is worth the search to find a good gym, being clear in your mind to define your requirements and staying with that definition until you find the gym that suits you best.

▼ **aerobic gym machines**
These can be the most popular machines in the gym. If you use these machines a lot, make sure that there are enough of them so that you do not have to wait around for one to become available.

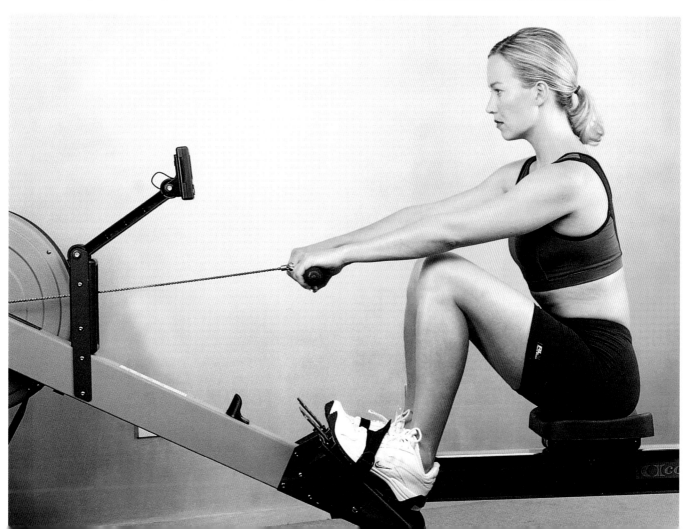

choosing a personal trainer

Years ago, only the rich and famous could afford the services of a personal trainer. Now, with more personal trainers around, this service has become accessible to a greater number of people to help them get fit and healthy. Working with a personal trainer is one of the best ways to ensure you get the most from your exercise routine. A good trainer should motivate you and inspire you to work toward new goals and perhaps even unexpected ones.

your personal requirements

What are your goals? If you want to learn to kickbox or train for a marathon, you will need a trainer with specialized knowledge. In most cases, it's best to look for a trainer who understands your goals and specific training needs, but who also has broad knowledge in general fitness. As you progress, your goals will change and it is better to have an all-around trainer to help you manage these changes effectively.

meet the trainer

It's absolutely essential to meet the trainer in person before you sign up for a course of sessions. Don't just rely on the recommendations of the gym manager or (even less reliable) those of the receptionist.

• Before the meeting, ask the trainer to take along an example of a program devised for another client who has goals that are similar to your own. This will help you to assess how successful the trainer is in enabling the client to achieve their goals. An effective trainer will devise a program of planned workouts for each individual client and there should be no problem in producing a copy for you. If the trainer can't or won't, your suspicions should be aroused.

• Check the trainer's qualifications and liability insurance. The overall reduction in quality is an unfortunate downside of the

huge expansion in the health and fitness industry. Trainers new to the business are not always licensed or adequately insured. In most countries there is no regulatory body that monitors personal trainers, so you will probably need to do some investigating of your own. A degree or qualification of similar standing in sports science or biomechanics is usually a reasonable indicator of quality. Don't choose a trainer because they were once good at sports; it does not necessarily follow that they know what will work for you personally.

• Ask for references from other clients to check whether the trainer is reliable and trustworthy.

• Don't hesitate to cross-examine a potential trainer. They want your business just as much as you want the help and expertise of an effective professional.

• A good trainer should interact with you to find out exactly what you want from your training program. Additionally, they should take you through a thorough assessment of your goals, fitness, suppleness and capabilities. Beware of a trainer who wants to start on a program right away.

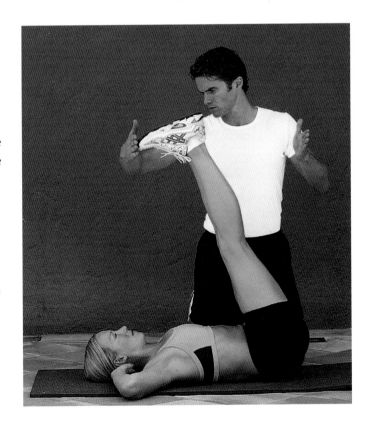

▶ **personal motivation**
With a good personal trainer's expert advice, fitness goals can be achieved far quicker than training on your own. By ensuring that you perform the exercises correctly, they increase the effectiveness of the workout as well as substantially reducing the risk of injury.

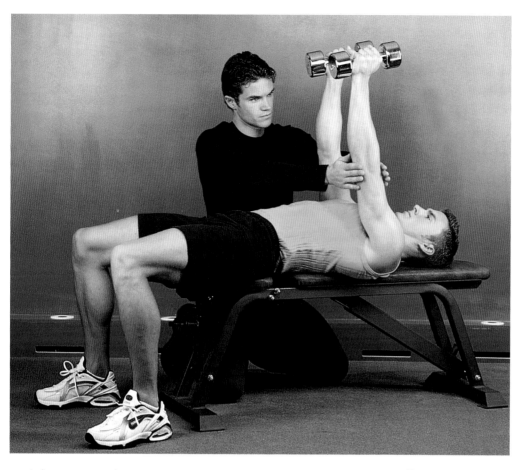

◄ **expert guidance**
A good personal trainer should
not only instruct you in the right
technique but should teach you
about your fitness program.
They should tell you what each
exercise is doing for you and
motivate you to move on to the
next level in your workouts.

match your needs

Even if the trainer has the correct qualifications, you will still want to consider the following questions.

• Does the trainer work out of a gym or come to your home? For most people it is more satisfactory – and you will probably achieve better results – to go to a gym or personal training studio for each session. In such a specialized environment, the enterprise becomes more challenging, is charged with a higher level of motivation, and gets you into a routine that is specifically about you, without the distractions of home. With the increasing number and availability of well-organized personal training centers, the days of the trainer who makes home visits are more or less past.

• How much of your work is going to be diet based? If you feel that this is a crucial part of your program – as it is for many people – you will need a trainer with expert, unbiased knowledge who can also offer you the necessary support. Find out if they have studied nutrition and ask for their opinion on diets in general. Read up on a few diets beforehand and see if the trainer is able to answer your questions.

personality

Consider whether you could spend three to four hours a week with your potential trainer. If you feel you may not get along well, your interest in seeing them will evaporate. You don't have to be bosom buddies, but it is better to choose someone you feel comfortable with: it will help you to enjoy working out.

cost

You should expect to pay the full cost for a course of sessions at the start but remember, the more sessions you pay for the greater the discount you should get; it never hurts to ask. In personal training you do generally get what you pay for. If a trainer is cheap, there is probably a good reason. Higher prices usually reflect a loyal client base and a schedule that is busy or booked up way in advance.

Once you have made the choice and have your personal trainer on board, use them as a constant source of information and expect to have regular reanalysis of your progress. This should be all part of the service that a good and professional trainer offers. So remember: if you don't get it, ask for it.

making the right choices

home exercise equipment

The last 20 years have seen an explosion in the home exercise equipment market. Some of these items are complicated, difficult to use, and promise instant results; more often than not, they will be left to gather dust within days of being bought. However, it is possible to buy several pieces of inexpensive, easy-to-store equipment that you can use to train a range of muscle groups and achieve a good overall workout.

simplicity is the key

For most people, the key to a good home gym is simplicity. The more complicated the equipment is to use or maintain, the more likely it is that you will avoid using it. The items here are simple to use, versatile, easy-to-store, and reasonably priced.

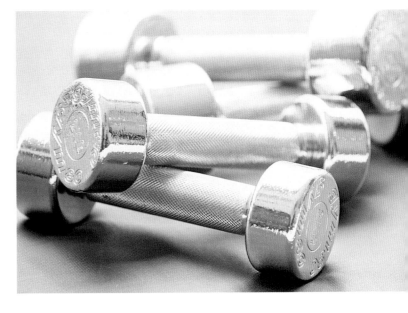

▲ dumbbells
Because of their versatility, dumbbells are an excellent purchase for home training. They can be used to work specific muscles or as a means of intensifying certain exercises.

◄ stability ball and medicine ball
These durable and relatively inexpensive items of gym equipment help to make training at home more interesting and varied.

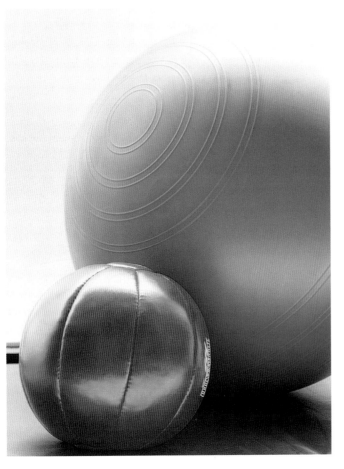

stability ball

This piece of equipment is popular in most gyms and provides a versatile base for a number of exercises.
• Although most commonly used for abdominal work, the stability ball is a great alternative "bench" for free-weight work and is particularly good for supported leg work exercises such as ball squats (see page 108).
• The stability ball can also be used to increase the intensity of some exercises and target more particular sets of muscles such as when used for ball push-ups (see page 85).

exertube

Although not as versatile as free weights, the exertube (also known as x-tube) is lightweight and takes up little space, so has a great advantage if you want to work out when you are away from the gym or traveling.

• The exertube is suitable for all fitness levels because it comes in a variety of thicknesses geared to different resistance levels.
• A minor disadvantage of this simple piece of equipment is that the exercise becomes progressively more difficult the farther the band is extended.

weights

Free weights and dumbbells for home use are very similar to what you would use in a gym; the only significant difference is that the gym probably has a far greater range of weights. If you like to use free weights for much of the time you spend in the gym, then these are an essential piece of equipment for your home training.
• Analyze your workout routine and determine the range of weights you most commonly exercise with. Choose a range of around five pairs of dumbbells, starting with a weight suitable for an exercise such as single-arm tricep extensions (*see page 101*) and going up to the maximum you would use for pec flys (*see page 82*) or bicep curls (*see page 96*).
• While adjustable dumbells might seem a more economical buy than a set, continually stopping to change weights will greatly reduce the effectiveness of the training. A good set of one-piece dumbbells should last a lifetime, and you can buy heavier dumbbells as your strength gradually increases.

▼ **exertube**
The exertube – a simple idea but no less effective for that – consists of two handles joined by a length of rubber tubing. Different levels of resistance are usually indicated by different colors.

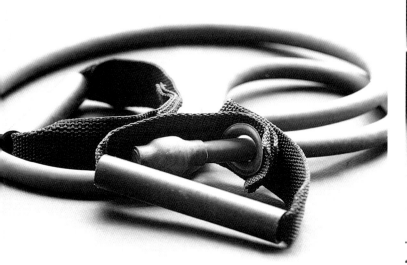

medicine ball

Not the most obvious choice for a piece of domestic exercise equipment. However, the medicine ball has a variety of uses in a home training program. It is useful for upper and lower body exercises, and can be used for work on the abdominals.
• Choose either a 6lb (3kg) or a 11lb (5kg) ball.
• The medicine ball can be used to perform exercises such as crunches (*see page 104*) and squats (*see page 107*) or even in circuit training. The exercises will be made harder and more intensive by carrying the ball. Throwing the ball with a partner (*see page 101*) or using it for overhead or rotational throws (*see page 174*) is a good way to develop upper body strength.

heart rate monitor

The heart rate monitor is one of the most important pieces of gym equipment whether in your gym bag or to use at home. It provides an instant and accurate display of the intensity of your workout at any stage.
• If you do not know how hard your heart (and therefore your body) is working, you will find it more difficult to improve the results of your exercise routine.
• Buy a monitor that performs the basic function of displaying your heart rate. More functions are not necessarily more useful and a pricier model may not be worth the investment.

▼ **heart rate monitor**
Some heart rate monitors have extra functions that allow you to store your training records or transfer data to your home computer, but it is probably better to get a model that simply measures your heart rate.

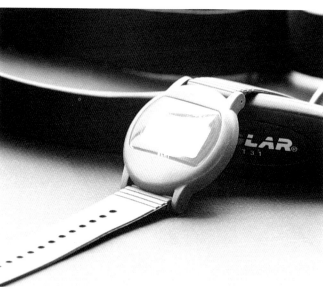

making the right choices

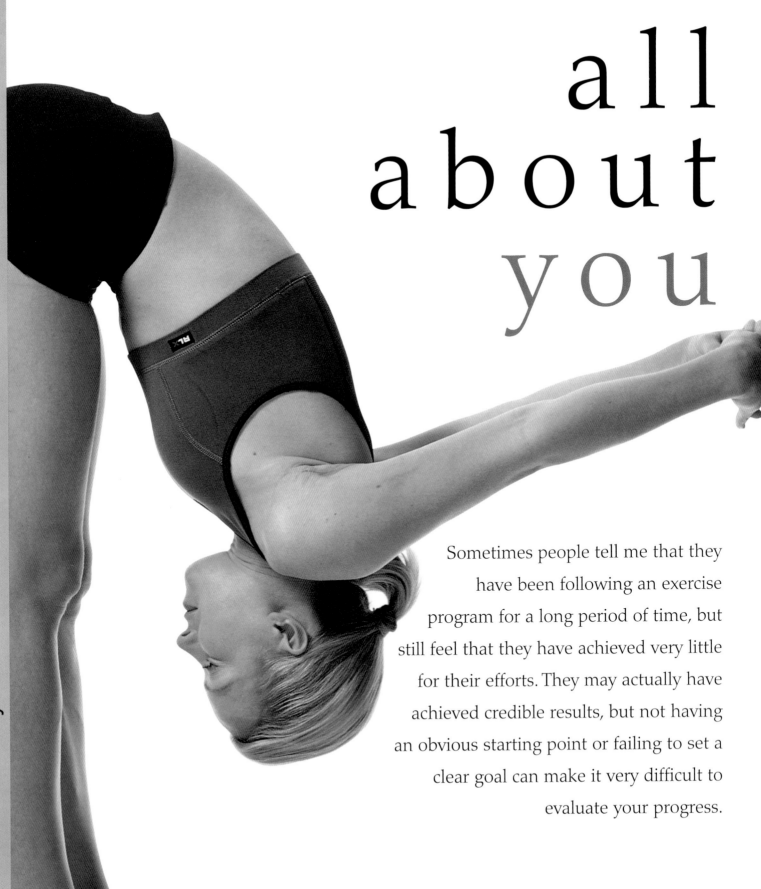

all
about
you

Sometimes people tell me that they have been following an exercise program for a long period of time, but still feel that they have achieved very little for their efforts. They may actually have achieved credible results, but not having an obvious starting point or failing to set a clear goal can make it very difficult to evaluate your progress.

questionnaire results

The questionnaires on pages 20–23 will help you to assess your diet and give an indication of your current level of fitness. They will establish your nutritional and physical starting points and will help you to get the most out of the programs in this book. Use the results of the questionnaires to highlight areas that need work. Once you have completed a program or attained a fitness goal, return to the questionnaires and retest yourself. Being aware of your progress will help to keep you motivated between programs. Don't be tempted to retest and change the fitness level at which you are working before you have completed a program. Each program has been especially designed with the different fitness levels in mind, and will guide you to your goal in the time it takes to complete it.

your score for the nutrition questionnaire

How to figure out your score:

a = 3 points,

b = 2 points,

c = 1 points

Your total score tells you how efficiently your digestive system functions and gives an indication of your body's acid/alkaline balance. The more alkaline your body the better; the nutritional guidelines in this book encourage a diet that is high in low-glycemic alkaline-forming foods.

A total of **26 points or fewer** indicates a good acid/alkaline balance in the body. If your score totals **more than 27 points**, you have an acid-forming body and you should increase your intake of alkaline food (*see pages 34–5*). If you score **more than 45 points**, a more alkaline diet together with an exercise program will radically improve your quality of life.

your score for the physical questionnaire

How to figure out your score:

a = 1 points,

b = 2 points,

c = 3 points

Your result establishes your level of fitness as either beginner, intermediate, or advanced. The programmes will work best for you if you exercise at the level most suited to your ability.

A score of **between 5 and 8 points** indicates the need for some serious changes to your lifestyle. You should follow the programs at the beginner fitness level. This level of fitness is probably the result of having ignored your fitness and health needs for many years. Choose a program with an appealing goal – perhaps you are about to go on vacation or you want to fit into a new outfit – and use it as a turning point. There are problems that you need to address, but the programs can help you, and now is the time to start.

A score of **between 9 and 13 points** indicates an average level of fitness. You should follow the program at the intermediate fitness level. You have probably been doing some form of exercise fairly regularly. Embarking upon a program now will reduce the likelihood of experiencing health problems later on in life.

A score of **between 14 and 18 points** indicates a high level of fitness. You should follow the program at the advanced fitness level. You are quite focused and have almost certainly been physically active on a regular basis for some time. Choose a program to suit your specific goals: it will help you to stay on course.

training and nutrition journals

One of the best ways to ensure that you realize your goals and maintain motivation levels along the way is to keep a training journal. Use these training journal templates to devise your own journal, or photocopy these blank examples and use them to chart your progress as you work toward your ultimate goal. Set yourself clear short- and long-term goals that will take you to your ultimate program goal. In your training journal, make a clear distinction between your aerobic and resistance goals. The purpose of the nutrition journal is to make you more aware of what you eat. People tend to conveniently forget the more unhealthy foods they eat. Keeping a written record can help motivate you to make changes.

training journal

aerobic goal	short term	long term
strength goal	short term	long term

ultimate program goal

date						**date**					
resistance	reps	sets	**aerobic**	time	intensity	**resistance**	reps	sets	**aerobic**	time	intensity

nutrition journal

date

daily water intake

daily fruit intake

daily vegetable intake

date	comments/energy levels
breakfast	
lunch	
dinner	
snacks	
drinks	
date	comments/energy levels
breakfast	
lunch	
dinner	
snacks	
drinks	

all about you

common sports injuries

Here I present some of the more common sports injuries with advice on how to identify them, treat them, and – ideally – prevent them in the first place. Generally, if you experience pain or discomfort when exercising, listen to your body and stop at once.

hip or thigh pain

The ITB (iliotibial band) is a band of fibrous tissue that runs from the top of the hip down the outside of the femur, or thigh bone. It maintains hip and knee stability when you are standing, and enables bending and straightening of the leg.

The ITB can become inflamed as a result of repeatedly bending the knee at angles of 20–30 degrees while also supporting heavy weight. This might happen when running, particularly if you run on cambered roads where your foot lands at an uneven angle, or if you rapidly increase speed and/or gradient. You might also strain your ITB if you wear unsuitable or wornout footwear that doesn't provide adequate support. Your ITB then compensates, and this can put it under unnecessary strain.

Anti-inflammatory creams can provide initial comfort, but to prevent recurrence of the complaint, adjust your running program accordingly and check the suitability and condition of your footwear. Wear and tear on the inside or outside edge of the sole means you land unevenly when you run, which puts you at greater risk of injury. Avoid running on uneven surfaces. Performing the glute stretch and the standing quadriceps stretch (*see page 46*) will help.

knee pain

Each of the quadriceps, the four main muscles at the front of each of the thighs, are attached to the hip. At the other end, they converge into a single tendon that runs into the kneecap and then attaches to the lower leg. Their main function is to enable powerful extensions of the knee, but they are also

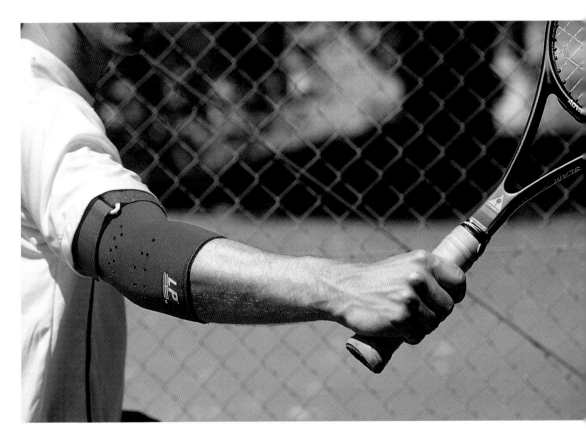

▶ tennis elbow
It's not just people who play tennis who get tennis elbow. Although nearly half of all tennis players will suffer from this uncomfortable condition at some point, they account for under 5 percent of all reported cases. The best treatment is to rest the arm.

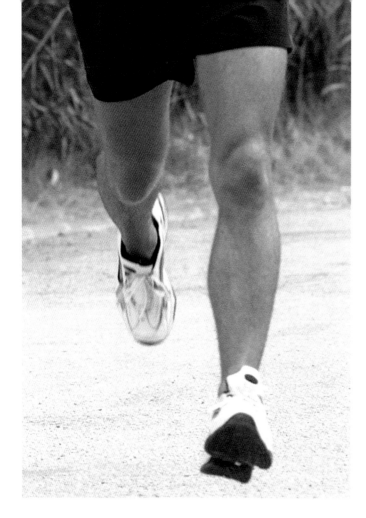

◄ running into problems
Great for gaining fitness and burning fat, running is also a high-impact sport that can put a lot of strain on the muscles and joints. Prevent injury by wearing good shoes that support your feet and ankles. Try to run on even ground wherever possible.

A combined bending and rotating movement of the lower arm is perfectly normal; that is, after all, how you bring food to your mouth. However, when you move your arm in the opposite way – the same motion as moving your hand away from your mouth – these muscles can rub against the bony part of the elbow. This action, combined with repetitive movements that increase tension and stress on the muscles in the wrist and elbow, causes what is known as tennis elbow. Tennis players suffer from tennis elbow as a result of the backhand stroke, which applies pressure to the tendons in their weakest position. You might experience pain when performing simple actions such as turning a door knob or shaking hands.

Treatment is to rest the elbow, and then to wear an elbow brace. Ease yourself back into exercise; perform the exercises in the tennis fitness program (*see page 167*).

shoulder pain

The shoulder girdle – the ball joint and the muscles that surround it – enables movement in the arms. It's important to take care of the muscles in your shoulders, especially when playing sports. People tend to focus on the superficial muscles of the chest and back when training, but the smaller deeper muscles enable the greatest mobility in the shoulder area. The group of four muscles in the shoulder is known as the rotator cuff. Their main function is to stabilize the shoulders, both for postural control as well as when moving the arms.

Injury to the rotator cuff can occur as a result of simple overuse or trauma. You overuse the muscles if you repeatedly perform an upward pressing action. Trauma usually occurs when you lift heavy weights while also bending and rotating the shoulder.

Pain occurs in the shoulder when the arm is bent at 90 degrees and the thumb is pointed toward the floor. Perform the inward rotator cuff and the outward rotator cuff exercises (*see page 93*), because these will strengthen the muscles in the shoulder and back. Avoid the overhead pressing action which puts the shoulder in the weakest position; applying pressure will do only more damage.

important for walking, any general movements of the leg, and postural control.

In most cases, pain in the front of the knee is caused by incorrect tracking of the patella over the knee, which in turn can be caused by muscular imbalances in the knee area. Putting too much weight on a flexed knee or sitting for long periods will aggravate the condition. Pain usually occurs just below the kneecap, but you may also feel it inside the knee, behind the kneecap.

Normal treatment is to strengthen the quadriceps. Try performing an inwardly rotated leg extension. This is just like a normal leg extension (*see page 110*) except with toes turned inward. Try also the hamstring stretches (*see page 46*). You might be advised to tape the patella to restrict movement.

tennis elbow

The elbow is a hinge joint, which means that you can move your lower arm backward and forward along one plane. However, a group of muscles that cross at the bony part of the elbow also enable rotation around the wrist and elbow.

glossary

Below is a list of terms used throughout this book, each of which is followed by a definition. Where a term, used as part of a definition, has its own full entry, that term is displayed in *italics*.

aerobic capacity The body's ability to take in and utilize oxygen. *Aerobic exercise* increases aerobic capacity.

aerobic exercise Exercise "with oxygen"; it builds heart and lung strength and enhances the body's ability to take in oxygen, feed oxygenated blood around the body, and create energy. The long-term effects of aerobic exercise are lower blood pressure, decreased risk of heart problems, and better circulation. It also helps to fight the onset and effects of aging.

abdominals These are the muscles of the stomach area. The muscle group extends from the rib cage to the pelvis and comprises three main muscles of importance: the rectus abdominus (the "six pack" muscles that run down the middle of the stomach), the obliques (the muscles on the outside of the stomach area) and the quadratus lumborum (the deep muscle that wraps around the mid-section of the torso and is important for posture).

anaerobic exercise Exercise "without oxygen"; fast explosive work that cannot be sustained for long periods of time. This form of exercise uses the less efficient anaerobic energy system that can be maintained for only short bursts.

antioxidants The collective name given to the nutrients and other substances that fight the buildup of *free radicals*.

body mass index (BMI) A good indicator of whether body size is in proportion to body structure. It measures weight in relation to frame size, taking into account total weight and body fat.

biceps The muscles at the front of the upper arms; used to bend the arms.

circuit training A training method where a series of exercises is performed, each for a short period of time. Circuit training can tone the muscles as well as having a heart-conditioning effect.

constant pace training A form of cardiovascular training that requires the heart rate being raised to the ideal level and then being maintained at that level for a specified period of time.

deltoids The three muscles of the shoulders, used in raising the arms up to the sides.

drop set A weight-training method where you fatigue the muscles, then drop the resistance to 75 percent of the first weight and continue until the muscle is fatigued once again.

free radicals The naturally occurring rogue oxygen molecules that roam around the body destroying cells. Poor diet, stress, and lack of exercise increase the buildup of free radicals. Many of the foods recommended in the book's nutritional program fight the buildup of free radicals.

glutes The muscles of the butt and hip area, which are used in the action of moving the leg backward.

hamstrings The muscles at the backs of the thighs; used to bend the legs.

hip flexor The muscles of the hip area; they are used in the action of bringing the knee up to the chest or raising the knee.

hip-to-waist ratio A figure that is arrived at by dividing the measurement of the waist by the measurement of the hip; used to assess a person's health in relation to their body fat distribution.

interval training A cardiovascular training method that works the heart within the optimum training zone. It works the heart in the higher range of the training zone, then uses the lower range as a recovery period; builds cardiovascular endurance.

lats / latissimus dorsi The large muscle of the back, which is used in all actions pulling down and toward the body.

maximum heart rate (MHR) The maximum level to which a person should raise their heart rate; it is determined by age and calculated in beats per minute (bpm).

optimum training zone The age-related heart rate training range that is ideal for burning fat and building cardiovascular strength; usually between 75 and 90 percent of *maximum heart rate*.

overloading The process of pushing the body beyond its usual physical limits, which helps to achieve greater results when exercising. You should aim to achieve overload whenever you work out.

pectorals The muscles of the chest area, used in moving the arms forward and pushing away from the body.

peripheral heart action (PHA) A resistance training technique that also conditions the heart. It concentrates exercises on the upper and lower body alternately, so the heart has to work hard to pump blood to the muscles at both ends of the body.

pronation / pronate With reference to the foot, this is a tendency to walk with body weight concentrated on the insides of the feet; shoes tend to wear on the inner sides of the soles. Wearing shoes suitable for your feet when exercising can help correct a tendency toward pronation.

pyramid training A training method that makes the body work harder with every set of exercises, therefore *overloading* the body to achieve greater improvement.

quads / quadriceps The muscles of the fronts of the thighs, used to straighten the legs.

repetition (rep) In *resistance training* a rep is one complete performance of an exercise, moving from the start position and back to the finish position. If you are asked to do 14 reps of an exercise, you should repeat that exercise 14 times before stopping.

repetition maximum (RM) The number of *repetitions* of a particular exercise to be performed to achieve *overload* on the muscles.

resistance training A training method that uses weights to tone and build the muscles.

saturated fat Oil and fat that is solid at room temperature; found in meat products and chemically processed foods. The unhealthiest form of fat, it has been linked to high blood pressure and heart disease.

set The number of repetitions you perform of an exercise in one attempt, without pausing. You are often asked to repeat sets, in which case you can take a short rest period between each set.

supination / supinate With reference to the foot, this is a tendency to walk with body weight concentrated on the outsides of the feet; shoes tend to wear on the outer sides of the soles. Wearing shoes suitable for your feet when exercising can help correct a tendency toward supination.

unsaturated fat Oil, such as olive oil, and fat that is liquid at room temperature; found in fish, nuts, seeds, and grains. The healthiest form of fat, it is essential for many of the functions of the body.

index

acknowledgments

author's acknowledgments

It seems that with each book you do, the list of those people who have a significant impact and support role gets greater. I was again lucky enough to have a fantastic team around me during every stage of the project, and I was again ecstatic with the final product. I want to thank all those who spent time on the project at Dorling Kindersley, in particular Mary Clare Jerram who always makes working on a project feel wonderfully straightforward. I need to move onto the "St. Tropez" set next with whom we spent a number of weeks shooting from early every morning until late into the night. Tracy Killick, the creative genius, managed to survive this shoot without hurting herself in any way (which was a first for the team), and about whom I am allowed to say nothing in relation to swimsuits and sarongs! Nasim Mawji, who managed to survive Tracy's driving each morning and still work tirelessly to do a fantastic editing job on the book. To this day I still don't know how she manages to turn my jottings of a mad man into the books they become. Izzy, Kevin, Spencer, and Hedwig, our wonderful models. Our amazing photographer, John Davis, had to work with clear blue skies, sunshine, heat, a lot of scantily clad women on the beach, and a St. Tropez setting! Tough life being a photographer John! Thanks to Clare and John, John's assistants, who had to put up with all of us!

I would also like to thank the Cinderella of the team, Gillian Roberts, who was not able to join us in the South of France, but who put in hours of work back at home.

I would like to give a special thank you to Sylvain Ercoli, general manager of the Byblos Hotel in St. Tropez, who allowed us to use the wonderful hotel as back drop for many of the shots. Thank you also to Patrick at Club 55 for allowing us to use this great venue for lunch, oops, I mean work!!

I once heard that a good book sells itself; personally I think it is also largely down to the fantastic sales team throughout the world that DK has gathered, and it is down to the great work of marketing and PR brains such as Fiona Allen, Katherine Bell, and Vivien Watten!

A very big thank you has to go to our wonderful case studies who were brilliant in lending themselves to me so that I could put them through their paces to achieve the various results that you can see in the book. Lastly, I would like to thank Helen Young and all the guys at Ralph Lauren who as ever gave us all the great clothing for the book and for their continued support.

And I, of course, have to give a special thank you to my brother Jon, with whom I wrote the book, who as always has worked tirelessly to pull together the project on my behalf and make it a success.

Thank you to Nik, Richard, Jason, Ayo, and all of my team in London who have played their own part in the book either through information, or just general support when it was needed – much appreciated guys! Thank you to Helen, for putting up with me throughout all of it!

Matt

publisher's acknowledgments

Dorling Kindersley would like to thank the five case studies: Charlotte Baker, Howard Cravitz, Sasha Castling, Tim Lewis, and Jo Craven, and the models: Kevin Dixon at DV8 Management, Hedwig Molin at Nevs Models, Spencer Hayler at MOT Models, Isabella Seibert at MOT Models, and Pam Nolan. Thanks also to Amanda Cross for hair and makeup; John Fenn and Claire Collins for assisting with photography; the Byblos Hotel in St Tropez for permitting us to photograph on their premises; Pierre et Vacances at Saint Pons Les Mures, Grimaud, for allowing us to use their tennis courts, golf course, and swimming pool for photography; Polo Sport for kindly supplying clothing from their new RLX range. Hugh Thompson and Lloyd Tilbury provided editorial and design assistance respectively; Valerie Chandler compiled the index. Particular thanks are due to Nasim Mawji for her commitment and dedicated work throughout this project.

Picture researcher: Cheryl Dubyk-Yates
Picture librarian: Hayley Smith
The publisher would like to thank the following for their kind permission to reproduce their photographs: (Abbreviations key: t=top, b=bottom, r=right, l=left, c=center)
Powerstock Photolibrary / Zefa: 192cl, 197cr.
Corbis Stock Market: John Henley 194bl; Rob Lewine 202br; Anthony Redpath 199bl.
All other images © Dorling Kindersley
For further information see: www.dkimages.com
Jacket Superstock Ltd/Joan Glase: inside front flap bl
Jacket DK Picture Library: inside front flap cl

Matt Roberts gyms can be found at:

matt roberts personal training
32–4 Jermyn Street
London SW1Y 6HS
UK
Tel: (44) (0)20 7439 8800

matt roberts at le saint géran
Poste de Flacq
île Maurice
Tel: (230) 401 1000

Matt Roberts is developing his own range of health- and fitness-related products. For a list of products and recommended retailers, contact the head office on (44) (0)20 7439 8800.

For more information about Matt Roberts Personal Training, visit:
www.personaltrainer.uk.com
www.healthhub.com